Critical Thinking in Contemporary Dermatology: Cognitive Essays

Somesh Gupta • Nikhil Mehta
Pankhuri Dudani
Editors

Critical Thinking in Contemporary Dermatology: Cognitive Essays

Springer

Editors
Somesh Gupta
Department of Dermatology and Venereology
All India Institute of Medical Sciences
New Delhi, India

Nikhil Mehta
Department of Dermatology and Venereology
All India Institute of Medical Sciences
New Delhi, India

Pankhuri Dudani
Department of Dermatology and Venereology
All India Institute of Medical Sciences
New Delhi, India

ISBN 978-981-97-0410-1 ISBN 978-981-97-0411-8 (eBook)
https://doi.org/10.1007/978-981-97-0411-8

This Springer imprint is published by the registered company Springer Nature Singapore Pte Ltd.
The registered company address is: 152 Beach Road, #21-01/04 Gateway East, Singapore 189721, Singapore

Foreword

Drs. Somesh Gupta, Nikhil Mehta, and Pankhuri Dudani are to be congratulated for editing this most thought-provoking textbook, *Critical Thinking in Contemporary Dermatology: Cognitive Essays*. The editors had successfully assembled a group of prominent dermatologists to discuss specific diseases and conditions from their personal perspective, including new thoughts and ideas. The final product is indeed a nice addition to the literature and a refreshing read on these topics.

The textbook started with a discussion of brain-skin interactions, followed by highlighting the interdependence of intrinsic and extrinsic aging processes, including the contributions of skin exposomes (UV, pollution, lifestyle, etc.). The idea of beauty and aesthetic enhancement was covered very thoughtfully in subsequent chapters. This was followed by essays on hair, nail, skin optics, and dermatologic diagnosis, the latter incorporating the fast and slow thinking concept described by Daniel Kahneman. The next section included provocative discussion on information processing by human brain, and essays on inflammatory and autoimmune skin diseases and new developments in therapy. Procedural dermatology was then covered, including an interesting perspective from a trainee's point of view. The importance of patient-centered care was discussed: teledermatology, managing patients' expectations, patient-reported outcome measures, holistic dermatology, and personalized medicine. An essay on the social determinants of health concluded the book, before the epilogue by the editors.

In contrast to traditional textbooks, this book is an easy read on topics that one would discuss at an after-dinner round table among friends and colleagues. It is a welcome addition to our dermatology library.

Henry W. Lim
Department of Dermatology
Henry Ford Health-Michigan State University
Detroit, MI, USA

Preface

This book is a collection of essays where selected global experts discuss current issues in Dermatology from their unique perspectives. While there is no dearth of disease-specific books and review articles, we know those to be comprehensive compilations, reshaping already known facts. There is little room for expression of new thoughts and ideas worth exploring. We believe that anyone working diligently for years together in any field notices patterns and develops an intuitive deep understanding about it, something that is difficult to convey and might be impossible to prove. Nevertheless, it is at the very least an intriguing perspective and might even be a revolutionary thought process. Einstein's paper on relativity was entirely theoretical, had no references, was built upon *thoughts*, and it was 14 years before it was proven, that too by someone else! An even more striking example is that of the evolution of the Atomic Theory; first proposed as a theory by the Greek philosopher Democritus (400 BC), a contemporary of Aristotle. His ideas were disregarded by the latter and subsequently majority of the scientific community, until it was modified and proven over 2000 years later by Dalton, Thomson, Rutherford, and others. The ideas acted as a seed for thoughts, and as science advanced, the ideas could be tested. It is interesting to note that Aristotle's ideas of all objects being made of the four elements was intriguing, aligns with ancient Indian philosophy, and may be true too; and may be proven in future by even more sophisticated tools.

We are a generation that has more writers than readers, and publications are being churned out at an unforeseen rate. While it is good for overall scientific advancement, we all know that negative findings rarely find eyeballs in a market coloured by confirmation bias; and even in-depth literature reviews cannot bring balance where such original studies are not easily accepted for publication. Peer-reviewed scientific literature follows a fixed pattern and often rejects ideas not fitting into already known patterns. A recent article in Nature suggests that there is a significant decline in the number of disruptive publications. This may be due to obsessions of journals, authors, and policy makers with matrices such as impact factor and cite score. Only those articles are likely to be cited more which are on the radar of popular but average information seekers. This means papers and articles based on novel ideas from real-life experiences may remain unpublished because they do not fit into publication priority of citation-hungry journals.

We need such a space for expression of personal experiences, original thoughts, observations, and *opinions* based on cognitive thinking. In this rapidly evolving scientific era, these may act as springboards for future scientists to come up with treatment regimens and cures for diseases that ail us today. We want this book to be able to create interest among our readers to look at the skin with wonder, to think laterally, and to question fundamentals.

We want to stimulate imagination because evidence can only confirm what is already known; it is imagination that is our guide to the future.

We hope you find it to be a refreshing change and exciting read irrespective of the number of years you've spent working with the skin.

Pick any part and read from anywhere! Your innate curiosity and playfulness are welcome.

New Delhi, India Somesh Gupta
New Delhi, India Nikhil Mehta
New Delhi, India Pankhuri Dudani

Contents

1 The Outer Brain: Ten Amazing Ways the Skin and Brain Connect

Robert Norman

Over the last several years, I have been working on a new book titled *The Outer Brain: The Power of the Brain-Skin Connection.* I have always been fascinated by this powerful connection and started from the beginning—the embryo—to explore what makes this all happen. Join me as I provide a brief springboard for further exploration of ten ways the brain and skin connect. In my book, I cover hundreds of avenues of brain-skin interactions and have chosen ten here that may be of particular interest to my readers. I have also created a series of YouTube videos that cover the Brain-Skin connections.

Reflecting on the texture of the skin and its intricate connections below the surface prompts the question: Why does the skin share such a profound link with the nervous system? Both the skin and the nervous system originate from the outermost layer of the embryo, known as the ectoderm, which serves as the initial covering for the embryonic body. While the primary role of the central nervous system is to keep the organism informed about external stimuli, it forms from the in-turned section of the embryonic body's surface.

Following the differentiation of the brain, spinal cord, and other central nervous system components, the remaining surface covering transforms into the skin along with its associated features, such as hair, nails, and teeth. The ectoderm is also responsible for generating the sensory organs for smell, taste, hearing, vision, and touch—essentially, everything related to external experiences. This perspective leads to the notion that the nervous system can be seen as a concealed aspect of the skin, and conversely, the skin can be considered the external nervous system.

These two organ systems establish an intimate connection from their initial stages of development and maintain this interconnectedness throughout an

R. Norman (✉)
Nova Southeastern University, Fort Lauderdale, FL, USA

Center for Geriatric Dermatology, Integrative Dermatology and Neuro-Dermatology, Tampa, FL, USA

S. Gupta et al. (eds.), *Critical Thinking in Contemporary Dermatology: Cognitive Essays*, https://doi.org/10.1007/978-981-97-0411-8_1

individual's life. Frederic Wood Jones, a notable English anatomist from the early twentieth century, aptly expressed this relationship, stating that true wisdom for a physician and philosopher lies in recognizing that when observing the external appearance of fellow humans, one is essentially studying the external nervous system rather than merely the skin and its appendages.

Skin defines our social identity and our medical identity as well. For more on the cultural imperative of the skin, see *The Blue Man and Other Stories of the Skin* [1].

Our skin also reflects critical changes to the way we think, feel, and perceive, as well as our ability to handle stress and make decisions. By knowing how to read its signals, the skin can reveal the beginning stages of depression, personality disorders, and dementias, including Alzheimer's disease and even Parkinson's, long before these diseases wreak personal havoc. What can we do right now to protect, enhance, and even reverse changes to both our inner and outer brains?

Here I will present ten brain and skin narratives. I will dive deep during certain inquiries and leave more room for questions in others.

1.1 How Does the Human Skin Microbiome Influence Our Brain and Mental Status?

Our skin reflects critical changes to the way we think, feel, and perceive. Both skin cells and brain cells develop from the same kind of embryonic tissue (ectoderm). The human skin, the body's largest organ, plays host to a community of beneficial microorganisms [2]. The skin microbiota is composed of millions of bacteria, fungi and viruses. The key roles of the skin microbiota, in a similar fashion to the gut microbiota, are to educate our innate and adaptive immune system, protect against invading pathogens, and break down natural products.

A diverse microbiota colonizes the skin and has evolved to utilize the nutrients available on the skin's surface. Although there are myriad environmental perturbations over time, the skin microbiota of a healthy adult remains largely stable. Altered microbial states can create or alter skin diseases.

How do the gut and skin microbiota differ? Microbial communities in the gut stabilize around 3 years, with most strains likely acquired from family members and close contacts.

Initial colonization of the newborn's skin depends on the way the baby first enters the world. Vaginal delivery allows bacteria colonization with the vagina, and Caesarian section babies acquire skin microorganisms.

Skin microbial species change during puberty due to a rise in hormones that fire up the sebaceous glands to produce more sebum. These changes result in marked variations in the bacterial and fungal landscape and predict which skin diseases will be more likely compared to the pre-pubertal period.

The gut is filled with all kinds of microbiota-friendly, juicy meals compared to the much less diversified and robust diet provided to the skin microbiota. For the skin microbiota, the issue of survival depends on a menu selection of basic proteins and lipids in an acidic, cool, and desiccated environment of sebum, sweat, and the stratum corneum.

Much has been written lately about the gut microbiome and the brain [3]. We have many unanswered questions. How does the human skin microbiome influence our brain and mental status? What is the crosstalk between the immune system, the brain, the mouth, the gut and the skin microbiota?

What about the effect of geographical location (for example, China vs the United States) on the microbiome? If the skin microbiome affects the brain, could different species inherent in different geographic regions affect brain function differently?

1.2 Touch: The Primary Brain-Skin Connection

How does the skin communicate with the brain through the sense of touch? Touch involves sensory receptors that decode physical or chemical stimuli into electrical impulses that travel from the outer brain to the inner brain, along the central nervous system, at over 200 miles per hour. These receptors can identify changes in pressure, pain, heat and cold. They are located in every part of the skin, with the hands, face, and mouth having the most. The tongue has more than 9000 sensory receptors, which is why babies first learn to explore their world with their tongues.

The brain has evolved two distinct but parallel pathways that process touch. The first is *the sensory pathway*, linking the skin to the primary somatosensory cortex. This is the region of the brain that decodes touch. The sensory pathway is also involved in creating memories from tactile experiences, which explains how touch not only conveys but also activates deep-seated emotions. Touch can be a powerful contributor to emotional well-being, and a lack of touch adds to the social isolation that goes hand-in-hand with epidemic depression. Each touch can play an important role in the development of self-esteem or unfortunately, with abuse, create a painful memory.

Why are certain touches experienced differently depending on the person or context of the interaction? For instance, a hug from your spouse or partner hopefully lights you up more than a hug from a casual acquaintance.

The second pathway that connects the brain with the skin is hormonal, referred to as *the neuroendocrine pathway*. This brain pathway signals the brain to release oxytocin, the love hormone, and is associated with social bonding and sexual pleasure. It also is the mechanism that creates the feedback loop of stress-related skin conditions like acne, atopic dermatitis, psoriasis, melasma (brown spots) and alopecia (hair loss), which is first triggered through the mast cells in the skin.

As we age, the skin loses its ability to decode touch. Every year following adulthood, we lose one percent of our tactile sense as the density of nerve endings in the hands and feet decreases: the nerves die off and don't return. The insulating material in the brain, called myelin, also coats nerve fibers in the skin, and as we age, myelin naturally breaks down, and the information that transfers from the skin to the brain along the two pathways moves more slowly. This is one of the reasons that the elderly are prone to falling: their brain is getting less information from the soles of their feet. A loss of touch perception also affects the elderly in other ways, especially those in bed for sustained periods. Because their brain does not receive the message of touch, it doesn't prompt them to move or turn in their beds, creating injuries and subsequent infections, including pressure ulcers.

Stimulation to the skin, through touch, enhances neurogenesis, the proliferation of new brain cells and neuronal connections throughout life. A 1986 study noted that massaged preterm infants gained 47% more weight than non-massaged infants, were more socially responsive, and were discharged 6 days earlier from the hospital. Yet I have unfortunately witnessed the deleterious effects of poor parenting, with infants showing failure to thrive and other debilitating problems due to a lack of parental touch. I recall the story of one 4-month-old boy that I examined who had been abandoned by his parents. He was finally adopted by his grandparents, who doted on him through their gentle touch. When I saw him just a few weeks later he seemed to have gained a much greater sense of mental stability.

The profound consequences of touch deprivation have been illustrated through several poignant narratives in the 2014 book "Romania's Abandoned Children" by Nelson, Fox, and Zeanah [4]. Focused on the aftermath of the 1989 fall of Romania's Ceausescu regime, which left approximately 170,000 children in dire conditions across 700 overcrowded institutions, the book delves into the far-reaching effects of early experiences on children's brain development, behavior, and psychological well-being.

The devastating impact of lack of responsive care, social interaction, stimulation, and psychological comfort deprivation is vividly portrayed in the accounts. The Bucharest Early Intervention Project (BEIP), initiated in 2000, played a crucial role in investigating this. This project conducted a meticulously controlled examination of foster care as an alternative to institutionalization. A group of 136 abandoned infants and toddlers were included in the study, with half placed in foster care specifically established for the project, while the other half remained in substandard Romanian institutions. Over twelve years, both groups underwent assessments covering physical growth, cognitive functioning, brain development, and social behavior. Data from a third group of children raised by their birth families were collected for comparison.

The study revealed severe impairments in IQ and various social and emotional disorders among institutionalized children, accompanied by changes in brain development. Importantly, the research highlighted a positive correlation between the age at which an institutionalized child entered foster care and the extent of their recovery, emphasizing the critical role of early intervention in mitigating the detrimental effects of institutionalization.

1.3 Phantom Vibration Syndrome and Hypervigilance

> We all understand the joys of our always-wired world—the connections, the validations, the laughs … the info. … But we are only beginning to get our minds around the costs.

Andrew Sullivan [5] It's a singularly modern problem but also one rooted deep in human biology: Sometimes people feel their cell phones vibrating on their skin when there is no cell phone around. You've probably felt it yourself. In one study, 89% of participants had experienced these phantom vibrations. Victims have started calling the response "vibranxiety" or "ringxiety." Given that more than half the people on our planet carry a cellular phone, vibrate-mode usage is quite common. For a certain percentage, moderate to severe symptoms of phantom vibrations will result in symptoms that may need treatment.

I also have a personal connection: I was treating Kevin G., a 27-year-old who saw me for skin issues, when he mentioned a problem that was driving him a bit batty. "I constantly feel my pocket vibrating, and when I check, I find that my cell phone is in another pocket, or sometimes it's still in my car. Is there something I can do about this?"

The answer is surprisingly complicated. For many researchers, including Jack Tsao, an assistant professor of neurology at the Uniform Services University in Maryland, the phenomenon has a physiological basis related to the phantom limb. Given that both skin cells and brain cells develop from the same kind of embryonic tissue (ectoderm), it makes sense that there are numerous ways that we can manifest those connections. In the case of an amputated leg, the neurons that control the leg's movement and sensation still exist in the brain. The brain can also provide vibrations to your right thigh like a phantom limb.

That addresses the how. As for the why, Jon Kaas, a professor of psychiatry at Vanderbilt University, studies phantom vibration using conditioning experiments. "People are rewarded when they are able to detect low amplitude vibrations, so they get better and better at responding," Kaas says. That behavior may create an automatic behavior that increases nerve-brain connections and forms new pathways. William Barr, chief of neuropsychology at NYU School of Medicine, describes cell phones as virtual appendages, part of the "neuromatrix" of the body. "It's an interesting technological statement about society that our machines are becoming part of us," he says. "If your cell phone is not there, you still feel like it is."

The objective of a 2010 cross-sectional study by Rothberg et al. of medical staff at an academic medical center was "to describe the prevalence of and risk factors for experiencing 'phantom vibrations,' the sensory hallucination sometimes experienced by people carrying pagers or cell phones when the device is not vibrating." Of 169 participants, 68% of cell phone users reported sometimes feeling the sensation of a vibrating cell phone when, in fact, the phone was not actually vibrating or not even being carried. Thirteen percent of the survey's respondents reported feeling phantom cell phone vibrations at least once per day. A cell phone in a breast pocket was more likely to create phantom vibrations than on a belt clip.

According to David Linden, a professor of neuroscience at the Johns Hopkins University School of Medicine, phantom cell phone vibrations are the products of expectation based on prior individual experience and "phantom cell phone vibration results from no stimulus at all and hence qualifies as a full-blown hallucination." He states that if the person was examined in the brain scanner, it's likely they would show activation of the appropriate site in the body map of the primary somatosensory cortex.

In Rothberg's study, the authors argue that the term "sensations" in the context of phantom vibrations is more accurately described as tactile hallucinations. In this phenomenon, the brain interprets a sensation that does not correspond to any actual external stimulus. Despite the association of the term "hallucination" with mental illness, the authors note that phantom vibration syndrome occurs in a majority of normal individuals. Given the widespread use of the term and to align with popular understanding, the authors suggest retaining the term "phantom vibration syndrome" even though it carries a connotation linked to mental health. These authors note that vibration syndrome may result from the cerebral cortex's misinterpretation of incoming sensory signals. They note, "To deal with the overwhelming amount of sensory input, the brain applies filters or schema based on what it expects to find, a process known as hypothesis-guided search." In the case of phantom vibrations, the brain anticipates a call and misinterprets sensory input via this preconceived hypothesis. The sensory stimulus may include muscle contractions, pressure from clothing, or other sensory stimuli.

As Rothberg et al. state, hallucinations, while sometimes indicative of pathology, are not exclusive to abnormal conditions; they frequently manifest in individuals considered normal and extend beyond vibrations. Instances of auditory hallucinations involving cell phone ringtones are also reported. The widespread occurrence of phantom vibrations suggests that this sensation is rooted in normal brain mechanisms. Why do certain individuals, such as younger people, experience phantom vibrations, and why are some body locations more susceptible? Rothberg et al. suggest that younger minds exhibit increased neural plasticity and more imaginary vibrations. The Rothberg study reflects that urgency may have a certain role in the answer. Pager vibrations require urgent attention. Just as new mothers can consistently imagine hearing their baby's monitor go off, certain people feel obligated to constantly check their phones and pagers. The vibrations stimulate the brain's creation of a sensory memory for that particular phone location, which continues when enforced.

Ultimately, phantom vibration reflects how the human body ignores certain stimuli and fixates on others. Sensations are not just sensations; expectations, experiences, and psychological states all influence the threshold for signal detection. As a result, there is no quick fix. The best strategy would be simply to disable vibrate mode and eliminate skin-phone contact, causing the skin-brain connections to diminish over time.

I suggested that tactic to Kevin. On follow-up, he reported fewer episodes of phantom vibration, but he still had occasional symptoms. Perhaps the vibrations were an anticipatory signal now embedded in his nervous system—a persistent symptom of our deep dependency on our devices.

Here's another possible sensory addiction to add to the mix. Haptics is the science and technology of transmitting and understanding information through touch [6]. In the case of a cell phone, a joystick, or a myriad of other devices, haptics are any type of technology that gives you a tactile response when you do something. A haptic touch is a specific form of haptic feedback that uses vibrations to mimic sensations like pressing a button or scrolling through a list when you do it on your screen. The click-click and vibration feel can make the user keep coming back for more and more.

Phantom vibration leads one to explore the trend in hypervigilance. In a recent Ofcom study the researchers found that the average person spends 8 h and 21 min sleeping in 24 h. But the average adult also clocks up an enormous 8 h 41 min actively connected to media or digital communication, indicating that many people spend more than half their waking hours peering into an electronic device.

How far does this high-tech hypervigilance go? According to a new HuffPost/YouGov survey, 63% of smartphone users aged 18–29 admitted to drifting to sleeping with a cell phone, smartphone or tablet in their bed. Why not substitute a significant other for a smartphone? Not only does it disrupt sleep, it leads to even more hypervigilance that can become addictive and disruptive.

Has the intoxicating noise of the phone as it demands your attention become a siren that draws you and your hypervigilant ego to its illuminated shores despite the danger it may hold? If you are tense and on high alert, it's tough to get restful sleep: "Subconsciously, you're expecting a call or text and this means your sleep will be lighter," explains sleep expert Dr. Neil Stanley.

1.4 How Did the Evolution of Hairlessness Help Us to Stay Alive and Create Bigger Brains?

Theories abound as to why we became relatively hairless compared to other species. One theory about our abandonment of fur includes the avoidance of parasites [7]. As we became less nomadic and inhabited caves and other dwelling sites for longer periods of time, we allowed more contact with parasites or other animals. One example is bat bugs, who feed on sleeping bats and crossed species onto early hairy humans, giving rise to bed bugs. Our sedentary and group lifestyle also provided a host for fleas and their transmissible diseases, such as the plague; hosting fleas is a singular fact to us and no other primates. Losing hair was a major buzz-kill.

The issue is survival and living long enough to mate. Even without vectors, hair favors the spread of disease. As with most dermatologists I have treated children and others with severe bacterial and fungal hair infections that may have resulted in mortality in our early ancestors.

Each of us possesses between two million and five million eccrine glands to discharge sweat. Hairless skin and watery sweat help humans eliminate excess heat more efficiently than collecting warmth in the fur found in all other primates.

The invention of clothing allowed us to change clothing to control our temperatures and protect the skin from other ectoparasites, such as ticks and lice. Due to weather patterns and dietary changes incorporating more meat, human hunters needed to travel greater distances for diminished food supplies. Losing hair along with increased ability to sweat to avoid overheating were life-saving adaptations. Combined with the fact that hairlessness helped prevent infections, the trait of being hairy eventually had more costs than benefits.

What about bigger brains? According to Nina Jablonski, "the loss of most of our body hair and the gain of the ability to dissipate excess body heat through eccrine sweating helped to make possible the dramatic enlargement of our most temperature-sensitive organ, the brain [8]." In Jablonski's research she noted that Australopithecines had a brain that was 400 cubic centimeters on average, and the modern brain is three times that size. The higher caloric intake of meat and other foods also contributed to the high energy demands of the growing brain. Losing our body hair, increasing the number of our eccrine sweat glands, and boosting our calories all contribute to our gray matter expansion. To answer your question, shaving off all your hair will *not* make you smarter.

1.5 How Can the Skin Provide a Way to Detect Brain Abnormalities?

Much of my interest and research over the last decade has been on the connection between the skin and the brain, including searching for skin biomarkers to detect Alzheimer's disease (AD) and the connection between Parkinson's disease (PD) and melanoma.

Neurodegenerative disorders are identified by the abnormal accumulation of protein aggregates in the brain. Notably, the occurrence of phosphorylated Tau protein (p-Tau) aggregates is a distinctive feature of Alzheimer's disease (AD) and other significant neurodegenerative conditions like corticobasal degeneration and frontotemporal dementia. These aggregates also play a role in conditions like Parkinson's disease (PD).

What is Tau? Traditionally, it was considered a cytoplasmic protein whose major biological function would be to stabilize microtubules and facilitate axonal transport. According to this view, in AD there is a hyperphosphorylation of Tau that leads to the intracellular accumulation of Tau in the form of neurofibrillary tangles. Now we know that Tau protects the nuclear and chromatin organization for proper gene expression throughout neuronal life. Tau protein transfer to the cytoplasm results in the loss of the protector role of nuclear Tau and subsequent global chromatin disorganization. Therefore, the cytoplasmic Tau protein accumulations that characterize AD have been completely reinterpreted, as it is the search for new therapeutic solutions.

Let me briefly and simply explain the two key disease players and what we have found. PD is a neurodegenerative disorder that triggers the death of dopaminergic neurons within the brain's substantia nigra. This disorder is characterized by intracellular inclusions primarily composed of proteinaceous α-synuclein amyloid fibrils. Melanocytes are the pigmented cells that give rise to skin, hair and eye color, and melanoma is a potentially deadly cancer arising from melanocytes. Interestingly, there is a significant coincidence of PD and melanoma that may suggest a shared pathophysiology [9].

Recently, we reported that PD and melanoma patients have increased staining for α-synuclein in their skin [10]. We think that neurons and melanocytes, both derived from neuroectodermal cells, may share protein synthesis and regulation pathways that become dysfunctional in PD and melanoma. Therefore, uncovering the behavior of α-synuclein in melanoma could both provide novel approaches for treating melanoma and insights into the role of α-synuclein in PD. As Dean and Lee (2021) noted, we should investigate how α-synuclein influences melanoma cell survival because this may reveal new insights into α-synuclein function that may be used to prevent dopaminergic cell death and subsequently PD.

Identifying PD has been limited by inadequate sensitivity and specificity. Various diagnostic tests have been utilized, including olfactory function testing, cardiovascular autonomic testing, biological fluids (including CSF and blood) testing and PET or SPECT imaging. According to Rodriguez-Leyva (2014, 2016) and Wang and collaborators (2021), skin deposition of misfolded α-synuclein is a potential biomarker for PD [11]. For Donadio (2019) "the autonomic skin innervation is a useful site for the search of abnormal α-syn aggregates since peripheral sympathetic nerves could be the earliest affected neural region and autonomic symptoms may precede the classical symptoms of synucleinopathy, such as motor dysfunction in PD [12, 13]."

While Tau protein was traditionally believed to be limited to the central nervous system, it has also been discovered in peripheral tissues. In 2017, my colleagues Maria E. Jimenez-Capdeville, Ildefonso Rodríguez-Leyva, William Eng, and I published our paper, which described our investigation into variation in Tau expression in oral mucosa cells according to the individual's cognitive impairment [9].

Immunocytochemistry and immunofluorescence analyses uncovered the existence of Tau and four phosphorylated Tau (p-Tau) forms within the cytoplasm and nucleus of oral mucosa cells. Subjects with cognitive impairment exhibited a higher positivity for both Tau and p-Tau in comparison to control subjects, showcasing a speckled pattern in both the nucleus and cytoplasm. Quantitative real-time polymerase chain reaction revealed elevated mRNA expression of Tau in subjects with cognitive impairment compared to the control group.

Our findings highlight an increased presence of p-Tau and Tau transcripts in the oral mucosa of cognitively impaired individuals when contrasted with healthy subjects. The feasibility of quantifying p-Tau using flow cytometry supports the potential use of oral mucosa analysis as a screening tool for proteinopathies in cognitively impaired patients. By employing oral swabs for specimen collection and identifying biomarkers for dementia, this research opens avenues for future investigations. It empowers patients to assess these crucial markers, facilitating informed health decisions.

As a clinician and researcher, I truly enjoy working with my colleagues who have inquisitive minds and are searching to unlock the mysteries of human life. Collaboration is a key to our progress and by sharing our important research and clinical findings, we can move ahead at a more effective and rapid pace.

Dementia, Parkinson's Disease, skin cancer and many other issues that may be helped by robust skin biomarkers and research are among the most important public health issues of our time. The sooner we can create new preventions and treatments based on the successful results of our collective hard work, the quicker we can alleviate the suffering of millions of diseased and debilitated co-inhabitants of our world.

1.6 Do Women and Men Feel and Remember Touch Differently?

Over the years, I have heard countless stories about touch and skin, told from myriad points of view, and I wonder about the gender derivation of the narratives.

Do sexual orientation and hormones affect the brain-skin connection? Men and women are genetically sculpted in different ways. What are the ways that female vs male touch interacts with the brain?

Females have a higher recall of emotional details. Criminologists know this. What about with touch?

Do epigenetics such as mothering style influence the brain-skin connection?

Rates of myelination differ. Childhood adversity and being more or less in touch with the world affect brain-skin validation.

Men think about sex more often—that's how we are genetically wired. We are all female in our first eight weeks of life until the brain in males is soaked with testosterone from the testes, and various brain areas change shape. How does this affect the perception and memory of touch? If a person "changes sex," does a change in touch and brain interaction accompany the new variations, if any?

In Dr. Louann Brizendine's books "The Female Brain" and "The Male Brain," she observes that women, on average, use around 20,000 words per day, while men use approximately 7000 words per day. According to Barton Goldsmith, this difference may result in men feeling talked out by the end of the day while women still have a surplus of words to express. Goldsmith suggests that men might be less inclined to engage in conversation because women tend to surpass them in verbal expression.

Goldsmith also notes that men and women exhibit distinct conversational styles. Women often speak more rapidly when excited and may interrupt their partners struggling to articulate their thoughts. In such situations, men may feel disconnected or shut down because they sense a disruption and find it challenging to express their feelings. Men, generally finding it more challenging to verbalize emotions, may encounter difficulty getting back on track in emotional conversations.

1.7 What Does the Skin Reveal About Psychiatric Disorders?

In what ways does the skin reveal brain changes? Perhaps the most important skin signs are seen with neuropsychiatric, addiction, pain and itch disorders.

Psychiatric disorders are central nervous system conditions with a neurobiological basis. They generally involve disturbances of emotion, cognition, motivation and socialization. Psychiatric disorders can either lead to psychocutaneous (skin) manifestations as a consequence or they may arise as a result of a chronic dermatological condition that impacts the patient's mental health.

What can be done about these troubling maladies? Treatment for neurodermatitis is multifocal. Initial treatment usually involves topical and systemic glucocorticoids. Glucocorticoids are used to decrease the itching and redness of affected areas. Additionally, treatment may be aimed at decreasing depression or any psychological ailments, if present. Counseling and Habit reversal therapy have been successful in encouraging the cessation of scratching.

Several studies have been launched to find ways to quiet the discomfort of prurigo nodularis (PN). Kiniksa Pharmaceuticals sponsor one to investigate the efficacy and safety of vixarelimab (KPL-716), a monoclonal antibody administered subcutaneously that targets oncostatin M (OSM) receptor-beta (OSMRβ) to inhibit two cytokine signaling pathways, interleukin-31 (IL-31) and OSM. This potentially disrupts the pruritus, inflammation, hyperkeratosis and fibrosis associated with PN. Many cases of PN are associated with depression, and perhaps utilizing psychiatric interventions with new injectable treatments might provide relief.

What skin diseases reflect neuroendocrine dysfunction? Neurocutaneous disorders include tuberous sclerosis, ataxia-telangiectasia, and Sturge-Weber syndrome.

Although itching and pain sensations were thought to be sent along the same nerve pathways at one time, researchers reported the discovery in 2003 of itch-specific nerve pathways. Nerve endings that are specifically sensitive to itching have been named *pruriceptors*.

Pruritus, commonly known as itch, initiates with external stimuli such as dust, touch, or a mosquito landing on the skin. It is an innate defense mechanism that alerts the body to potential harm. When the stimuli surpass a certain threshold and scratch the skin's surface layer, dermal skin receptors promptly send a signal through skin fibers to the spinal cord and then to the cerebral cortex in the brain, triggering the urge to scratch. While scratching may provide temporary relief, a persistent itch can lead to a chronic itching and scratching cycle.

The term "itch" has taken on various connotations in our society. Research indicates that catchy songs can become stuck in our heads due to a "brain itch" or "cognitive itch," akin to histamines that induce an itching sensation in the brain. The only way to alleviate this cognitive itch is by repeatedly replaying the tune. Consequently, songs like "Who Let The Dogs Out?" can be likened to an auditory itch that has the potential to drive a person to the brink of frustration.

'Senile pruritus' refers to the dry skin of aging. I never liked that term, although it dates back to when the term senile had a more benign connotation, perhaps like misplacing your keys instead of feeling your mind slip into the shadows.

1.8 What Are the Connections Between Touch, Sight, Hearing, and Mental Illness?

The research is provocative but still inconclusive. How do touch, vision, and the brain interact with mental illness? Are there levels of brain-tactile dysfunctions in a continuum just as there is with autism and schizophrenia? No congenitally blind person has been shown to have schizophrenia. Why do psychopaths have such high pain thresholds?

According to ScienceDaily, USC scientists have identified a "mind's touch" to complement Shakespeare's famous reference to "the mind's eye [14]." The researchers found that, as a person observes an object, the brain not only processes its visual appearance but also retains the memory of what it feels like to touch that object. This connection is so robust that a computer, analyzing data solely from the brain's touch-processing region, can predict the object the person is looking at.

Building on prior research that demonstrated a similar connection between the visual and auditory regions of the brain, the research group led by Antonio and Hanna Damasio at the USC Dornsife Brain and Creativity Institute used magnetic resonance brain scans and specially programmed computers to investigate the interaction between memory and the senses. The study's findings were published in the journal Cerebral Cortex.

The Damasio research team conducted an experiment in which participants watched five video clips featuring hands touching different objects. They utilized functional magnetic resonance imaging (fMRI) to scan the region of the participants' brains responsible for processing touch sensations. The data generated by the scan was then fed into a specially programmed computer.

Surprisingly, the computer accurately predicted, based solely on how the "tactile" part of the cerebral cortex had responded, which of the five video clips the participants had viewed [15]. Kaspar Meyer, the lead author of the study, explained that when individuals were asked to imagine the sensation of touching contrasting objects, such as a cold, slick piece of metal versus the warm fur of a kitten, they often reported experiencing these sensations in their "mind's touch." The study demonstrated that this mental touch sensation activated the same brain regions as actual physical touch.

The ScienceDaily author notes, "Human brains capture and store physical sensations, and then replay them when prompted by viewing the corresponding visual image."

I spoke with my friend Chelsea, who is a blind massage therapist who had attended the Florida School for the Deaf and the Blind (FSDB). After she graduated, she went to a technical college. I asked her about her school and work. "We learned anatomy, physiology, science, body mechanics and did massage for seven months," Chelsea said.

"You said you close your eyes when you work on clients. Does that help you with your tactile ability and concentration?" I asked. "I know with a sighted person like myself many times, for example, when I listen to music, I like to close my eyes because I don't want all the distractions of looking around the room. I just want to sense and feel the music. Is this a similar feeling?"

"Yes, I think closing my eyes gives me extra concentration and focus," Chelsea said. "I think I bring a positive energy to my clients. I always try and be in a good mood and happy focusing on then," she said. "Sometimes I have my eyes open; it just depends. I usually keep the room dim or low lighting. I like to do a verbal consultation before each client but we have all things documented with an iPad."

Not all blind people are completely blind; some can see light or images that may interfere with a full tactile sensation. I asked her about Braille, and she replied, "I do read Braille. I think our fingertips and touch strength are a little bit better because when you lose your sight, your other senses become stronger. You become more aware of your other perceptions and you become more focused and more in tune."

"Do you take care of all kinds of clients?" I asked.

"I have worked on thousands of people from seven years old up to 93 years old. I have also become stretch certified. I like to check in with them throughout the session to make sure everything is good. Today I had six clients, five women and one male. They all were 1-h sessions. Sometimes I do 90-min sessions. And a variety of people and muscle issues."

What do we know about the connection between touch and vision? Which blind people are more adept at Braille? What is the relationship between color vision and tactile perception? Do color-blind people have heightened or decreased tactile sensation? "You can't trick a color-blind person into seeing color." Are there tricks between the skin and the brain?

The sense of touch allows us to make a better connection between sight and hearing and therefore helps adults to learn to read [16]. These results should improve learning methods, both for children learning to read and adults learning foreign languages.

1.9 How Does Aging Skin Contain Clues About Aging Brains?

The aging process occurs concurrently with the buildup of stress. Aging is described as a gradual deterioration over time in living organisms, driven by an increased vulnerability to diseases and adverse circumstances. This results in diminished viability and physiological functions. In simpler terms, aging is marked by an individual's diminished capacity to respond effectively to stress.

Both skin cells and brain cells develop from the same kind of embryonic tissue (ectoderm). A brain biopsy to detect brain tissue aging is impractical, but a skin biopsy is readily attainable and can provide an experimental model for aging research on the brain. The skin and brain age in similar ways. Influences include inherited genes, diet, environmental factors, sleep, exercise, and hormones. As we age, skin becomes dry and thin due to hormone decline.

How does the brain-skin interaction change as time goes on? What brain-skin magic can be done to help decrease the assault on both the brain and the skin?

As highlighted in a publication by Chen and Lyga, the skin serves as the primary sensory organ for external stressors, encompassing factors like heat, cold, pain, and mechanical tension [17]. Three categories of receptors—thermoreceptors for temperature, nociceptors for pain, and mechanoreceptors for mechanical stimuli—play a role in transmitting external signals to the spinal cord and subsequently to the brain. Cutaneous sensory fibers also relay information regarding changes in temperature, pH, and inflammatory mediators to the central nervous system (CNS). The nerve terminals are often associated with these receptors, indicating a close interaction. In response to these signals, the brain influences stress responses in the skin.

Arguably, the body's immune system is the most crucial element for enduring challenging conditions and resisting the fragility associated with aging. Beyond its role in eliminating antigens, the immune system plays a pivotal role in maintaining the body's internal balance. It actively monitors for aberrant reactions that could lead to unchecked malignancies, aids in the body's reshaping and rebuilding in adaptation to stressors, and ensures physiological well-being (2). The diminished capacity to handle stressors supports the idea that aging, inherently associated with progressing into "elderly" status, signifies a state of increased vulnerability to diseases and an inability to withstand stresses typically managed by the immune system. This diminished resilience implies that aging itself can be considered a disease state (3). The weakening of the human immune system's efficiency and the reduced dynamic interaction between the brain and the skin contribute to this state of vulnerability in the face of physiological challenges.

In their concluding remarks, Chen and Lyga assert, "Recent research has revealed that the skin is not merely a recipient of signals from psychological stress; it actively engages in the stress response through a local HPA axis, peripheral nerve endings, and various local skin cells such as keratinocytes, mast cells, and immune cells. Moreover, intricate feedback mechanisms and communication exist between the brain and the skin, with pro-inflammatory cytokines and neurogenic inflammatory pathways playing significant roles in mediating these responses." The authors emphasize the impact of major pathways and effector cells on skin functions and diseases, highlighting how chronic stress can adversely influence the skin's aging process.

We live in a time with a "silver tsunami" of aging, an unprecedented number of older people due to increased life expectancy and survival. Investigating how and when we age, immunity, and dermatological manifestations in our elderly is a complex and challenging task.

1.10 How Can We Deliver Life-Enhancing Therapy to the Brain via the Skin?

What are topical nootropics (brain-enhancing drugs)? How does transdermal drug delivery work? What are common drugs delivered via the skin? How will this change in the future?

Being the largest organ in the body, the skin constitutes about 10% of an individual's body mass. Its extensive surface area makes it a practical portal for administering potent drugs for systemic effects.

In an article by Prausnitz and Langer, it is stated that "Transdermal delivery offers an appealing alternative to oral drug delivery and is positioned to serve as an alternative to hypodermic injections. Throughout history, people have applied substances to the skin for therapeutic purposes, and in modern times, various topical formulations have been developed to address local conditions. The first transdermal system for systemic delivery, a 3-day patch delivering scopolamine to combat motion sickness, received approval in the United States in 1979. A decade later, nicotine patches achieved transdermal blockbuster status, significantly elevating the profile of transdermal delivery in both medicine and the public sphere [18]."

"Presently, numerous transdermal delivery systems exist for drugs like estradiol, fentanyl, lidocaine, and testosterone. There are combination patches containing multiple drugs for contraception and hormone replacement, as well as iontophoretic and ultrasonic delivery systems for analgesia. It is estimated that over one billion transdermal patches are currently manufactured annually for cosmetic, topical, and transdermal delivery applications."

Addressing brain cancers that originate as metastases from skin cancer represents a challenging scenario. Promising results have been seen in preclinical models involving the utilization of stem cells loaded with oncolytic viruses.

In a study conducted at Brigham and Women's Hospital and reported in PNAS, researchers have proposed a potential solution for eliminating tumor cells that have spread to the brain. The team has devised cancer-killing viruses capable of being delivered via stem cells through the carotid artery, and they have applied this approach to metastatic tumors in the brains of clinically relevant mouse models [19].

Metastatic brain tumors, commonly originating from lung, breast, or skin cancers, constitute the most frequently observed tumors within the brain and contribute to around 40% of advanced melanoma metastases. According to Khalid Shah, MS, PhD, the director of the Center for Stem Cell Therapeutics and Imaging (CSTI) in the BWH Department of Neurosurgery and the leader of the study, the current therapeutic options for such patients are limited, especially when there are numerous metastases. Their results represent the first insights into targeting multiple brain metastatic deposits using stem-cell-loaded oncolytic viruses designed to selectively eliminate dividing tumor cells.

How can lasers be used on the skin for drug delivery? Employing lasers as a drug permeation-enhancement method proves effective in facilitating drug delivery into or across the skin [20]. This involves the controlled disruption and ablation of the stratum corneum (SC), the primary barrier for drug delivery. Lin et al. discussed in their article the mechanisms behind laser-assisted drug permeation, including direct ablation of the skin barrier, optical breakdown via a photomechanical wave, and a photothermal effect. Ablative approaches for enhancing drug transport offer advantages such as increased bioavailability, rapid treatment time, prompt recovery of SC integrity, and the absence of a need for skin surface contact.

The combination of transdermal stem cells and laser techniques for treating both the skin and brain has garnered increasing attention and is expected to continue growing in significance over time.

1.11 Summary

I appreciate your readership and any insights you can provide on the power of the Brain-Skin connection.—drrobertnorman@gmail.com

References

1. Norman R. The blue man and other stories of the skin. California: University of California Press; 2014.
2. Byrd A, Belkaid Y, Segre J. The human skin microbiome. Nat Rev Microbiol. 2018;16:143–55. https://doi.org/10.1038/nrmicro.2017.157.
3. https://www.getquip.com/blog/your-oral-microbiome-explained
4. Nelson F, Zeanah. Romania's abandoned children. Cambridge: Harvard University Press; 2014.
5. Sullivan, A (2016). 'I used to be a human being', New York Magazine, 19 September. Available at: https://nymag.com/intelligencer/2016/09/andrew-sullivan-my-distraction-sickness-and-yours.html (Accessed 11 April 2024).

6. Fredembach B, de Boisferon AH, Gentaz E. Learning of arbitrary association between visual and auditory novel stimuli in adults: the "bond effect" of haptic exploration. PLoS One. 2009;4(3):e4844.
7. Dunn R. The wild life of our bodies: predators, parasites, and partners that shape who we are today. New York: Harper; 2011.
8. Jablonski N. https://www.scientificamerican.com/article/the-naked-truth/
9. Arredondo LF, Aranda-Romo S, Rodríguez-Leyva I, Chi-Ahumada E, Saikaly SK, Portales-Pérez DP, González-Amaro R, Salgado-Bustamante M, Enriquez-Macias L, Eng W, Norman RA, Jimenez-Capdeville ME. Linking Parkinson's disease and melanoma: interplay between α-synuclein and Pmel17 amyloid formation. Tau protein in oral mucosa and cognitive state: a cross-sectional study. Front Neurol. 2017;8:554.
10. Rodriguez-Leyva I, Chi-Ahumada E, Mejía M, Castanedo-Cazares JP, Eng W, Saikaly SK, Carrizales J, Levine TD, Norman RA, Jimenez-Capdeville ME. The presence of alpha-synuclein in skin from melanoma and patients with Parkinson's disease. Mov Disord Clin Pract. 2017;4(5):724–32.
11. Wang Z, Becker K, Donadio V, Siedlak S, Yuan J, Rezaee M, Incensi A, Kuzkina A, Orrú CD, Tatsuoka C, Liguori R, Gunzler SA, Caughey B, Jimenez-Capdeville ME, Zhu X, Doppler K, Cui L, Chen SG, Ma J, Zou WQ. Skin α-synuclein aggregation seeding activity as a novel biomarker for Parkinson disease. JAMA Neurol. 2020;78(1):1–11. https://doi.org/10.1001/jamaneurol.2020.3311. Epub ahead of print. Erratum in: JAMA Neurol. 2021;78:120.
12. Rodríguez-Leyva I, Chi-Ahumada EG, Carrizales J, Rodríguez-Violante M, Velázquez-Osuna S, Medina-Mier V, Martel-Gallegos MG, Zarazúa S, Enríquez-Macías L, Castro A, Calderón-Garcidueñas AL, Jiménez-Capdeville ME. Parkinson disease and progressive supranuclear palsy: protein expression in skin. Ann Clin Transl Neurol. 2016;3:191–9.
13. Rodríguez-Leyva I, Calderón-Garcidueñas AL, Jiménez-Capdeville ME, Rentería-Palomo AA, Hernandez-Rodriguez HG, Valdés-Rodríguez R, Fuentes-Ahumada C, Torres-Álvarez B, Sepúlveda-Saavedra J, Soto-Domínguez A, Santoyo ME, Rodriguez-Moreno JI, Castanedo-Cázares JP. α-synuclein inclusions in the skin of Parkinson's disease and parkinsonism. Ann Clin Transl Neurol. 2014;1:471–8.
14. https://www.sciencedaily.com/releases/2011/09/110908141443.htm
15. Meyer K, Kaplan JT, Essex R, Damasio H, Damasio A. Seeing touch is correlated with content-specific activity in primary somatosensory cortex. Cerebral Cortex. 2011;21:2113. https://doi.org/10.1093/cercor/bhq289.
16. https://www.sciencedaily.com/releases/2009/03/090318112937.htm
17. Chen Y, Lyga J. Brain-Skin connection: stress, inflammation and skin aging. Inflamm Allergy Drug Targets. 2014;13(3):177–90.
18. Prausnitz M, Langer R. Transdermal drug delivery. Nat Biotechnol. 2008;26:1261–8.
19. Du W, Seah I, Bougazzoul O, Choi G, Meeth K, Bosenberg MW, Wakimoto H, Fisher D, Shah K. Stem cell-released oncolytic herpes simplex virus has therapeutic efficacy in brain metastatic melanomas. Proc Natl Acad Sci U S A. 2017;114:E6157–65.
20. Lin CH, et al. Lasers as an approach for promoting drug delivery via skin. Expert Opin Drug Deliv. 2014;11:599–614.

Skin Aging

2

Nikhil Mehta and Somesh Gupta

Skin aging, like all aging, is a natural time-bound process. It is characterized by skin thinning and atrophy, pigmentary changes, pallor, changes in skin texture, xerosis, loss of tensile strength and elasticity, increased laxity and wrinkles, increased fragility and decreased healing, alopecia, dysplastic changes, and decreased thermoregulatory control [1]. Skin aging does not occur in isolation and often correlates well with aging and mortality. It is often said that *skin mirrors your internal health*. Older-looking twins die earlier, have lesser physical and cognitive function, and have shorter telomere length [2]. "Looking older for one's age" indeed correlates with early mortality [3], and more vascular age [4]. Therefore, restricting skin anti-aging treatments to fillers and toxins while ignoring general health measures is short-sightedness.

Skin aging is conventionally divided into intrinsic and extrinsic types. Intrinsic aging is the natural chronological aging programmed into the genetic code of an organism. *Nothing is permanent*, and change in the form of aging with time is the only constant. Adult human skin has 35 billion cells that are rapidly proliferating and are thus exposed to the accumulation of imperfections, as explained by the second law of thermodynamics, the law of entropy. These imperfections contribute to intrinsic aging. In comparison, extrinsic skin aging encompasses changes ascribed to external environmental factors like sun exposure, smoking, air pollution, lifestyle, and metabolic factors. Predominant extrinsic skin aging is due to photoaging.

Despite the conventional separation, any extrinsic factor causes changes, and aging, by influencing the expression of various genes and hastening the pathways responsible for intrinsic aging. It is impossible to study intrinsic aging in isolation in humans, as there's invariably an impact of external factors. Intrinsic aging is

N. Mehta · S. Gupta (✉)
Department of Dermatology and Venereology, All India Institute of Medical Sciences, New Delhi, India
e-mail: someshgupta@aiims.edu

S. Gupta et al. (eds.), *Critical Thinking in Contemporary Dermatology: Cognitive Essays*, https://doi.org/10.1007/978-981-97-0411-8_2

influenced by many factors and variables external to the genetic code and can be tweaked. Smoking, diabetes, metabolic factors, and an individual's microbiome are all internal factors that can impact intrinsic aging. The twin who smokes or is unmarried looks older [5]. Although the biological clock keeps on ticking independently, we can make it run slightly faster or slower.

2.1 Clinical Features and Pathology

The changes in chronological aging include epidermal, dermal, and subcutaneous fat atrophy, loss of tensile strength and elasticity, increased laxity, fragility, and wrinkles. The epidermis becomes thinner, and the dermo-epidermal junction flattens and weakens, increasing fragility on tangential pressure and wrinkling. There is a decrease in basal layer division, epidermal turnover, and transfer of nutrition to the epidermis. There's decreased hair and nail growth and decreased hair density. The density of melanocytes also decreases. Dermis also undergoes atrophy, a decrease in fibroblasts, cellularity, and vasculature, with a decrease in collagen and elastin. This results in decreased tensile strength and elasticity, increased skin laxity and wrinkles, fragility, and decreased wound healing. Glycosaminoglycans are also altered, leading to decreased average hydration of the skin. Despite sebaceous hyperplasia, there's decreased sebum output, hence xerosis of the skin. Sweat glands reduce in number and size, and thermoregulatory control decreases [1].

In photoaging, too, there's wrinkling, decreased fibroblasts, and collagen, similar to chronological aging. Dissimilarities include increased proliferation and turnover of the epidermis, along with dysplastic changes, hence the development of seborrheic keratosis, actinic keratosis, and basal and squamous cell carcinomas, due to the effect of ultraviolet radiation (UVR) on deoxyribose nucleic acid (DNA). There's acanthosis, and the skin acquires a rough leathery texture and sallow yellow color in photoaging in contrast to the thinned-out look of non-exposed aged skin. There's activation and proliferation of melanocytes. Many pigmentary changes occur, including freckles, lentigines, dyspigmentation in the form of spotty/mottled hyperpigmentation and hypopigmentation, and idiopathic guttate hypomelanosis. And lighter skin types are predisposed to melanomas. Instead of decreased elastin, there's elastosis, but as the increased elastic tissue is dysfunctional, there's still decreased elasticity, hence laxity and wrinkles. The dermis has dilated vessels which manifest as telangiectasis and has perivascular inflammatory infiltrate [6, 7]. Some workers consider melasma to be a photoaging disorder [8].

2.2 Genetics

How much variation exists in the speed of this clock amongst humans? Are there fast and slow agers? Various single nucleotide polymorphisms (SNPs) and allelic variants have been demonstrated to be longevity-associated. However, few of them have been consistent, and those too have a very modest effect size [9].

Table 2.1 Factors and mechanisms of aging

Extrinsic factors that hasten aging	Mechanisms of aging
Photo exposure	DNA damage and premature senescence
Smoking	Extracellular matrix (ECM) degradation
Pollution	Oxidative stress and inflammaging
Stress	Advanced glycation end products (AGEs)
Lifestyle	Neuroendocrine system
Metabolic factors	Sirtuins
	Epigenetics
	Dysbiosis

Genome-wide association studies (GWAS) have established common conserved pathways in various age-related diseases, like cardiovascular diseases, metabolic diseases, cancer, and neurodegenerative diseases [10]. Studies analyzing SNPs and GWAS in skin aging have also found associations of specific alleles with specific signs of skin aging. SNPs of pigmentation genes are significantly associated with facial pigmented spots [11, 12], and SNPs of other genes are significantly associated with wrinkles [13].

The role of genetics in extrinsic skin aging is made more apparent by how different races photoage. Different ethnic populations have different frequencies of alleles of melanogenic and other pathways, which have differential activity, hence differential types of photoaging. Caucasian skin has smaller and clustered melanosomes, less UV protection, and thinner stratum corneum and dermis. Hence Caucasian skin photo-ages earlier, has more atrophy and decrease in skin elasticity, has earlier and more wrinkles, and more skin laxity. Asians and Africans have large melanosomes, thicker stratum corneum, thicker and more compact dermis, with larger and a greater number of fibroblasts. Hence, during photoaging, they have more pigmentary manifestations like dyspigmentation but delayed wrinkles [14, 15]. Africans also have more and larger fibroblasts in the dermis and more skin dryness, acanthosis, and textural changes due to photoaging than other races. The equivalent sun protection factor of the African epidermis is 13.4, compared to 3.4 for the Caucasian epidermis [16]. Chinese women have an onset of wrinkles about 10 years later and much more pigmentary spots than French women with similar photo exposure [17]. South Indians show fewer signs of skin aging (including wrinkles and laxity markers) than north and east Indians [18] (Table 2.1).

2.3 Mechanisms

2.3.1 DNA Damage and Premature Senescence

Intrinsic and extrinsic skin aging have many common pathways and mechanisms. Cells normally accumulate DNA damage as they age. This rate is increased significantly due to DNA damage, directly by ultraviolet B (UV-B) and indirectly by oxidative stress due to increased reactive oxygen species (ROS) by ultraviolet-A

(UV-A) and UV-B. As this accumulated damage can result in tumorigenesis if the DNA repair systems are overwhelmed, another way by which tumor suppressor genes mitigate carcinogenesis is by inducing premature senescence [19]. Premature senescence is growth arrest and functional inactivation of cells without cell death. DNA damage decreases epidermal and mesenchymal stem cells [20] and causes premature senescence in dermal fibroblasts [21], which leads to the premature aging phenotype of epidermal and dermal atrophy.

Telomeres shorten with each cell division. A critical level of shortening of telomeres with age triggers physiological replicative senescence, which resembles the stress-induced senescence triggered by DNA damage [22]. Shorter telomeres are a marker of aging and skin aging, and premature telomere shortening may result from DNA damage and oxidative stress [22, 23]. Factors causing DNA damage, premature aging, and skin aging, such as smoking, air pollution, lifestyle, and metabolic factors, are associated with shorter telomeres [24]. Sun-exposed skin has shorter telomeres than non-exposed skin [25]. Many premature aging syndromes have defects in the DNA repair pathway and telomer maintenance [19].

2.3.2 Extracellular Matrix (ECM) Degradation

Apart from premature senescence of fibroblasts, another factor responsible for decreased extracellular matrix of the dermis is the enzyme imbalance, which involves decreased collagen production, decreased activity transforming growth factor-βand increased activity of matrix metalloproteinases (MMPs), without any increase in the tissue inhibitors of MMPs (TIMPs). This is done by mediators like transcription factor activator protein-1 (AP-1) and nuclear factor-κB (NF-κB), which are in turn activated downstream to mitogen-activated protein kinase (MAPK) and mammalian target of rapamycin (mTOR) pathways. Extrinsic causes of aging, like UV-A radiation, oxidative stress, and smoking, activate the MAPK [26] and mTOR [27] pathways to initiate these downstream effects. They also cause a proinflammatory milieu and influx of neutrophils and macrophages, which secrete and elastase, degradation of elastin, and replacement by abnormal non-functional highly branched elastic tissue [26].

Besides enzymatic damage through various pathways, UV radiation, through the formation of reactive oxygen species (ROS), directly damages protein structure and carbohydrate side chains of ECM components collagen, elastin, and glycosaminoglycans [26].

2.3.3 Oxidative Stress and Inflammaging

Persistent low-grade inflammation is a common feature of various lifestyle and metabolic diseases, including obesity and metabolic syndrome, diabetes, atherosclerosis, and cardiovascular diseases, which are considered age-related chronic diseases and manifestations of accelerated aging [28]. The persistent inflammation is thought to be an evolutionary response to the state of nutritional excess mediated by gut microbiota, leading to faster aging. Photoaging also has a persistent inflammation mediated by ROS and oxidized lipids [29]. These persistent inflammatory cells increase MMPs and matrix degradation, leading to further ROS production [30]. Topical anti-inflammatory agents like ibuprofen and naproxen are photoprotective and decrease wrinkle formation and visible skin sag in mice [31]. Topical diclofenac is useful for treating actinic keratosis due to the inhibition of cyclooxygenase [30].

2.3.4 Advanced Glycation End Products (AGEs)

AGEs are the products of non-enzymatic glycation of proteins and lipids, distinct from enzymatic glycosylation. After glycation, further chemical reactions, like oxidation and molecular rearrangements, form the advanced end products. The non-enzymatic glycation is normally present at low levels in vivo and is increased by high blood sugar levels. Glycated hemoglobin is a well-known AGE that is a useful marker of average sugar levels for a relatively long period. AGEs aren't just formed in vivo but are also ingested through the diet. AGEs directly and indirectly cause harmful effects by binding to receptors for AGEs (RAGE), further activating downstream MAP Kinase and NFκB pathways and leading to a proinflammatory state. Removal of AGEs requires glutathione-dependent enzymes, leading to a decrease in antioxidant levels. The level of AGEs increases with chronological aging, and this accumulation rate is further increased in diabetes and other disorders of aging. Sun exposure also leads to increased localized levels of AGEs compared to non-exposed skin [32].

AGEs cause decreased proliferation and increased senescence of keratinocytes and fibroblasts. They bind directly to extracellular matrix proteins and alter their mechanical and chemical properties. Glycated collagen has decreased flexibility and increased stiffness, and glycated elastin has decreased elasticity. The degradation and turnover of these aberrant matrix proteins are also decreased. AGEs also lead to oxidative stress and a proinflammatory state through indirect action. These are also the features of aging and photoaging. AGEs are a known biomarker to predict diabetes-related complications and a proposed biomarker to predict skin aging [32].

2.3.5 Neuroendocrine System

Brain-endocrine systems, through cortisol and catecholamine pathways, mediate the response to psychological and other forms of stress [33]. Stress has been shown to cause decreased epidermal proliferation [34], dermal atrophy, compromised barrier function, increased TEWL, wrinkling [35] melanogenesis, earlier skin neoplasms [36], and poor wound healing [37] in murine models and humans. Many of these changes are similar to topical steroid application [33]. Some of them, including decreased epidermal proliferation and decreased barrier function, can be reversed using steroid antagonists [38] and barrier repair creams [39].

Another important mediator is insulin-like growth factor-1 (IGF-1). Levels of IGF-1 in serum decrease with aging, perceived aging, and wrinkling [40]. IGF-1's proposed anti-aging and anti-cancer mechanisms include the protection of keratinocytes and fibroblasts from UV-induced DNA damage and premature senescence [41], and the reduction of ECM degradation [40].

2.3.6 Dysbiosis

Dysbiosis refers to the imbalance or maladaptation of the microbiome on or in an organism. The gut microbiome profile is emerging as a biomarker of aging. People with age-related disorders have a gut different microbiome than controls [42]. *Bifidobacterium*, considered responsible for immune tolerance, is a marker of longevity in aged individuals, while proinflammatory species like those belonging to *Enterobacteriaceae* and *Clostridium* are considered bad for health. An abundance of *Firmicutes* phylum over *Bacteroidetes* phylum is considered a marker of dysbiotic microbiome [43]. Using artificial intelligence, a gut microbiome profile-based clock has been created to predict age with a mean error of a few years [44]. However, whether this association between microbiome and longevity translates to a causative role is yet to be answered. There is much indirect evidence. Calorie restriction, Metformin, and Rapamycin have all been demonstrated to increase life span in animal models. Alteration of the microbiome is considered one of the main mechanisms behind this effect [43]. Although controversial due to a retracted paper, the Mediterranean diet is also associated with increased longevity and alteration in the microbiome. Microbial transplants have caused weight loss and better glycemic control in animal models. Different microbiome causes many epigenetic changes, which may influence aging [42].

Like the gut microbiome, older people have a different skin microbiome than younger people [45]. The gut microbiome becomes less diverse with aging [42]. Still, studies on the change in the diversity of the skin microbiome with aging have heterogeneous results and the variability in data might be due to the use of different sites [45, 46]. A different artificial intelligence system found skin microbiome to be a better predictor of age than gut microbiome [47]. It is well known that an altered skin microbiome is a characteristic of a variety of inflammatory skin diseases like atopic dermatitis, seborrheic dermatitis, acne, psoriasis, and bacterial vaginosis, and evidence is accumulating that correcting this dysbiosis can reduce the severity of these diseases [48].

2.3.7 Epigenetics

Various premature aging syndromes that involve prematurely aged skin have similar changes as chronological aging. Skin cells from patients of these diseases have reduced expression of many genes, mediated by epigenetic changes of DNA and histone methylation and acetylation [49]. Many environmental factors may act by changing gene expression through epigenetic changes. Monozygotic twins, having the same genotype and almost identical epigenetic patterns at birth, acquire a different DNA methylation pattern as they age, suggesting that different phenotypes can result from the same genotype due to epigenetic changes, which in turn, are caused by environmental factors [49]. Inheritance of the impact of environmental factors on the previous generation to the next generation is usually ascribed to epigenetic changes. However, such a change has not been elucidated yet with regard to skin aging.

2.3.8 Sirtuins

Sirtuins are a family of proteins that reduce the transcription of genes through histone deacetylation. In animal models, their overactivity causes increased longevity, and decreased activity decreases lifespan. They are conserved in human species too, and immunological and molecular studies suggest that they are involved in pathways similar to those in these animal models in humans. These studies show that their effects are induced by oxidative stress, and in response, they affect the transcription of key genes, decreasing oxidative stress [50]. They also have antioxidant, anti-inflammatory, anti-senescence, and DNA reparative effects on the skin. They decrease UV-induced ECM degradation in the skin [51]. They can also serve as biomarkers of aging as their expression decreases with age and increases with calorie restriction. Apart from oral antioxidants, Metformin, Resveratrol, and other drugs increasing sirtuin activity all have been proposed as longevity agents in animal models. However, there's no direct evidence yet showing that they increased the human lifespan or prevented skin aging [50, 51].

2.4 Extrinsic Factors and Their Mechanisms Leading to Skin Aging

Sun exposure causes skin aging through DNA damage, premature senescence, increasing oxidative stress and inflammation, ECM degradation [52], and accumulation of AGEs. Smoking [53] and air pollution [54] hasten premature skin aging primarily through oxidative stress and ECM degradation. Oxidative stress also causes DNA damage and inflammation. Many of their effects on skin aging are mediated by aryl hydrocarbon receptors [55]. Lifestyle factors and diseases, such as obesity, diabetes mellitus type-2, and metabolic syndrome, cause a variety of age-related diseases. Premature skin aging in them is characterized by inflammaging, oxidative stress, and excess accumulation of AGEs. Looking old for one's age due to excessive stress can be explained by neuroendocrine axis. All of these extrinsic factors are associated with markers of premature senescence, like premature shortening of telomeres. How dysbiosis and epigenetics tie into the mechanisms of these factors is yet to be elucidated (Fig. 2.1).

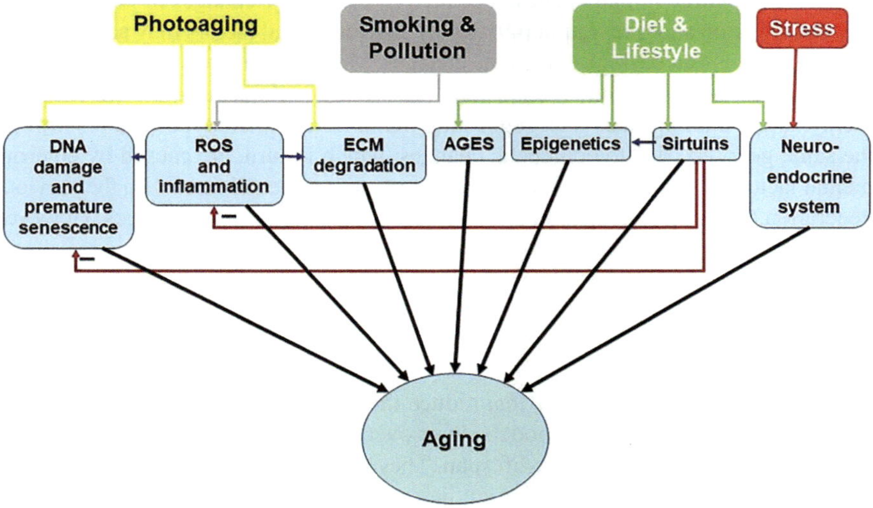

Fig. 2.1 Pathogenesis of aging

2.5 Prevention and Treatment of Skin Aging

Biometric twin studies and comparisons using monozygotic and dizygotic twins ascribe 60% of skin aging to genetic factors and 40% to environmental factors [3], while other workers believe that environmental factors play the dominant role in skin aging. The latter is a more optimistic point of view, as environmental factors are more tweakable, implying that a major component of skin aging is preventable. The nature vs nurture debate might lean more towards nurture. The average life expectancy of humans has more than doubled in a century, largely due to the change in how we adapt to environmental factors. Many workers consider aging to be a disease that is treatable and potentially curable in the future. Perhaps, human civilization can make similar advances in delaying skin aging, as the same factors are responsible for aging and skin aging.

The management of skin aging has two conventional aspects: general measures to retard skin aging and therapeutic measures to decrease and reverse the signs of already-aged skin. Many therapies do both.

2.6 Prevention of Skin Aging

2.6.1 Photoprotection and Sunscreens

As photoaging is the dominant extrinsic aging, appropriate photoprotection is a very effective and essential way to delay and decrease the signs of skin aging. Guidelines for fair-skinned population groups recommend using a broad-spectrum sunscreen with at least 30 sun protection factors (SPF) and a critical wavelength over 370 nm. Consistent use of a broad-spectrum sunscreen has been demonstrated to significantly decrease, and even reverse, the signs of photoaging on the face [56, 57]. Other ways of protection include staying indoors or in shade, using a broad-brimmed hat or umbrella, and using a dark, thickly woven cloth or one with a high UV protection factor (UPF) to cover the face. The use of tinted glasses in vehicles and pigmented foundations as make-up are other photoprotective measures.

2.6.2 Antioxidants

In recent years, many agents have been touted to have photoprotective effects of their antioxidant and anti-inflammatory properties. But robust evidence regarding these 'oral sunscreens' to manage photoaging has been lacking so far. Many of these agents have been shown to scavenge free radicals, inhibit endogenous ROS-producing enzymes, decrease inflammatory markers, increase UV tolerance in the form of increased minimum erythema dose, decrease UV-induced ECM damage, and decrease DNA damage and photo-carcinogenesis, in in vitro studies, animal models and even human studies [58]. However, the demonstration of these effects on molecular markers has rarely translated into a demonstration of clinical benefit in humans. This might be due to the inherent difficulty of clinical trials but can also be a reflection of the modest effect size of these agents. Oral nicotinamide prevents actinic keratosis [59] and non-melanoma skin cancers [60], while topical nicotinamide reverses the aged skin appearance, pigmentary changes, and wrinkles [61]. In small, open, uncontrolled trials, oral *polypodium leucotomos* extract lessened the severity of photodermatoses [62]. Topical forms of Vitamin C and E have been shown to have anti-skin aging effects [63], but not oral supplementation. Direct clinical studies of these agents to study their effects on skin aging are lacking.

2.6.3 Dietary and Lifestyle Measures

Calorie restriction, appropriate weight, exercise, healthy diet, stress avoidance and cessation of smoking are all interventions that are well established to prevent various age-related disorders like diabetes, atherosclerosis, cardiovascular diseases, and frailty and are overall associated with longevity. Many of these interventions have been shown to enhance life span in animal models, human epidemiological association studies, case-control, and cohort studies. It is intuitional that these lifestyle measures also prevent skin aging. It is well known and observed that cessation of smoking partially reverts the older appearance to the younger self. Exercise can lead to younger skin even if started late in life. Overall, good health is associated with healthy skin.

2.7 Treatment of Skin Aging

2.7.1 Retinoids

Topical retinoids are the only drugs that have consistently demonstrated significant reversal in signs of aging. Apart from treatment, they are also useful in the secondary prevention of skin aging and retard further changes associated with skin aging. Topical tretinoin in various concentrations, isotretinoin, tazarotene, retinol, retinaldehyde, and adapalene, have been shown to have a good effect in treating photoaged skin [64]. Through downstream effects of their action on retinoid receptors, they increase epidermal proliferation, decrease collagen degradation and increase GAGs. They primarily increase epidermal thickness, lead to compact stratum corneum, and decrease wrinkles through dermal ECM effects that occur when used for long term [64]. Not just wrinkling, but pigmentary changes also improve, albeit to a lesser extent. Topical tretinoin 0.02% is FDA-approved for photoaging.

2.7.2 Botulinum Toxins, Fillers, and Rejuvenation Procedures

Botulinum toxin A is an effective temporary procedure to lessen skin wrinkles and laxity. A single session is effective for 3–9 months, subject to variations of procedure and person. Fillers help correct subcutaneous volume loss that occurs during aging. Botox and fillers are akin to long-term cosmetic camouflage as they don't correct the underlying basic pathology and its mechanisms but treat only the symptoms. But they give immediate results. On the other hand, skin rejuvenation involves inducing controlled trauma to the dermis and collagen to stimulate neocollagenesis, resulting in tighter and smoother skin. Needling, lasers, radiofrequency devices, and high-frequency ultrasound are the ways of inducing skin rejuvenation.

2.8 Conclusion

Skin aging is a natural process, but looking older than one's chronological age can be disadvantageous and carries an opportunity cost. Looking older for one's age, or "aging poorly," correlates with less longevity. The methods to prevent premature skin aging are the same that prevent various age-related disorders and maintain a healthy life, with the addition of photoprotection and topical retinoids. People not motivated for calorie restriction and diet control, healthy diet, exercise, and smoking cessation, despite their obvious and proven advantages on overall health, can also be offered the additional incentive of looking younger with these interventions.

References

1. Fenske NA, Lober CW. Structural and functional changes of normal aging skin. J Am Acad Dermatol. 1986;15(4 Pt 1):571–85.
2. Christensen K, Thinggaard M, McGue M, Rexbye H, Hjelmborg JVB, Aviv A, et al. Perceived age as clinically useful biomarker of ageing: cohort study. BMJ [Internet]. 2009 [cited 2020 Dec 29];339. https://www.ncbi.nlm.nih.gov/pmc/articles/PMC2792675/.
3. Christensen K, Iachina M, Rexbye H, Tomassini C, Frederiksen H, McGue M, et al. "Looking old for your age": genetics and mortality. Epidemiology. 2004;15(2):251–2.
4. Kido M, Kohara K, Miyawaki S, Tabara Y, Igase M, Miki T. Perceived age of facial features is a significant diagnosis criterion for age-related carotid atherosclerosis in Japanese subjects: J-SHIPP study. Geriatr Gerontol Int. 2012;12(4):733–40.
5. Rexbye H, Petersen I, Johansens M, Klitkou L, Jeune B, Christensen K. Influence of environmental factors on facial ageing. Age Ageing. 2006;35(2):110–5.
6. Han A, Chien AL, Kang S. Photoaging. Dermatol Clin. 2014;32(3):291–9, vii.
7. Yaar M, Gilchrest BA. Photoageing: mechanism, prevention and therapy. Br J Dermatol. 2007;157(5):874–87.
8. Passeron T, Picardo M. Melasma, a photoaging disorder. Pigment Cell Melanoma Res. 2018;31(4):461–5.
9. Soerensen M. Genetic variation and human longevity. Dan Med J. 2012;59(5):B4454.
10. Johnson SC, Dong X, Vijg J, Suh Y. Genetic evidence for common pathways in human age-related diseases. Aging Cell. 2015;14(5):809–17.
11. Jacobs LC, Hamer MA, Gunn DA, Deelen J, Lall JS, van Heemst D, et al. A genome-wide association study identifies the skin color genes IRF4, MC1R, ASIP, and BNC2 influencing facial pigmented spots. J Invest Dermatol. 2015;135(7):1735–42.
12. Law MH, Medland SE, Zhu G, Yazar S, Viñuela A, Wallace L, et al. Genome-wide association shows that pigmentation genes play a role in skin aging. J Invest Dermatol. 2017;137(9):1887–94.
13. Liu Y, Gao W, Koellmann C, Le Clerc S, Hüls A, Li B, et al. Genome-wide scan identified genetic variants associated with skin aging in a Chinese female population. J Dermatol Sci. 2019;96(1):42–9.
14. Vierkötter A, Hüls A, Yamamoto A, Stolz S, Krämer U, Matsui MS, et al. Extrinsic skin ageing in German, Chinese and Japanese women manifests differently in all three groups depending on ethnic background, age and anatomical site. J Dermatol Sci. 2016;83(3):219–25.
15. Markiewicz E, Idowu OC. Personalized skincare: from molecular basis to clinical and commercial applications. Clin Cosmet Investig Dermatol. 2018;11:161–71.
16. Kaidbey KH, Agin PP, Sayre RM, Kligman AM. Photoprotection by melanin—a comparison of black and Caucasian skin. J Am Acad Dermatol. 1979;1(3):249–60.
17. Nouveau-Richard S, Yang Z, Mac-Mary S, Li L, Bastien P, Tardy I, et al. Skin ageing: a comparison between Chinese and European populations. A pilot study. J Dermatol Sci. 2005;40(3):187–93.
18. Shome D, Vadera S, Khare S, Ram MS, Ayyar A, Kapoor R, et al. Aging and the Indian face: an analytical study of aging in the Asian Indian face. Plast Reconstr Surg Glob Open [Internet]. 2020 [cited 2020 Dec 31];8(3). https://www.ncbi.nlm.nih.gov/pmc/articles/PMC7253281/.
19. Nakanishi M, Niida H, Murakami H, Shimada M. DNA damage responses in skin biology—implications in tumor prevention and aging acceleration. J Dermatol Sci. 2009;56(2):76–81.
20. Panich U, Sittithumcharee G, Rathviboon N, Jirawatnotai S. Ultraviolet radiation-induced skin aging: the role of DNA damage and oxidative stress in epidermal stem cell damage mediated skin aging. Stem Cells Int [Internet]. 2016 [cited 2020 Dec 31];2016. https://www.ncbi.nlm.nih.gov/pmc/articles/PMC4842382/.

21. Chen W, Kang J, Xia J, Li Y, Yang B, Chen B, et al. p53-related apoptosis resistance and tumor suppression activity in UVB-induced premature senescent human skin fibroblasts. Int J Mol Med. 2008;21(5):645–53.
22. Kosmadaki MG, Gilchrest BA. The role of telomeres in skin aging/photoaging. Micron. 2004;35(3):155–9.
23. Buckingham EM, Klingelhutz AJ. The role of telomeres in the ageing of human skin. Exp Dermatol. 2011;20(4):297–302.
24. Shammas MA. Telomeres, lifestyle, cancer, and aging. Curr Opin Clin Nutr Metab Care. 2011;14(1):28–34.
25. Ikeda H, Aida J, Hatamochi A, Hamasaki Y, Izumiyama-Shimomura N, Nakamura KI, et al. Quantitative fluorescence in situ hybridization measurement of telomere length in skin with/without sun exposure or actinic keratosis. Hum Pathol. 2014;45(3):473–80.
26. Kammeyer A, Luiten RM. Oxidation events and skin aging. Ageing Res Rev. 2015;21:16–29.
27. Choi YJ, Moon KM, Chung KW, Jeong JW, Park D, Kim DH, et al. The underlying mechanism of proinflammatory NF-κB activation by the mTORC2/Akt/IKKα pathway during skin aging. Oncotarget. 2016;7(33):52685–94.
28. Franceschi C, Garagnani P, Parini P, Giuliani C, Santoro A. Inflammaging: a new immune-metabolic viewpoint for age-related diseases. Nat Rev Endocrinol. 2018;14(10):576–90.
29. Zhuang Y, Lyga J. Inflammaging in skin and other tissues—the roles of complement system and macrophage. Inflamm Allergy Drug Targets. 2014;13(3):153–61.
30. Thornfeldt CR. Chronic inflammation is etiology of extrinsic aging. J Cosmet Dermatol. 2008;7(1):78–82.
31. Bissett DL, Chatterjee R, Hannon DP. Photoprotective effect of topical anti-inflammatory agents against ultraviolet radiation-induced chronic skin damage in the hairless mouse. Photodermatol Photoimmunol Photomed. 1990;7(4):153–8.
32. Gkogkolou P, Böhm M. Advanced glycation end products. Dermatoendocrinol. 2012;4(3):259–70.
33. Chen Y, Lyga J. Brain-skin connection: stress, inflammation and skin Aging. Inflamm Allergy Drug Targets. 2014;13(3):177–90.
34. Tsuchiya T, Horii I. Epidermal cell proliferative activity assessed by proliferating cell nuclear antigen (PCNA) decreases following immobilization-induced stress in male Syrian hamsters. Psychoneuroendocrinology. 1996;21(1):111–7.
35. Aioi A, Okuda M, Matsui M, Tonogaito H, Hamada K. Effect of high population density environment on skin barrier function in mice. J Dermatol Sci. 2001;25(3):189–97.
36. Saul AN, Oberyszyn TM, Daugherty C, Kusewitt D, Jones S, Jewell S, et al. Chronic stress and susceptibility to skin cancer. JNCI J Natl Cancer Inst. 2005;97(23):1760–7.
37. Cole-King A, Harding KG. Psychological factors and delayed healing in chronic wounds. Psychosom Med. 2001;63(2):216–20.
38. Choi EH, Demerjian M, Crumrine D, Brown BE, Mauro T, Elias PM, et al. Glucocorticoid blockade reverses psychological stress-induced abnormalities in epidermal structure and function. Am J Physiol Regul Integr Comp Physiol. 2006;291(6):R1657–62.
39. Choi EH, Brown BE, Crumrine D, Chang S, Man MQ, Elias PM, et al. Mechanisms by which psychologic stress alters cutaneous permeability barrier homeostasis and stratum corneum integrity. J Invest Dermatol. 2005;124(3):587–95.
40. Noordam R, Gunn DA, Tomlin CC, Maier AB, Griffiths T, Catt SD, et al. Serum insulin-like growth factor 1 and facial ageing: high levels associate with reduced skin wrinkling in a cross-sectional study. Br J Dermatol. 2013;168(3):533–8.
41. Lewis DA, Travers JB, Somani AK, Spandau DF. The IGF-1/IGF-1R signaling axis in the skin: a new role for the dermis in aging-associated skin cancer. Oncogene. 2010;29(10):1475–85.
42. Bana B, Cabreiro F. The microbiome and aging. Annu Rev Genet. 2019;53:239–61.
43. Kim M, Benayoun BA. The microbiome: an emerging key player in aging and longevity. Transl Med Aging. 2020;4:103–16.
44. Galkin F, Mamoshina P, Aliper A, Putin E, Moskalev V, Gladyshev VN, et al. Human gut microbiome aging clock based on taxonomic profiling and deep learning. iScience. 2020;23(6):101199.

45. Shibagaki N, Suda W, Clavaud C, Bastien P, Takayasu L, Iioka E, et al. Aging-related changes in the diversity of women's skin microbiomes associated with oral bacteria. Sci Rep [Internet]. 2017 [cited 2021 Jan 7];7. https://www.ncbi.nlm.nih.gov/pmc/articles/PMC5585242/.
46. Ying S, Zeng DN, Chi L, Tan Y, Galzote C, Cardona C, et al. The influence of age and gender on skin-associated microbial communities in urban and rural human populations. PLoS One [Internet]. 2015 [cited 2021 Jan 7];10(10). https://www.ncbi.nlm.nih.gov/pmc/articles/PMC4624872/.
47. Huang S, Haiminen N, Carrieri AP, Hu R, Jiang L, Parida L, et al. Human skin, oral, and gut microbiomes predict chronological age. mSystems. 2020;5(1):e00630–19.
48. Yu Y, Dunaway S, Champer J, Kim J, Alikhan A. Changing our microbiome: probiotics in dermatology. Br J Dermatol. 2020;182(1):39–46.
49. Orioli D, Dellambra E. Epigenetic regulation of skin cells in natural aging and premature aging diseases. Cells [Internet]. 2018 [cited 2021 Jan 14];7(12). https://www.ncbi.nlm.nih.gov/pmc/articles/PMC6315602/.
50. Grabowska W, Sikora E, Bielak-Zmijewska A. Sirtuins, a promising target in slowing down the ageing process. Biogerontology. 2017;18(4):447–76.
51. Garcia-Peterson LM, Wilking-Busch MJ, Ndiaye MA, Philippe CGA, Setaluri V, Ahmad N. Sirtuins in skin and skin cancers. Skin Pharmacol Physiol. 2017;30(4):216–24.
52. Fisher GJ, Kang S, Varani J, Bata-Csorgo Z, Wan Y, Datta S, et al. Mechanisms of photoaging and chronological skin aging. Arch Dermatol. 2002;138(11):1462–70.
53. Morita A. Tobacco smoke causes premature skin aging. J Dermatol Sci. 2007;48(3):169–75.
54. Schikowski T, Hüls A. Air pollution and skin aging. Curr Environ Health Rep. 2020;7(1):58–64.
55. Parrado C, Mercado-Saenz S, Perez-Davo A, Gilaberte Y, Gonzalez S, Juarranz A. Environmental stressors on skin aging. Mechanistic insights. Front Pharmacol [Internet]. 2019 [cited 2021 Jan 11];10. https://www.ncbi.nlm.nih.gov/pmc/articles/PMC6629960/.
56. Hughes MCB, Williams GM, Baker P, Green AC. Sunscreen and prevention of skin aging: a randomized trial. Ann Intern Med. 2013;158(11):781–90.
57. Randhawa M, Wang S, Leyden JJ, Cula GO, Pagnoni A, Southall MD. Daily use of a facial broad spectrum sunscreen over one-year significantly improves clinical evaluation of photoaging. Dermatol Surg. 2016;42(12):1354–61.
58. Parrado C, Philips N, Gilaberte Y, Juarranz A, González S. Oral photoprotection: effective agents and potential candidates. Front Med (Lausanne) [Internet]. 2018 [cited 2021 Jan 13];5. https://www.ncbi.nlm.nih.gov/pmc/articles/PMC6028556/.
59. Surjana D, Halliday GM, Martin AJ, Moloney FJ, Damian DL. Oral nicotinamide reduces actinic keratoses in phase II double-blinded randomized controlled trials. J Invest Dermatol. 2012;132(5):1497–500.
60. Chen AC, Martin AJ, Choy B, Fernández-Peñas P, Dalziell RA, McKenzie CA, et al. A phase 3 randomized trial of nicotinamide for skin-cancer chemoprevention. N Engl J Med. 2015;373(17):1618–26.
61. Bissett DL, Miyamoto K, Sun P, Li J, Berge CA. Topical niacinamide reduces yellowing, wrinkling, red blotchiness, and hyperpigmented spots in aging facial skin. Int J Cosmet Sci. 2004;26(5):231–8.
62. Caccialanza M, Percivalle S, Piccinno R, Brambilla R. Photoprotective activity of oral polypodium leucotomos extract in 25 patients with idiopathic photodermatoses. Photodermatol Photoimmunol Photomed. 2007;23(1):46–7.
63. Rattanawiwatpong P, Wanitphakdeedecha R, Bumrungpert A, Maiprasert M. Anti-aging and brightening effects of a topical treatment containing vitamin C, vitamin E, and raspberry leaf cell culture extract: a split-face, randomized controlled trial. J Cosmet Dermatol. 2020;19(3):671–6.
64. Mukherjee S, Date A, Patravale V, Korting HC, Roeder A, Weindl G. Retinoids in the treatment of skin aging: an overview of clinical efficacy and safety. Clin Interv Aging. 2006;1(4):327–48.

The Concept of Beauty and Its Evolutionary Basis

3

Henriette De La Garza and Neelam A. Vashi

3.1 Introduction

Beauty has been defined by the Oxford Dictionary as *a combination of qualities, such as shape and color, that pleases the senses, especially the sight* [1]. Even though beauty may be difficult to define, it is easily recognizable. The fascination with aesthetics dates back from the ancient Greek times through the Renaissance to modern surgical practice. The classical position that attributes beauty to a few key specifics, such as symmetrical proportions, has been a matter of debate [1]. Human aesthetic judgment is a complicated mixture of objective, subjective, and sociocultural factors or trends. The subjective component of beauty is influenced by the individual beholder and goes beyond symmetric measurements [2]. David Hume argued that beauty is entirely subjective, a matter of feelings and emotion [3]. What is beautiful to one observer may not be so to another. Immanuel Kant also believed that aesthetic judgment is based on feelings of pleasure that depend on personal taste [4]. Plato and Aristotle viewed beauty as objective in the sense that it is not localized in the eyes of the beholder. Plato believed that beauty resides in the domain of the forms, not in the observer's experience [3, 5]. Aristotle held a similar view and considered beauty to be defined by characteristics such as symmetry, order, balance, and proportion [3]. This chapter explores perceptions of beauty over time across different cultures, the research behind evolutionary theories, and the reasoning behind beauty ideals.

H. De La Garza · N. A. Vashi (✉)
Department of Dermatology, Boston University Cosmetic and Laser Center, Boston University School of Medicine, Boston, MA, USA
e-mail: nvashi@bu.edu

S. Gupta et al. (eds.), *Critical Thinking in Contemporary Dermatology: Cognitive Essays*, https://doi.org/10.1007/978-981-97-0411-8_3

3.2 Divine Proportions

Aristotle defined beauty as "an imprecise sense of harmonious or aesthetically pleasing proportionality [6]." Since then, various aesthetic proportions have been proposed, such as the 1:1 ratio, the axial facial division into thirds, and the golden ratio [6]. The Golden ratio, also known as the Greek letter Phi, is the most alluring and is seen worldwide. This numerical value equal to approximately 1.618 can be found by dividing a line such that the ratio of the short segment to the long segment is equivalent to the ratio of the long segment to the entire line [7]. It has been referred to as the "divine proportion" and can be found throughout nature, from the structure of DNA and nautilus seashells to Da Vinci's Mona Lisa [8]. Marquardt attempted to scientifically analyze the mathematics of perfect facial features by developing the Phi mask, which claims to represent the ideal facial archetype based entirely on the golden ratio (Fig. 3.1). According to Marquardt, as the face comes closer to this ratio, it is perceived as more beautiful. He performed cross-cultural surveys on beauty in modern and historical times and found that beauty is related to

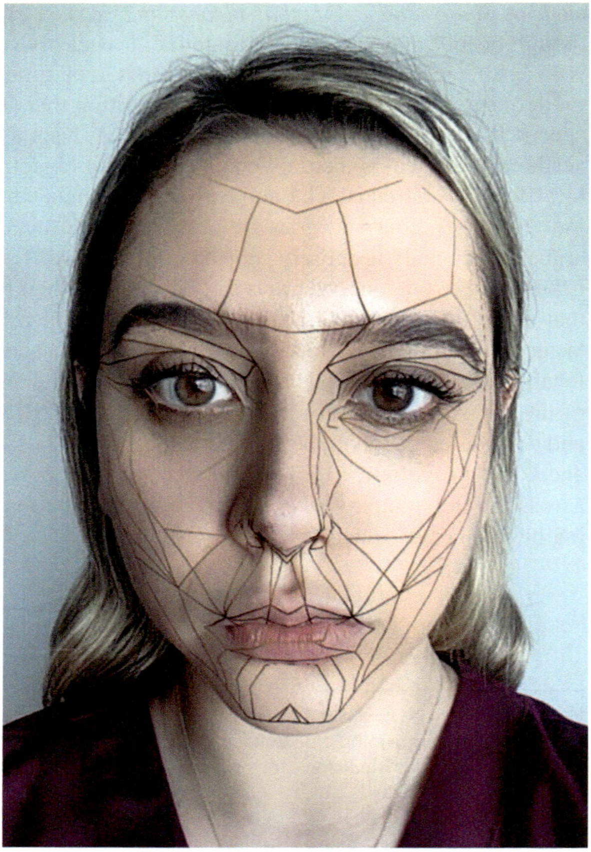

Fig. 3.1 Golden ratio mask

the golden ratio and is the same for both genders and all races and cultures [8]. However, a recent study found that modern facial proportions of beauty do not entirely match the golden ratio [9]. Moreover, Chinese, Arabian, Turkish, Croatian, Korean-American, and Greek studies did not conform to the neoclassical facial canons [10–15]. Race is not the only factor that may alter the proportions related to the Golden Ratio; it has been found that certain facial measurements, such as the distance between the mouth and nose, tend to expand with age. As we age, we lose fat around the eyes, cheekbones, inner jawline, and cheeks, allowing our face to lose volume. With age, even faces previously considered symmetrical deviate from the golden ratio, which may explain why we perceive younger faces as more beautiful.

3.3 Perceptions Across Cultures

The appreciation of human aesthetics is deeply rooted in our historical past and has evolved. Beauty is characterized as an individual assessment of attractiveness that is influenced by societal or cultural standards. The definitions and perceptions of beauty vary within different cultures, from the Kayan tribes, who believe that long giraffe-type necks are the ultimate sign of beauty, to several parts of Asia where white skin is considered a sign of beauty and affluence [16]. Caucasian beauty ideals include round eyes, narrow faces, small noses, high cheekbones, small lips, and white skin [17]. Asians view an oval face shape with a delicate and defined chin and larger eyes as beautiful features [18]. Interestingly, although most of the Asian population has a small or absent supratarsal crease, they perceive the presence of an upper eyelid crease as more attractive [19]. Due to the high interethnic variability in African Americans, it is difficult to establish specific facial features that are considered attractive in this population. However, some facial features are more represented, such as full lips, increased facial convexity, a broader nasal base with decreased nasal projection, bimaxillary protrusion, and orbital proptosis [20]. Studies have shown that African Americans perceive thinner women with lower facial adiposity as more attractive. They also consider lighter, yellow-toned skin more beautiful [21]. Hispanics also have wide ethnic variations. Common features within these populations include thick nasal skin, bimaxillary protrusion, prominent malar eminences, and noses with a broad base and wider tip. Hispanics, particularly Latin Americans, distinguish attractiveness by decreased nasal prominence, less protrusive lips, and less bimaxillary protrusion [22].

While facial norms and measurements of one ethnicity are generally not applied to another, there seems to be an agreement on what is considered beautiful across different cultures. Symmetry is a universal component of facial attractiveness [23]. One study evaluated beauty ideals within cosmetic advertisements across 18 countries and found that symmetry was the common characteristic among all models [24]. Similarly, studies have shown a positive correlation between averageness and perceived attractiveness despite ethnicity [6]. Evenness of skin tone is also considered a cross-cultural beautiful facial trait. In an eye-tracking study, facial stimuli with even skin tones were judged more attractive and received more visual attention

[25]. A study of 170 female facial skin images concluded that color homogeneity influences perceptions of age, attractiveness, health, and youth [26]. A youthful appearance is also highly valued as an attractive feature across all ethnicities. This may be related to the fact that as we age, we lose facial fat, our skin gets thinner, and we get wrinkles and dark spots, all of which deviate from the universal traits of beauty. A multi-center study with participants from several countries observed a decline in perceived attractiveness with aging across all nationalities [22]. Morphologic characteristics of each sex, also known as sexual dimorphism, are also highly associated with increased attractiveness. The visual dissimilarity between men and women is largely attributable to differences in body fat and muscle distribution, along with conspicuous differences in body hair and facial hair distribution. A woman with feminine features is considered more attractive. The feminine beauty ideal is constructed on the notion that physical attractiveness, including a feminine body shape and facial features, is one of women's most important assets. These ideals may have originated because of the belief that feminine features correlate with fertility and health. A large study including 28 countries supported these ideals, reporting an overall preference for feminine faces, with another study further corroborating that men prefer feminine features [27, 28].

3.4 How Beauty Standards Have Changed Through History

The quest for beauty has been as old as time itself; women across the world have been experimenting with different attires, weights, hairdos, makeup, and beauty aids since time immemorial. Every era has held its own standards of what is considered beautiful. Over time, our concept of beauty seems to fluctuate; what is considered beautiful today may be ridiculed tomorrow, or just like with fashion, it may come back in trend. Table 3.1 describes the perception of the "ideal beautiful woman" throughout time.

Table 3.1 Ideal woman and beauty perceptions throughout time

Time	Perceptions of beauty
Ancient Egypt (1292–1069 B.C.)	Slender figure Narrow shoulders Narrow hips High waist Symmetrical face Youthful Yellow or "golden" skin [29]
Ancient Greece (500–300 B.C.)	Plump figure Wide hips Nipped waist Fat on lower stomach Big buttocks Golden-red hair Blue eyes Light skin [30]

Table 3.1 (continued)

Time	Perceptions of beauty
Han dynasty (206 B.C.–220 A.D.)	Slim figure Narrow waist Large eyes Small feet Dark hair Red lips Slim eyebrows White skin [31]
Italian Renaissance (1400–1700)	Round figure Ample bosom Rounded stomach Full hips Blonde hair Rosy lips Thin eyebrows Fair skin [32]
Victorian England (1837–1901)	Plump figure Cinched waist (hour-glass figure) Dark eyes Rosy cheeks Fair skin [33]
Roaring twenties (1920s)	Slim figure Boy-like figure Flat chest Downplayed waist Short bob hairstyle Red lips with accentuated cupid bow Fair skin [34]
Golden Age of Hollywood (1930s–1950s)	Curvy figure (hour-glass) Slim waist Large breasts Curly hair Blue eyes Plucked high-arched eyebrows Blonde Pronounced cheekbones Pale skin [35]
Swinging sixties (1960s)	Slim figure Long, thin legs No waist definition Nude/light pink lips Lights skin [36]
Supermodel era (1980s)	Athletic figure Tall Toned arms Big hair Thick eyebrows [37]

(continued)

Table 3.1 (continued)

Time	Perceptions of beauty
Heroin Chic (1990s)	Extremely thin figure Androgynous Thin eyebrows Full lips Sucked in cheeks Translucent skin [38]
Postmodern beauty (2000s–today)	Skinny figure Flat stomach Large breasts and buttocks Thigh gap Tanned skin [39]

3.5 Why Do We Care About Beauty?

Attractiveness elicits positive emotional reactions in perceivers, creating desires to establish close relationships. When we think about our ideal romantic partner, we think of someone with characteristics like a good sense of humor, intelligence, kindness, and good looks. Research has shown that we rank most or all of these traits as more important than good looks [40]. But how do we reach these conclusions when aesthetic judgments are formed in less than 1/10th of a second [41]? The world of dating is rapidly changing due to the increasing use of dating applications. Making a good first impression has never been more important than using a mobile dating app due to the opportunity to find a potential mate and be chosen based on a profile. This phenomenon has been called "love at first swipe." When looking at a person's profile, the first thing that is judged is one's appearance. Research shows that having more feminine, baby-like, and happy faces is perceived to be more trustworthy [42]. Similarly, it has been demonstrated that having objective components of beauty such as symmetry, averageness, skin homogeneity, youthfulness, and emotional resemblance all impact the perception of beauty [43]. Beauty is important because we associate other positive qualities with a pleasing appearance. For example, attractive individuals are expected to be happier and to have more likeability, social competence, and intelligence than unattractive individuals [44]. Studies have shown that beauty influences the admission process in graduate education and that attractive people are more frequently hired, promoted, and earn a higher income [45]. Aided by these advantages, attractive people are expected to enjoy higher success and better lives, contributing to the notion that "beauty is power." Furthermore, it has been established that what is "beautiful is good [46]." Even our brain unconsciously elicits positive emotions when exposed to attractive faces, which stimulate activity in the medial orbitofrontal cortex, a region known to represent rewarding stimuli [47].

3.6 Beauty and Reproductive Success

People show more interest in establishing romantic relationships with attractive partners not only because of these feelings and perceptions but also because beauty is thought to be a phenotypic reflection of genetic superiority, thereby increasing sexual selection preference [8]. According to this evolutionary perspective and the good genes theory, physical attractiveness is a cue for mate quality and reproductive value [48]. Women look for masculine features such as a defined jaw, prominent brow, and muscular build because these traits are often associated with other traits such as strength and higher fertilizing ability, which would be advantageous to pass on to their offspring and would mean that the man can provide and protect his family [49]. Interestingly, research has shown a positive linear correlation between penis size and perceived attractiveness [50]. A recent study showed that semen quality is positively predicted by masculinity, suggesting that masculinity may be a signal of male fertility [51]. While women's attraction is focused on a man's ability to provide for his family, men put more emphasis on signs of fertility and youth. Physical appearance provides a strong set of cues: an hour-glass figure, large breasts, "child-bearing" hips, full lips, white teeth, and clear, smooth, and unblemished skin are signs of health and youthfulness that help men ensure that their genes will be passed on to his offspring [52]. There is a general association of attractiveness with youthfulness, health, and reproductive success [53]. The goal is to appear physically desirable to attract the most suitable mate as a provider for one's yet-unborn progeny. People look for certain traits in their potential mates, which guide them to choose partners who will provide the best chance of their own genes surviving. Physical attractiveness is not only related to the offspring's quality but also to the quantity. In fact, studies have shown that attractive women were found to have more biological offspring than less attractive women [54]. One study showed that very attractive women had 16% more children than their less attractive counterparts [49]. The process of sexual selection is in our nature and can even be found in animals. For example, male peacocks compete to attract mates through the beauty of their appearance and their brightly colored iridescent tails. Interestingly, studies have proven that peacocks with large tails have higher survival rates [55]. Similarly, the silver backs of adult male gorillas serve as an advertisement of high social status that attracts females and also confers other advantages of status, such as access to food. However, sexual selection in humans is more complex as we are characterized by mutual mate choice in which both men and women scrutinize the desirability of potential mates. Charles Darwin proposed a theory of sexual selection in which he described mate preferences as a "taste for the beautiful." He hypothesized that attractive traits enhance mating success by either attracting mates or intimidating rivals [56]. Evolutionary theories view individuals as signalers and perceivers. In essence, the signalers display signs, and the receivers recognize these signals, which help them identify attractive features and ultimately attract them to another person. Attractiveness appears to be associated with a person's preferences and desires. Just like the silverback of gorillas, attractiveness in humans is related to higher socioeconomic status, which may also play an important role when selecting a mate. Thus, it has been hypothesized that certain features are considered attractive because of their benefits, which may be material and/or genetic. It is the fundamental assumption that physical attractiveness gives reliable cues to genetic quality, health, reproductive potential, and a higher quality of life. Beauty appears to play a significant role in choosing a mate; the effectiveness of these seductive signals is and will always be an important driver in our pursuit of beauty.

3.7 Malleability of Beauty

The importance of beauty not only lies in how others view us and the consequences of these perceptions, but it significantly impacts how we view ourselves. Beauty and self-confidence go hand in hand. People who consider themselves beautiful are more confident. Confident people are perceived as more charming, and research has found that they also have more chances of marrying equally beautiful partners [46]. Beauty and confidence are associated with upward economic mobility and improved interpersonal relations. This concept is supported by a meta-analysis of more than 900 studies, which proved that people are treated differently based on how physically attractive they are perceived to be [17]. Unattractive people or those with facial disfigurement are often stigmatized and can be targets of discrimination. In popular culture, facial disfigurement, scars, hyperpigmentation, and rhytides are often used to portray evil characters [57]. This may contribute to a tendency toward prejudice and the attribution of the "what is beautiful is good" stereotype that is associated with people's desires to seek plastic surgery and cosmetic procedures. The skin is a practical parameter to evaluate health, beauty, and perceived age. Consequently, dermatologists constantly receive patients who seek to improve their skin condition and overall appearance, spending millions of dollars on cosmetic procedures. In 2019, Americans spent $8.2 billion on cosmetic procedures, and the beauty and cosmetic industry revenue was estimated to be approximately 49.2 billion dollars in 2019 [58]. Data from the American Society of Plastic Surgeons report that they performed more than 3.3 million surgical and 13.2 million minimally invasive cosmetic procedures in the United States in 2020 [59]. Given beauty's profound influence on our everyday lives, it is not surprising that people seek procedures to alter their appearance to conform to societal expectations and boost their self-confidence. A study of 101 women found that body dissatisfaction, physical appearance, teasing, and media influence were related to their desire to have cosmetic surgery [60]. Another study of 332 university students showed a strong correlation between participants' self-rated attractiveness and self-esteem [61]. Research investigating the relationship between changes in physical attractiveness and changes in self-esteem has shown that cosmetic procedures have a positive impact on patients' quality of life (QoL). A study of 105 patients who underwent elective cosmetic surgery found significant improvements in QoL 6 months after surgery compared to baseline measurements. Patients reported improvement in depression and overall mood as well as positive changes in their social and sex life, friendships, and leisure activities [62]. The lack of self-confidence is typically connected to a specific physical feature that a person dislikes about themselves. If this concern is removed, self-esteem can be restored, enhancing social competence and interactions. While some forms of body dissatisfaction are quite the norm, practitioners must remain alert for those with an unhealthy sense of self or body dysmorphic disorder. Although the Golden ratio and its applications in the anatomy of the face and body can facilitate the decision-making process of surgical and cosmetic procedures, optimum aesthetic results can only be accomplished when the patient's psychological expectations and cultural background are considered.

3.8 Social Media Influence

Social media platforms have become increasingly popular forms of communication and information transmission, which can also represent an alternate reality. Social media has introduced certain criteria for establishing beauty and increased our interest in attractiveness and perfect looks [63]. The human need to advertise beauty, health, and well-being has been fueled by the increasing use of social media, which has also potentiated what we today deem as beauty standards. The content on these platforms often projects a perfect image of oneself enhanced by photo editing. While filters of the past focused on color changes to black and white or sepia, today's filters are more advanced, allowing the easy alteration of one's physical appearance. They contour the face, plump lips, and add makeup (Fig. 3.2). Thousands of social media users, even celebrities, have been victims of the pressures of social media, posting heavily photoshopped and edited images that make themselves appear thinner or seemingly more attractive. When others view such images, they often compare themselves to what is projected on these platforms, negatively impacting their own self-esteem. These habits and portrayals may lead to unrealistic and unattainable expectations for viewers and can lead them to seek body or face-altering procedures. Social media has had a significant impact on behavioral aspects of body image and facial features through the focus on specific traits as being more beautiful. For example, full lips have gained particular attention and are seen in multiple celebrity, model, and influencer accounts. Kylie Jenner, who is the fifth-most followed Instagram user in the world with over 242 million followers, confessed in 2015 that she had received a soft-tissue augmentation of her lips, and within 24 h, there was a 70% rise in inquiries for lip-fillers on the internet [64]. In fact, the American Society of Plastic Surgeons reported that more than 27,000 Americans had lip augmentation treatment during that year [65]. With the increasing use of social media and marketing of fuller lips, these numbers continue to rise by the day, with over 3,410,730 soft-tissue filler procedures performed in 2020 [65]. Research suggests that people are more likely to follow successful individuals' choices and are more likely to be influenced by the choices of attractive individuals than unattractive individuals [66]. These biases may explain the impact of social media content on social learning for human mate preferences as followers emulate the choices of others, greatly influencing sexual selection. The choices of those individuals with the highest popularity or admiration may carry a great weight,

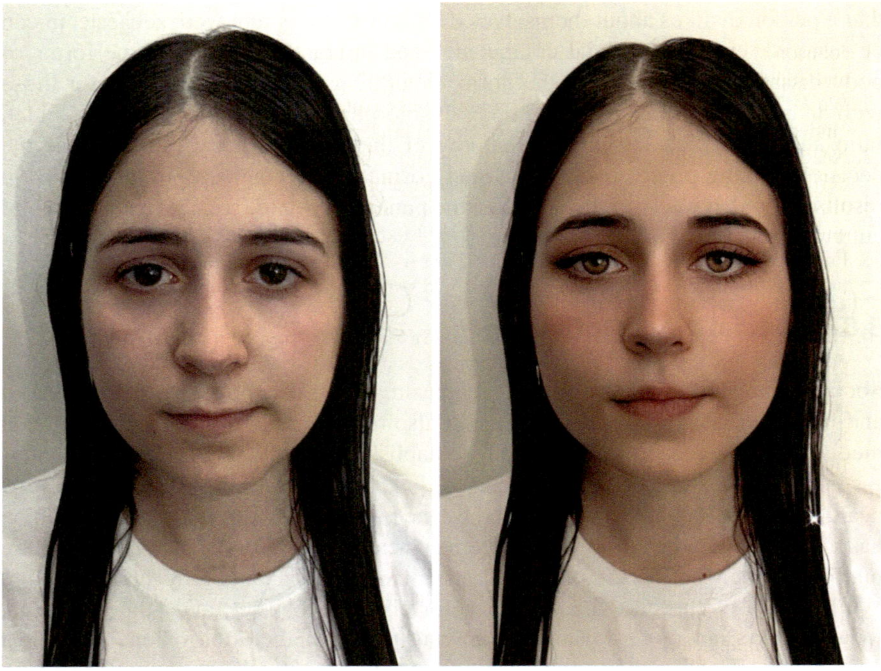

Fig. 3.2 Modern social media filters. Without (left) and with (right) filter

rapidly generating agreement in preferences within a population and allowing social learning to be more influential. The type of pictures that we see also affect our perceptions of people. A study showed that women rate men as more desirable when they post pictures surrounded by women than when shown alone or with other men [67]. Similarly, studies have demonstrated that positive characteristics are attributed more frequently to men who are paired with attractive women [68]. Both men and women find a face paired with an attractive partner to be more attractive, alluding to the notion that an attractive partner helps to radiate beauty [69]. The plethora of dating apps has led millions of people to seek partners online, becoming a modern version of sexual selection. Social media platforms have become an important intermediary for couple formation, whereby individuals with internet access are substantially more likely to have a romantic partner. This furthers the pressures to have an online presence and paint a picture of beauty and indulgence, enhancing one's appearance with the hopes of attracting and retaining mates. The twenty-first century has seen the rise of new forms of visual self-improvement. With photo editing, cosmetic procedures, and makeup, beauty has the potential to be easily crafted and deceived. In the competition of beauty, people use self-signaling to indicate their own worth and for mate selection. The desire to be beautiful continues to be a strong driving force in our daily lives. With the ever-changing beauty norms, pursuing beauty seems to be an everlasting quest.

References

1. Prokopakis EP, Vlastos IM, Picavet VA, et al. The golden ratio in facial symmetry. Rhinology. 2013;51(1):18–21. https://doi.org/10.4193/Rhino12.111.
2. Sutherland CAM, Liu X, Zhang L, Chu Y, Oldmeadow JA, Young AW. Facial first impressions across culture: data-driven modeling of Chinese and British perceivers' unconstrained facial impressions. Pers Soc Psychol Bull. 2018;44(4):521–37. https://doi.org/10.1177/0146167217744194.
3. Sartwell C. "Beauty". In: Zalta EN, editor. The Stanford encyclopedia of philosophy (Winter 2017 edition), https://plato.stanford.edu/archives/win2017/entries/beauty/.
4. Guyer P. The psychology of Kant's aesthetics. Stud Hist Phil Sci. 2008;39(4):483–94. https://doi.org/10.1016/j.shpsa.2008.09.010.
5. Synnott A. The beauty mystique. Facial Plast Surg. 2006;22(3):163–74. https://doi.org/10.1055/s-2006-950173.
6. Little AC, Jones BC, DeBruine LM. Facial attractiveness: evolutionary based research. Philos Trans R Soc Lond B Biol Sci. 2011;366(1571):1638–59. https://doi.org/10.1098/rstb.2010.0404.
7. Perez JC. Codon populations in single-stranded whole human genome DNA are fractal and fine-tuned by the Golden ratio 1.618. Interdiscip Sci. 2010;2(3):228–40. https://doi.org/10.1007/s12539-010-0022-0.
8. Singh P, Vijayan R, Mosahebi A. The Golden ratio and aesthetic surgery. Aesthet Surg J. 2019;39(1):NP4–5. https://doi.org/10.1093/asj/sjy240.
9. Burusapat C, Lekdaeng P. What is the Most beautiful facial proportion in the 21st century? Comparative study among Miss Universe, Miss Universe Thailand, neoclassical canons, and facial Golden ratios. Plast Reconstr Surg Glob Open. 2019;7(2):e2044. https://doi.org/10.1097/GOX.0000000000002044.
10. Ricketts RM. Divine proportion in facial esthetics. Clin Plast Surg. 1982;9(4):401–22.
11. Al-Sebaei MO. The validity of three neo-classical facial canons in young adults originating from the Arabian Peninsula. Head Face Med. 2015;11:4. https://doi.org/10.1186/s13005-015-0064-y.
12. Karaca Saygili O, Cinar S, Gulcen B, Ozcan E, Kus I. The validity of eight neoclassical facial canons in the Turkish adults. Folia Morphol (Warsz). 2016;75(4):512–7. https://doi.org/10.5603/FM.a2016.0028.
13. Pavlic A, Trinajstic Zrinski M, Katic V, Spalj S. Neoclassical canons of facial beauty: do we see the deviations? J Craniomaxillofac Surg. 2017;45(5):741–7. https://doi.org/10.1016/j.jcms.2017.01.029.
14. Choe KS, Sclafani AP, Litner JA, Yu GP, Romo T 3rd. The Korean American woman's face: anthropometric measurements and quantitative analysis of facial aesthetics. Arch Facial Plast Surg. 2004;6(4):244–52. https://doi.org/10.1001/archfaci.6.4.244.
15. Zacharopoulos GV, Manios A, De Bree E, et al. Neoclassical facial canons in young adults. J Craniofac Surg. 2012;23(6):1693–8. https://doi.org/10.1097/SCS.0b013e31826b816b.
16. Beauty around the world. 2008. https://www.oprah.com/style/beauty-around-the-world/5. Accessed 19 July 2020.
17. Langlois JH, Kalakanis L, Rubenstein AJ, Larson A, Hallam M, Smoot M. Maxims or myths of beauty? A meta-analytic and theoretical review. Psychol Bull. 2000;126(3):390–423. https://doi.org/10.1037/0033-2909.126.3.390.
18. Samizadeh S, Wu W. Ideals of facial beauty amongst the Chinese population: results from a large national survey. Aesthetic Plast Surg. 2020;44(4):1173–83. https://doi.org/10.1007/s00266-020-01815-x.
19. Hwang HS, Spiegel JH. The effect of "single" vs "double" eyelids on the perceived attractiveness of Chinese women. Aesthet Surg J. 2014;34(3):374–82. https://doi.org/10.1177/1090820X14523020.

20. Talakoub L, Wesley NO. Differences in perceptions of beauty and cosmetic procedures performed in ethnic patients. Semin Cutan Med Surg. 2009;28(2):115–29. https://doi.org/10.1016/j.sder.2009.05.001.
21. Coetzee V, Faerber SJ, Greeff JM, Lefevre CE, Re DE, Perrett DI. African perceptions of female attractiveness. PLoS One. 2012;7(10):e48116. https://doi.org/10.1371/journal.pone.0048116.
22. Voegeli R, Schoop R, Prestat-Marquis E, Rawlings AV, Shackelford TK, Fink B. Cross-cultural perception of female facial appearance: a multi-ethnic and multi-centre study. PLoS One. 2021;16(1):e0245998. https://doi.org/10.1371/journal.pone.0245998.
23. Rhodes G, Yoshikawa S, Clark A, Lee K, McKay R, Akamatsu S. Attractiveness of facial averageness and symmetry in non-western cultures: in search of biologically based standards of beauty. Perception. 2001;30(5):611–25. https://doi.org/10.1068/p3123.
24. Spyropoulou GC, Pavlidis L, Herrmann S, et al. Can cosmetics' advertisements be an indicator of different perceptions of beauty amongst countries? Aesthetic Plast Surg. 2020;44(5):1871–8. https://doi.org/10.1007/s00266-020-01679-1.
25. Fink B, Matts PJ, Klingenberg H, Kuntze S, Weege B, Grammer K. Visual attention to variation in female facial skin color distribution. J Cosmet Dermatol. 2008;7(2):155–61. https://doi.org/10.1111/j.1473-2165.2008.00382.x.
26. Matts PJ, Fink B, Grammer K, Burquest M. Color homogeneity and visual perception of age, health, and attractiveness of female facial skin. J Am Acad Dermatol. 2007;57(6):977–84. https://doi.org/10.1016/j.jaad.2007.07.040.
27. Marcinkowska UM, Kozlov MV, Cai H, et al. Cross-cultural variation in men's preference for sexual dimorphism in women's faces. Biol Lett. 2014;10(4):20130850. https://doi.org/10.1098/rsbl.2013.0850.
28. Kleisner K, Tureček P, Roberts SC, et al. How and why patterns of sexual dimorphism in human faces vary across the world. Sci Rep. 2021;11(1):5978. https://doi.org/10.1038/s41598-021-85402-3.
29. Tour Egypt. 2021. http://www.touregypt.net/featurestories/beauty.htm. Accessed 13 July 2021.
30. Wichmann A. Would you be considered beautiful in ancient Greece? 2021. https://greekreporter.com/2021/06/24/ancient-greek-beauty-standards-beautiful-greece/. Accessed 13 July 2021.
31. Pham T. Beauty of ancient Chinese. 2018. https://hst124.trampham.bergbuilds.domains/women/beauty-of-ancient-chinese/. Accessed 13 July 2021.
32. Hering E. Portraiture and the female ideal in renaissance art. 2020. https://e-hering.medium.com/portraiture-and-the-female-ideal-in-renaissance-art-bd0b4db2ffe8. Accessed 13 July 2021.
33. Victorian makeup guide & beauty history. 2015. https://vintagedancer.com/victorian/victorian-makeup-beauty-guide/#:~:text=The ideal Victorian beauty was,these problems of the skin.&text=Flowers were soaked in water and made into a nice face wash. Accessed 13 July 2021.
34. Beauty ideal over the decades, part 11: the 20's. 2020. https://www.idealiststyle.com/blog/beauty-ideal-over-the-decades-part-11-the-20s. Accessed 13 July 2021.
35. Beauty ideal over the decades, part 10: the 30's. 2020. https://www.idealiststyle.com/blog/beauty-ideal-over-the-decades-part-10-the-30s. Accessed 13 July 2021.
36. Beauty ideal over the decades, part 7: the 60's. 2020. https://www.idealiststyle.com/blog/beauty-ideal-over-the-decades-part-7-the-60s. Accessed 13 July 2021.
37. Beauty ideal over the decades, part 5: the 80's. 2020. https://www.idealiststyle.com/blog/beauty-ideal-over-the-decades-part-5-the-80s. Accessed 13 July 2021.
38. Beauty ideal over the decades, part 4: the 90's. 2020. https://www.idealiststyle.com/blog/beauty-ideal-over-the-decades-part-4-the-90s. Accessed 13 July 2021.
39. Beauty ideal over the decades, part 3: the 2000's. 2020. https://www.idealiststyle.com/blog/beauty-ideal-over-the-decades-part-3-the-2000s#:~:text=Sexy was the look,in,layered hairstyles were very popular. Accessed 13 July 2021.
40. Apostolou M. Parent–offspring conflict over mating: domains of agreement and disagreement. Evol Psychol. 2015;13(3):1–12. https://doi.org/10.1177/14747049156045.

41. Willis J, Todorov A. First impressions: making up your mind after a 100-ms exposure to a face. Psychol Sci. 2006;17(7):592–8. https://doi.org/10.1111/j.1467-9280.2006.01750.x.
42. Buckingham G, DeBruine LM, Little AC, et al. Visual adaptation to masculine and feminine faces influences generalized preferences and perceptions of trustworthiness. Evol Hum Behav. 2016;27(5):381–9. https://doi.org/10.1016/j.evolhumbehav.2006.03.001.
43. Zebrowitz LA. First impressions from faces. Curr Dir Psychol Sci. 2017;26(3):237–42. https://doi.org/10.1177/0963721416683996.
44. Eagly AH, Ashmore RD, Makhijani MG, Longo LC. What is beautiful is good, but…: a meta-analytic review of research on the physical attractiveness stereotype. Psychol Bull. 1991;110:109–28. https://doi.org/10.1037/0033-2909.110.1.109.
45. Elder GH Jr. Appearance and education in marriage mobility. Am Sociol Rev. 1969;34(4):519–33.
46. Lemay EP Jr, Clark MS, Greenberg A. What is beautiful is good because what is beautiful is desired: physical attractiveness stereotyping as projection of interpersonal goals. Pers Soc Psychol Bull. 2010;36(3):339–53. https://doi.org/10.1177/0146167209359700.
47. O'Doherty J, Winston J, Critchley H, Perrett D, Burt DM, Dolan RJ. Beauty in a smile: the role of medial orbitofrontal cortex in facial attractiveness. Neuropsychologia. 2003;41(2):147–55. https://doi.org/10.1016/s0028-3932(02)00145-8.
48. Grammer K, Fink B, Møller AP, Thornhill R. Darwinian aesthetics: sexual selection and the biology of beauty. Biol Rev Camb Philos Soc. 2003;78(3):385–407. https://doi.org/10.1017/s1464793102006085.
49. Jokela M. Physical attractiveness and reproductive success in humans: evidence from the late 20 century United States. Evol Hum Behav. 2009;30(5):342–50. https://doi.org/10.1016/j.evolhumbehav.2009.03.006.
50. Mautz BS, Wong BB, Peters RA, Jennions MD. Penis size interacts with body shape and height to influence male attractiveness. Proc Natl Acad Sci USA. 2013;110(17):6925–30. https://doi.org/10.1073/pnas.1219361110.
51. Tazzyman SJ, Seymour RM, Pomiankowski A. Fixed and dilutable benefits: female choice for good genes or fertility. Proc Biol Sci. 2012;279(1727):334–40. https://doi.org/10.1098/rspb.2011.0633.
52. Jasieńska G, Ziomkiewicz A, Ellison PT, Lipson SF, Thune I. Large breasts and narrow waists indicate high reproductive potential in women. Proc Biol Sci. 2004;271(1545):1213–7. https://doi.org/10.1098/rspb.2004.2712.
53. Pflüger LS, Oberzaucher E, Katina S, Holzleitner IJ, Grammer K. Cues to fertility: perceived attractiveness and facial shape predict reproductive success. Evol Hum Behav. 2012;33(6):708–14. https://doi.org/10.1016/j.evolhumbehav.2012.05.005.
54. Vashi NA. Evolutionary basis of attraction BT—beauty and body dysmorphic disorder: a clinician's guide. In: Vashi NA, editor. Springer International Publishing. 2015. pp. 45–62. https://doi.org/10.1007/978-3-319-17867-7_3.
55. Pike TW, Petrie M. Offspring sex ratio is related to paternal train elaboration and yolk corticosterone in peafowl. Biol Lett. 2005;1(2):204–7. https://doi.org/10.1098/rsbl.2005.0295.
56. Prum RO. Aesthetic evolution by mate choice: Darwin's really dangerous idea. Philos Trans R Soc Lond Ser B Biol Sci. 2012;367(1600):2253–65. https://doi.org/10.1098/rstb.2011.0285.
57. Croley JA, Reese V, Wagner RF Jr. Dermatologic features of classic movie villains: the face of evil. JAMA Dermatol. 2017;153(6):559–64. https://doi.org/10.1001/jamadermatol.2016.5979.
58. Plastic surgery statistics. 2020. https://www.plasticsurgery.org/news/plastic-surgery-statistics. Accessed 20 July 2021.
59. Beauty industry: revenue in the U.S. 2020. 2020. https://www.statista.com/statistics/243742/revenue-of-the-cosmetic-industry-in-the-us/. Accessed 20 July 2021.
60. Markey CN, Markey PM. Correlates of young women's interest in obtaining cosmetic surgery. Sex Roles. 2009;61:158–66. https://doi.org/10.1007/s11199-009-9625-5.
61. Swami V, Chamorro-Premuzic T, Bridges S, Furnham A. Acceptance of cosmetic surgery: personality and individual difference predictors. Body Image. 2009;6(1):7–13. https://doi.org/10.1016/j.bodyim.2008.09.004.

62. Rankin M, Borah GL, Perry AW, Wey PD. Quality-of-life outcomes after cosmetic surgery. Plast Reconstr Surg. 1998;102(6):2139–47. https://doi.org/10.1097/00006534-199811000-00053.
63. Maymone MBC, Laughter M, Dover J, Vashi NA. The malleability of beauty: perceptual adaptation. Clin Dermatol. 2019;37(5):592–6. https://doi.org/10.1016/j.clindermatol.2019.05.002.
64. Kylie Jenner's lip confession leads to huge increase in cosmetic surgery enquiries. 2015. https://www.independent.co.uk/life-style/fashion/news/kylie-jenner-lip-filler-confession-leads-70-rise-enquiries-procedure-10232716.html. Accessed 10 Aug 2021.
65. A brief history of lip augmentation. 2018. https://www.dazeddigital.com/beauty/head/article/42623/1/history-lip-augmentation#:~:text=KylieJenner confessed she'd,lip augmentation treatment in 2015. Accessed 10 Aug 2021.
66. Little AC, Jones BC, Debruine LM, Caldwell CA. Social learning and human mate preferences: a potential mechanism for generating and maintaining between-population diversity in attraction. Philos Trans R Soc Lond Ser B Biol Sci. 2011;366(1563):366–75. https://doi.org/10.1098/rstb.2010.0192.
67. Hill SE, Buss DM. The mere presence of opposite-sex others on judgments of sexual and romantic desirability: opposite effects for men and women. Pers Soc Psychol Bull. 2008;34(5):635–47. https://doi.org/10.1177/0146167207313728.
68. Sigall H, Landy D. Radiating beauty—effects of having a physically attractive partner on person perception. J Pers Soc Psychol. 1973;28:218–24. https://doi.org/10.1037/h0035740.
69. Little AC, Burriss RP, Jones BC, DeBruine LM, Caldwell CA. Social influence in human face preference: men and women are influenced more for long-term than short-term attractiveness decisions. Evol Hum Behav. 2008;29:140–6. https://doi.org/10.1016/j.evolhumbehav.2007.11.007.

4 Cosmetic Enhancement Should Be Need-Based, Not Greed-Based

Jaishree Sharad

Minimally invasive Cosmetic procedures are on the rise as the need to look a certain way in today's era and age has become a person's priority.

In a survey conducted in 2017 by the American Society for Dermatologic Surgery, the percentage of consumers considering cosmetic treatment increased from 30% to 70% [1].

The most common treatments people opted for were laser and light therapies, fillers and neuromodulator injections, chemical peels, and body sculpting [2].

It has always been thought that people seek cosmetic procedures either due to vanity or psychological reasons. However, in recent studies, it was found that there are many more reasons behind the motivation to look good [3–8]. In a survey on why people wanted to improve their cosmetic appearance, 88.5% of patients wanted to look better, prettier, or more attractive for themselves rather than for others, 81.4% of patients wanted younger, fresher, and clearer-looking skin, and 68.2% wanted treatments to look better in photographs, suggesting the increasing significance of virtual reality in people's lives. Other reasons to get cosmetic procedures done were to increase their self-confidence, improve their quality of life or feel happier or rewarded. Many also wanted to look good when running into people they knew or look good for social events and make a better first impression. Procedures like injectables, thread lifts, and skin tightening are often preferred by people who want to look a certain way for themselves and impress others. Patients who opted for acne and acne scar treatments or procedures for rosacea or hyperpigmentation mostly wanted to be make-up-free. Non-surgical procedures scored over surgery due to cost and convenience. When it came to selecting their physicians, the reputation of the dermatologist and the facility were of prime importance.

J. Sharad (✉)
Skinfinitii Aesthetic Skin and Laser Clinic, Mumbai, India

S. Gupta et al. (eds.), *Critical Thinking in Contemporary Dermatology: Cognitive Essays*, https://doi.org/10.1007/978-981-97-0411-8_4

4.1 When Does It Become Greed-Based and Not Need-Based for Patients?

Social media, makeover shows and reality shows on television, the increasing number of beauty pageants, and various makeover advertisements are common influences on cosmetic surgical procedures. In one of the American shows, the protagonist not only morphed into a beauty queen after a slew of plastic surgery procedures, but she competed in a beauty pageant and won the title as well. A study by Quittkat et al. found that women were more dissatisfied with their bodies than men [9].

Social media has a huge influence on women paying more attention to their appearance. Social media refers to using Instagram, Facebook, Twitter, Snapchat, YouTube, etc., to create and share content or participate in social networking. Social media plays a key role today in setting the ideal beauty standards for all genders globally. It has been seen that this affects the self-esteem of people with regard to their concept of body image and body modification and what they think of themselves in society [10]. Social media is one of the most important factors contributing to the mental, emotional, physical and spiritual health of an individual.

Body image refers to a person's perception of their physical body and the positive or negative thoughts that come along with it. Social media has had a major impact on the perceptual, affective, cognitive and behavioral aspects of body image [11].

Instagram, for example, is a free social networking platform that encourages people to post photos and videos based on which the person gets followers, likes, and comments. The urge to have more followers, positive comments, and words of praise, as well as people liking their photos and videos, is almost like a behavioral addiction. This is attributed to dopamine, the pleasure hormone and is very similar to other substance use. Seeking feedback on social networking sites often results in people comparing themselves with their friends and colleagues and even wanting to impress the opposite gender, resulting in the desire to improve their facial features. Hence, one's physical appearance becomes important for the person. Instagram also allows people to use various filters to improve their image, sharpen facial features, lighten skin tone, contour the face, remove eyebags, give them a pout, etc. A number of times, people use these filters and eventually aim to look as they appear in the filters. That brings them to a dermatologist or cosmetic surgeon. Other times, selfies that distort facial features haunt the person, making them run to the physician for a cosmetic correction [12]. Many young girls and women also want to look like their favorite celebrities or influencers. Sometimes, viewing pictures of celebrities on Instagram has also led to women feeling depressed and embarrassed about their bodies [13]. The American Academy of Facial Plastic and Reconstructive Surgery reported increased requests for surgery due to social media photo sharing [14]. Rhinoplasty, Botox, and facelifts were the most commonly requested procedures.

Often, young girls compare themselves to other females on social media and become dissatisfied, resulting in greater engagement with appearance-changing strategies such as cosmetic surgery [15]. Media exposure and conversations with friends about appearance can influence women's attitudes towards cosmetic surgery

[16]. In a survey on the purchase of beauty products, 72% of millennials procure beauty products based on Instagram posts and other social networks [17]. In another study by Jang-Soon and Hye-Jin on 240 teenage males, cosmetics improved their appearance and resulted in their social success [18]. With bloggers constantly advertising on social media, skincare and cosmetic products have gained popularity. The expectations from individuals are thus rising in beauty and self-care. Imperfections are removed by airbrushing and using other digitized apps to sculpt faces, remove double chin, make lips bigger, slim waists, and reduce sizes to meet unreal beauty standards. This further leads to negative consequences such as low self-esteem, body dissatisfaction, and the urge to undergo cosmetic procedures.

In another study, women who did not get rid of body hair were labeled as being "dirty" and "gross." Hair removal in all genders is almost a compulsion to meet societal acceptance's beauty standards [19]. In 2010, there was an online wave of the living dolls concept where women aimed and practiced to look like dolls. These women would use wide-rimmed contact lenses, hair extensions, corsets, photo editing, and surgery, including eye-widening, breast implants, liposuction, and rib removal, to enhance their beauty. Despite knowing the risks of false eyelashes and acrylic nails, women chose to indulge in these to be accepted in society [20].

Physical dissatisfaction has a negative impact on the patient's self-image, interpersonal relationships, employability and social status. Depression and certain health conditions also result in people opting for cosmetic surgery [21, 22]. The perception of what is considered "cosmetic" has changed over the years, and awareness has increased. It has been found that body satisfaction and pursuit of beauty have a greater impact on patients opting for cosmetic procedures than social factors, like building good interpersonal relationships or having a high social standing [23].

Body Dysmorphic Disorder (BDD) is another reason for people to undergo cosmetic procedures and surgeries. It is estimated that 7–15% have BDD out of the many who seek cosmetic consultations [15]. Media, social environment and peers have a significant influence on individuals' desire to look a certain way or undergo cosmetic procedures.

An attempt to understand the person's personality before addressing their cosmetic concerns often helps in deciding whether to do a particular procedure or deny it, and it also allows the physician to provide treatment options that match one's personality.

Personality is described as a way of perceiving and relating the environment to oneself, and is affected by both genetics and the acquired environment. According to Eysenck, personality encompasses three major dimensions. Extraversion refers to sociability, vivacity, enthusiasm, and impulsivity. Neuroticism epitomizes depression, anxiousness, and emotional instability. Psychoticism signifies solitude, coldness, aggressiveness, and egocentricity [24]. Identifying the association between personality profiles and cosmetic treatment decisions would be worthwhile. Personality differences lead to diverse choices, which are significant references for doctors and beauty seekers regarding the recovery period, postoperative expectations, and operation design [25].

A physician must provide the right guidance on whether or not the person should actually undergo the cosmetic procedure and what the realistic results would be.

Psychological screenings of cosmetic surgery patients can make a huge difference to patients who are influenced by social media, peers, and external forces. More often than not, the patient is dissatisfied after having undergone a cosmetic procedure if they aimed to look like someone they have seen on social media [26]. It would be worthwhile to implement tools to screen patients to identify patient expectations. Patients with unrealistic expectations can be discouraged from undergoing treatments. We can improve their psychosocial functioning by alerting these women to the influence that online images can have on their behavior and body image. Training women on media literacy can improve their self-esteem and decrease their inclination towards elective cosmetic surgery [27].

In an interesting study by Fletcher, patients who came for cosmetic procedures had to fill out a questionnaire, which helped to determine the psychological motivators for treatment (Tables 4.1 and 4.2) [28]. People who opted for questions like "I want to look perfect," "I want to look 20 again," and "I want to look perfectly symmetrical" were considered as red flags. These categories of people were given another questionnaire, which consisted of a modified Cosmetic Procedure Screening Questionnaire (COPS) (Table 4.3) [29], in which patients were asked to describe features of biggest concern in order of highest priority and eight simple questions assessing the impact of those concerns on multiple aspects of daily life. This helped to assess whether or not the person had BDD. Those with BDD were politely refused treatment or sent to a mental health specialist.

When people who are extremely self-critical or have a distorted view of what they really look like opt for surgical or non-surgical procedures, they must be denied any treatment. They should be counseled and sent to a mental health expert. Changing their looks will certainly not solve their problems as they will always find flaws in themselves or be dissatisfied with their treatments. Identifying patients with unrealistic expectations and deferring them from treatments by counseling them will eventually benefit both the patient and the doctor.

People should be encouraged to follow qualified professionals who give authentic, honest advice on skincare and cosmetic procedures to create awareness. Instagram and Facebook often have stories of individuals who have fought hard to

Table 4.1 A questionnaire with a mix of healthy and unhealthy motivators. Fletcher [28]

• Look less saggy	• Look more masculine
• Look more attractive	• Look younger
• Look healthier	• Look like I can compete in the workplace
• Look slimmer	• Look perfectly symmetrical
• Look perfect	• Look more vibrant
• Look less angry/more approachable	• Look like I didn't spend days in the sun
• Look sexier	• Look less tired
• Look less like my older relatives	• Fix one particular flaw
• Look 20 again	• Look happier
• Look more feminine	

Table 4.2 Selected red flags for patients at risk of BDD during cosmetic consultation [28]

• Visiting multiple offices without success
• Showing a particular interest in one flaw to "fix"
• Camouflaging the areas of concern, excessive "cover-ups," such as makeup, hats, scarves, etc.
• Obsessively looking in the mirror during visit
• Inability to look at their own photographs taken at the clinic
• Showing practitioner multiple photographs of themselves that they like (that may be altered)
• Showing practitioner celebrity photographs they would like to emulate
• Coming prepared with a checklist of items to correct
• Confessing to "stalking" practitioner's social media channels

Table 4.3 Modified cosmetic procedure screening questionnaire [29]

Avoid looking at my feature(s)
Frequency of checking feature(s)
How ugly, unattractive or 'not right' feature(s)
Distress caused by feature(s)
Avoid situations or activities because of feature(s)
Preoccupation with feature(s)
Interference with relationship/dating
Interference with sexual relationship
Inability to work/study due to feature(s)
Interference with social life
Noticeability of feature(s) to other people
Frequency of comparing feature(s) to other people
Trying to please oneself or others by having the procedure
Amount of discouragement from having the procedure
Understanding from family/friends about feature(s)
Importance of appearance in defining who you are

change beauty standards through sheer dedication and hard work, be it exercising, eating healthy or building self-esteem and body acceptance through support groups and communities found online. One can reinforce confidence in people of all genders globally by blocking body shamers.

4.2 When Is It Need-Based for Physicians?

Seeking cosmetic correction for a disease, injury, wound, congenital deformity, or hereditary deformity is usually need-based and improves the quality of life.

Structural changes consisting of dermal thinning, fat loss and redistribution, muscle thinning, weakening of ligaments and skeletal resorption are a part of facial aging. This leads to changes, such as flattening of forehead, hooding of brows, hollow temples, hollow cheeks, tear trough deformity, thinning of lips, prominence of nasolabial folds, formation of jowls and marionette lines, ill-defined jawline, retruded chin as well as sagging of nose.

In a study by Fried et al., patients felt less anxious and had increased confidence and happiness after being injected with poly-L-lactic acid to make them look younger [30]. These patients also ate healthier, exercised, and were more comfortable with others.

When we talk of need-based cosmetic procedures, these are procedures that will genuinely make the patient feel happy and confident. These can be done to turn back the clock by a few years and make the person look youthful. Fillers for sunken eyes that make one look tired or for very thin lips or botulinum toxin for strong masseter muscles can also be done in youngsters to improve their facial expressions.

Sometimes people turn to us to correct a physical defect to feel more comfortable and confident in their own skin. There are case reports of fillers being done for facial asymmetries and deformities in cases of localized scleroderma, lipodystrophy, and traumatic scars. These give the patients immense confidence and boost their self-esteem and are certainly need-based treatments.

Acne scars can also cause depression and psychological imbalance. Treatments for acne scars can change a person's life, instilling in them a new sense of hope and joy as well as boosting their morale.

"Cosmetic" does not always mean "unimportant." It is indeed naïve to think that appearance doesn't matter. It matters in every walk of life. Even the ancient Egyptians, free of social media influences, regarded beauty as a sign of holiness, going to considerable lengths to procure Kohl and malachite for their eyes and red ochre for cheeks.

A person who feels they look tired all the time due to sunken eyes can be given fillers to look refreshed. A person who feels that the permanent frown on their forehead makes them look angry all the time can be advised to take botulinum toxin injections or even low G-prime fillers in case of static lines to erase the frown lines and make them look happier. Modern medicine has the tools to help many such conditions, sometimes making a person look like a better version of themselves. Patients should be given the benefits in all honesty and realistically so.

4.3 Physician Greed-Based Treatments

Self-aggrandizing doctors who opt for misleading marketing over medical ethics damage the reputation of the treatment as well as the profession.

Pillow-face syndrome was on the rise a few years ago. Filling the face with hyaluronic acid just to plump the face or creating duck lips with no aesthetics in mind, either due to lack of knowledge and judgment or greed to inject more fillers. Injecting more syringes of fillers could be due to three reasons. First, the pharma-driven teaching has imparted the knowledge of "more is better." Second, pharma companies promise to make you "star injectors" if you inject more. Third, you earn more money when you inject more. However, all these reasons are by far unethical and only selfish motives for injecting the patient. While most qualified physicians would not do this, there are unqualified, uninformed, and untrained people who often follow these policies.

Sometimes, when one invests in an expensive device, one wants to overcome the costs soon. That is when everything on the face or body should not look like a nail just because one has a hammer.

Sometimes young boys and girls want to opt for surgeries such as liposuction, wanting an easy way out. They could be advised to exercise and eat healthy instead of looking for an easy way out unless it is a condition like gynaecomastia.

A doctor's profession should not be driven by greed and ego; one must remember that the patient is not a commodity that can be exploited. Prioritizing profits or convenience over patient outcomes is unethical and wrong. Patient interaction should be about the patient, not a business model where targets need to be achieved for revenue generation.

Making exaggerated, baseless claims or coercing patients into unnecessary or inappropriate procedures is criminal for a doctor who has taken the Hippocrates oath.

Many dermatological or plastic surgery societies are now working on identifying the right patient from the self-obsessive one to tackle this issue. Patient screening tools and a training curriculum to help doctors understand the links between mental health, body image and cosmetic procedures are being introduced, which is a positive step forward.

World over, unregulated cosmetic clinics with unqualified professionals performing procedures ranging from neurotoxins, fillers, lasers to even breast and nose jobs, tummy tucks, and facelifts are on the rise. Slick websites promise the world quick and painless makeovers that will help them have the face and body they've dreamt of.

Offering discounted or free treatments to some celebrities to use their images on social media or for digital and print marketing has become another way of luring the commoner into cosmetic procedures and surgeries even when they do not need them.

Cosmetic dermatology and surgery are rapidly expanding practice sectors and are now available as popular services from being a niche market in the past. Aesthetic interventions can have a significant impact on the patient's well-being and mental psyche. Patient safety should be a doctor's priority. The centers for cosmetic procedures should be ethical, and the doctors performing these procedures should have the right skill and knowledge. Their skills should be upgraded from time to time to give the patient the best possible outcome. The products being used for the procedure should be safe and of good quality. Cheap, unregulated products or devices should not be used to compromise on the cost or make larger profits.

It is important to identify the patient's needs as much as to recognize the procedure's limitations or the doctor's competence. Should the person opt for a treatment, a proper discussion should be held regarding the procedure's benefits, risks, and the outcome. The patient should be given time to reflect so they can make the right decision. It is extremely important to consider the patient's vulnerabilities and psychological needs before jumping into a procedure. Detailed, honest informed consent should be taken. No procedure should be performed out of financial or commercial interest. Succumbing to greed for money or fame can be eventually detrimental not just to the patient but to the doctor as well.

References

1. American Society of Dermatologic Surgery. 2017 ASDS consumer survey on cosmetic dermatologic procedures. 2017. https://www.asds.net/Medical-Professionals/Practice-Resources/ASDS-Consumer-Survey-on-Cosmetic-Dermatologic-Procedures. Accessed 10 Jan 2018.
2. American Society of Dermatologic Surgery. 2016 ASDS consumer survey on cosmetic dermatologic procedures. 2016. https://www.asds.net/Medical-Professionals/Practice-Resources/ASDS-Survey-on-Dermatologic-Procedures. Accessed 10 Jan 2018.
3. Haas CF, Champion A, Secor D. Motivating factors for seeking cosmetic surgery: a synthesis of the literature. Plast Surg Nurs. 2008;28(4):177–82.
4. Von Soest T, Kvalem IL, Skolleborg KC, Roald HE. Psychosocial factors predicting the motivation to undergo cosmetic surgery. Plast Reconstr Surg. 2006;117(1):51–62; discussion 63–4.
5. Ferraro GA, Rossano F, D'Andrea F. Self-perception and self-esteem of patients seeking cosmetic surgery. Aesthetic Plast Surg. 2005;29(3):184–9.
6. Milothridis P, Pavlidis L, Haidich AB, Panagopoulou E. A systematic review of the factors predicting the interest in cosmetic plastic surgery. Indian J Plast Surg. 2016;49(3):397–402.
7. Sarwer DB, LaRossa D, Bartlett SP, Low DW, Bucky LP, Whitaker LA. Body image concerns of breast augmentation patients. Plast Reconstr Surg. 2003;112(1):83–90.
8. Imadojemu S, Sarwer DB, Percec I, Sonnad SS, Goldsack JE, Berman M, Sobanko JF. Influence of surgical and minimally invasive facial cosmetic procedures on psychosocial outcomes: a systematic review. JAMA Dermatol. 2013;149(11):1325–33.
9. Quittkat HL, Hartmann AS, Düsing R, Buhlmann U, Vocks S. Body dissatisfaction, importance of appearance, and body appreciation in men and women over the lifespan. Front Psychiatry. 2019;10:864.
10. Henriques M, Patnaik D. Social media and its effects on beauty. In: Levine MP, Santos JS, editors. Beauty—cosmetic science, cultural issues and creative developments. IntechOpen. 2020. https://doi.org/10.5772/intechopen.93322. https://www.intechopen.com/chapters/73271.
11. Aparicio-Martinez P, Perea-Moreno AJ, Martinez-Jimenez MP, Redel-Macías MD, Pagliari C, Vaquero-Abellan M. Social media, thin-ideal, body dissatisfaction and disordered eating attitudes: an exploratory analysis. Int J Environ Res Public Health. 2019;16(21):4177.
12. Walker CE, Krumhuber EG, Dayan S, et al. Effects of social media use on desire for cosmetic surgery among young women. Curr Psychol. 2021;40:3355–64.
13. Holland G, Tiggemann M. A systematic review of the impact of the use of social networking sites on body image and disordered eating outcomes. Body Image. 2016;17:100–10.
14. American Academy of Facial Plastic and Reconstructive Surgery. 2013. https://www.prnewswire.com/news-releases/new-survey-finds-social-media-is-a-major-influence-on-elective-surgery-191992411.html. Accessed 12 Apr 2019.
15. Crerand CE, Franklin ME, Sarwer DB. Body dysmorphic disorder and cosmetic surgery. Plast Reconstr Surg. 2006;118(7):167e–80e.
16. Sharp G, Tiggemann M, Mattiske J. The role of media and peer influences in Australian women's attitudes towards cosmetic surgery. Body Image. 2014;11(4):482–7.
17. Social media influence on sales [Internet]. 2017. https://www.forbes.com/sites/andrewarnold/2017/12/22/4-ways-social-media-influencesmillennials-purchasing-decisions/#3cdd48ea539f.
18. Jang-Soon P, Hye-Jin K. Perception about makeup influence on man's makeup and their success. J Korea Converg Soc. 2017;8(4):231–7.
19. Toerien M, Wilkinson S. Gender and body hair: constructing the feminine woman. Women's Stud Int Forum. 2003;26(4):333–44.
20. Elias AS, Gill R, Scharff C. Aesthetic labour: rethinking beauty politics in neoliberalism. London: Macmillan Publishers; 2017.
21. Nerini A, Matera C, Stefanile C. Psychosocial predictors in consideration of cosmetic surgery among women. Aesthetic Plast Surg. 2014;38(2):461–6.

22. Cheraghian B, Fereidooni-Moghadam M, Babadi H, Dashtbozorgi B. Psychological and personality characteristics of applicants for facial cosmetic surgery. Aesthetic Plast Surg. 2020;44(3):780–7.
23. Babadi H, Fereidooni-Moghadam M, Dashtbozorgi B, Cheraghian B. Investigating psychosocial causes of the tendency for facial cosmetic surgery. Aesthetic Plast Surg. 2018;42(4):1157–63.
24. https://courses.lumenlearning.com/boundless-psychology/chapter/trait-perspectives-on-personality/.
25. Qian H, Ling Y, Wang C, Lenahan C, Zhang M, Zheng M, Shao A. A correlative study between personality traits and the preference of site selection in cosmetic treatment. Front Psychiatry. 2021;12:648751.
26. Lee HH, Damhorst ML, Paff Ogle J. Body satisfaction and attitude theory: linkages with normative compliance and behaviors undertaken to change the body. Fam Consum Sci Res J. 2009;37(4):466–88.
27. Khazir Z, Dehdari T, Mahmoodi Majdabad M, Pournaghash TS. Psychological aspects of cosmetic surgery among females: a media literacy training intervention. Glob J Health Sci. 2015;8(2):35–45.
28. Fletcher L. Development of a multiphasic, cryptic screening protocol for body dysmorphic disorder in cosmetic dermatology. J Cosmet Dermatol. 2021;20(4):1254–62.
29. Veale D, Ellison N, Werner TG, Dodhia R, Serfaty MA, Clarke A. Development of a cosmetic procedure screening questionnaire (COPS) for body dysmorphic disorder. J Plast Reconstr Aesthet Surg. 2012;65(4):530–2.
30. Fried R, Werschler WP, Cenci J, Sternberg L, Dhanaraj P, Tolas D, Withrow S. Patient-perceived emotional and functional benefits of poly-L-lactic acid (PLLA) for the treatment of facial volume loss. J Clin Aesthet Dermatol. 2018;11(7):40–3.

5 Chasing Attractiveness: The Growing Obsession with Aesthetic Standards in Dermatology—Are We Promoting an Illusion of Beauty?

Mansak Shishak

The realm of dermatology is a highly visual science, with visual perception and aesthetics being closely intertwined. Dermatology aesthetics deals with design and learning to align the images in our brains with patients' bodies, using the face or other structures as biological manipulation models. It has little or nothing to do with functionality. Cosmetic procedural interventions have always emphasized on the ideal proportions and "golden ratios" of beauty. While a lot of it is largely influenced by history and art through the ages, and physicians dealing with cosmesis are by no means the only ones responsible for the perpetuation of aesthetic dogma in medicine, it appears that in trying to reach "perfection," we have become single-mindedly visual, quantitative, and robotic. Seeking only to align symmetry, iron out creases and fill out the beautiful troughs, such as of hands; not allowing sinewy surfaces; and becoming master craftsmen, attempting to achieve a specific beauty image for all our patients.

Are we at fault, or are we helpless?

In two decades or so, the anti-aging and cosmetic market has burgeoned from a few staple products to a never-ending glut of products, devices, injectables and pills that promise, often menacingly, to restore youthful vitality. Aggressive marketing aims to encourage chasing the appearance of youth as long as possible, disallowing any sagging or bagginess or any evidence of "age," such as fine lines and rhytides.

The growing obsession with cosmesis is getting more glaring with every passing day. Digital manipulation of photographs is far too accessible and easy. The great relishing of beautifying apps with a seemingly endless plethora of filter options is an open secret. Traces of freckles, solar lentigines, actinic damage or under-eye laxity are quite easily gone in a single swipe! Augmented reality makes structural facial modifications possible, with more chiseled jawlines, accentuated and lifted eyebrows, contoured cheekbones, and the "snatched" trend becoming a reality. This

M. Shishak (✉)
ISIC Multispecialty Hospital, New Delhi, India

S. Gupta et al. (eds.), *Critical Thinking in Contemporary Dermatology: Cognitive Essays*, https://doi.org/10.1007/978-981-97-0411-8_5

filtered form of oneself becomes the social perception and eventually a means of self-identity. Social interactions involving the metaverse may soon take over on a large scale. A global majority, particularly the young, are in a continuous loop of dopamine chase-and-reward cycle due to social media pressure.

What has led to this? And why is there such a consumption of beauty-related news?

What is beauty? Why are beauty stereotypes perpetuated through centuries? Is it environmental conditioning of stereotypes to classify something as attractive or unattractive? Or are we naturally hard-wired to get attracted to the so-called universal attributes of beauty?

Gestalt psychology, stemming from the school of Gestalt beliefs, is fundamental to understanding the principles of aesthetic designs. Gestalt principle explains that to process a lot of information, the mind tries to simplify matters and can process "holism" better than the sum of individual parts [1]. Putting it in context, we tend to process a face as a whole rather than the sum of its individual parts, such as eyes or nose. This provides a cognitive shortcut or bias to conclude on attributes of attractiveness; the mind takes shortcuts to conclude whether something is beautiful or not.

Some of the principles include:

1. Simplicity (praägnanz): The law of simplicity explains that the mind perceives things in its simplest form. Perhaps multiple textural changes on a single skin surface, such as a face with a combination of "open pores," rolling type acne scars and naevi, is more difficult to cognitively comprehend, which is the reason the mind automatically prefers a smoother appearance free of textural irregularities, which is simpler to process.
2. Similarity: This Gestalt principle suggests that similar items are grouped together based on color, size etc. Is this why color homogeneity is strongly preferred [2, 3] and conditions like vitiligo and melasma confuse the perception?
3. Continuity and symmetry: The law of continuity says that the human eye follows the smoothest paths while viewing lines, irrespective of how the lines were drawn. The mind also seeks symmetry in an attempt to simplify information processing. A beaked and deviated nose will not fall in the line of visual continuity and thus be prone to cognitive bias, placing it as "unattractive." Developmental anomalies are often associated with asymmetries and are not considered attractive. In body dysmorphic disorder (BDD), research has shown that there is abnormal information processing, with greater local processing compared to global processing. Interestingly, global processing efficiency correlates inversely with BDD severity [4].

Attraction may also be influenced by familiarity. The more we encounter faces with a certain feature or cosmetic procedure, the more attractive and desirable it may appear. The more common it gets, the more it forms a beauty trend and becomes aspirational. Current trends include "glass skin" and K-beauty: plump, rosy lips, dewy, hydrated skin and glossy, luscious dark hair—all examples of color contrast, which have been associated with youth and beauty [5].

Ramsey et al. argue that beauty stereotypes are ingrained in the brains early on and found that 6-month-old infants gazed longer at faces judged by adults as attractive and spent less time looking at faces judged as unattractive [6].

Using that argument, do we have a starting disadvantage when dealing with beauty stereotypes?

Is it easier, after all, to flow along evolutionary signals, allow nature to follow basic instincts, and let dermatological science build upon the structure of ideal beauty proportions?

Or are we playing the science of deception?

Darwin, in his theory of sexual selection, hypothesized mate choice as an active selection by species based on innate preferences and "taste for the beautiful" and "aesthetic faculty," giving importance and attention to ornaments using sensory and cognitive preference.

In his book "Sex, Evolution and Consumer Behavior," Geoffrey Miller explains attractiveness, evolutionary traits and "Costly Signals." As a part of evolution and natural selection, the brain has focused on features of attractiveness and beauty because they reliably measure health and fitness, implying greater reproductive success and absence of disease. More importantly, they are difficult to fake. Such features that genuinely signal reproductive fitness are known as Costly Signals [7]. But humans have devised ways by which others can be deceived by faking Costly Signals [8].

Are we complicit in the science of deception?

To what extent are we willing to go in a bid to "restore" Costly Signals?

We are privy to cosmeceutical advancements and covet the latest cosmetic products and machines.

We speak not of the craft and the vast terrain of dermatology with its amazing bounty of infectious, immunological and interventional procedures but seek validation from glossy magazines and awards handed out by celebrities where bills and cheques often exchange hands.

It has long spiraled out of control, but the end doesn't seem near.

We were told to point out lines and jowls and promise "10 years younger" treatments to patients. And so we did.

We continue pointing out lines and jowls, and tell them the wrinkles make them appear tired and angry. Their necks had to look like Queen Nefertiti's. We gasp when we see the effects of the toxin being worn off after a few months and readily suggest a retouch.

We have gladly jumped onto the bandwagon of social media and its filtered obsession. We have endorsed artificial beauty and glorified it.

By endorsing hyper-realistic images and concepts to the patient, we clearly have a strong role in driving the narrative.

The driving force for suggesting treatment modalities in aesthetics has commercial interests at play besides falling prey to global marketing giants. Misconceptions of beauty are perpetuated; glutathione injections are secretly and sometimes not-so-secretly administered. The global skin-lightening industry is expected to reach USD 16.6 billion in 2030 (Emergen Research, Aug 2022), despite the awareness and resistance movements against the terribly flawed misconception that glorifies lighter skin tones.

We don't educate patients about timely sun exposure and its benefits, but usher people into rooms filled with red and blue lights, offering more collagen production and anti-gravity skin effects.

The art of microblading for the eyebrows is a great tool for those with physiological or systemic sparseness of brows. But in doing so, we quickly infringed upon the territory of make-up artists by adding more strokes, pigment, arches, and, most disparagingly, offering to one and all. The lines between these industries are very poorly drawn and continuously shifting.

Patients presenting with unrealistic expectations have become the norm. We rarely care to pursue why a particular patient's insecurities are triggered. What is making them seek treatment? Many use cosmetic procedures as a conduit to reach a place of safety and feeling wanted. But do we care at all about their journey and destinations?

We are only the cheerleaders, not their coaches or guides.

Have we become a case of the blind leading the blind?

Are we all living in an illusionary space?

The growing obsession with appearances alone, chasing an illusion, a façade, has been created and propagated by advertisements and algorithms.

We must learn the art of dissuasion vs persuasion, of impacting lives for the better through our skills and tools vs feeding the insecurities and dilemmas of a person, and we must look at the anatomy of the skin and morphology of the face as windows of internal manifestations and not structures of manipulation alone. We need to understand our privilege of being the providers of "beauty" restoration or the restoration of "Costly Signals" in cases where it has been depleted because of trauma, disease, or aging [9]. Additionally, we are responsible for exercising caution and restraint when overstepping the boundaries of faking the signals. We must hold the mirrors ourselves first, rectify and learn to self-regulate when unhealthy trends and practices dominate.

References

1. Gabrieli G, Lee A, Setoh P, Esposito G. An analysis of the generalizability and stability of the halo effect during the COVID-19 pandemic outbreak. Front Psychol. 2021;12:631871.
2. Fink B, Matts PJ, Klingenberg H, Kuntze S, Weege B, Grammer K. Visual attention to variation in female facial skin color distribution. J Cosmet Dermatol. 2008;7(2):155–61.
3. Samson N, Fink B, Matts PJ. Visible skin condition and perception of human facial appearance. Int J Cosmet Sci. 2010;32(3):167–84.
4. Li W, Arienzo D, Feusner JD. Body dysmorphic disorder: neurobiological features and an updated model. Z Klin Psychol Psychother (Gott). 2013;42(3):184–91.

5. Porcheron A, Mauger E, Russell R. Aspects of facial contrast decrease with age and are cues for age perception. PLoS One. 2013;8(3):e57985.
6. Ramsey JL, Langlois JH, Hoss RA, Rubenstein AJ, Griffin AM. Origins of a stereotype: categorization of facial attractiveness by 6-month-old infants. Dev Sci. 2004;7(2):201–11.
7. Miller G. Spent: sex, evolution and consumer behavior. New York: Penguin Group; 2009.
8. Yarosh DB. Perception and deception: human beauty and the brain. Behav Sci (Basel). 2019;9(4):34.
9. Gupta S. It is the cooperation, stupid! J Cutan Aesthet Surg. 2016;9(4):274–7.

Hair Loss in the Naked Ape

6

Venkataram Mysore

Homo sapiens, despite being the most hairless among apes, places profound importance on the limited hair they possess due to its role in sexual identification and identity [1]. This has led to a surge in the market for hair-care products and management techniques in the last two decades, accompanied by a renewed interest in the physiology, pathology, and management of hair. This chapter critically examines various aspects, including the pathophysiology and psychology of hair loss, and provides an overview of the current state of management.

Trichologists note a perceived increase in the number of patients experiencing hair loss, particularly in patterned hair loss. This observation aligns with the findings of an Australian survey, revealing that 98.6% of men and 64.4% of women reported bitemporal hair loss [2]. The rise in patient numbers may be attributed to increased awareness, the availability of treatment options, and easy access to care. Additionally, the link between Androgenetic alopecia (AGA) and metabolic syndrome, a condition on the rise in the last few decades, could contribute to this trend [3–9]. Trichologists have also observed a shift in the age group of patients, with present-day individuals experiencing hair loss at a younger age than their predecessors.

Alopecia, or hair loss, is not just a physical concern but also has significant psychological impacts, causing emotional distress and leading to personal, social, and work-related challenges [10, 11]. A substantial percentage of individuals with alopecia report marital and career problems as a consequence [12]. The heightened concern for hair has resulted in a global increase in hair-related procedures. According to The International Society of Hair Restoration Surgery (ISHRS), approximately 635,189 hair restoration procedures were performed worldwide in 2016, marking a substantial 60% increase from 2014. Asia, as the largest

V. Mysore (✉)
Venkat Center for Advanced Skin, and Plastic Surgery and Postgraduate Training, Bangalore, India

S. Gupta et al. (eds.), *Critical Thinking in Contemporary Dermatology: Cognitive Essays*, https://doi.org/10.1007/978-981-97-0411-8_6

contributor with 195,284 surgeries, experienced a 36% surge. The total number of hair restoration patients (surgical and medical) worldwide in the past year reached 1,838,946, reflecting a staggering 74% increase from 2014 [13].

The apparent lack of hair in humans stands in stark contrast to the significant concern and attention given to hair-related issues, and it warrants discussion. Three distinctive and interconnected traits set humans apart from other primates: bipedality, practical nakedness, and the family reproductive unit, and these characteristics are interrelated [14]. Unlike other primates, humans are unique in their inability to carry babies without relying on their hands. A hairless bipedal mother, for instance, would need to stand and walk upright to hold her baby, severely limiting her activities. In this scenario, the male partner would take on the responsibility of collecting and bringing food to her to prevent their baby from starving, fostering a sense of responsibility and care.

As a reward for such responsible behavior, including care and providing food, the mother might have been more likely to accept her partner sexually at any time. This potential for sexual relations beyond oestrus cycles could have strengthened the pair's bond. Consequently, hairless and upright pairs would have been better positioned to establish strong family units. This unique trait opened up alternative reproductive strategies, such as the development of a larger pelvis with a substantial birth canal to accommodate a baby with a larger head or the delivery of an immature baby with post-birth rearing. The combination of practical nakedness and bipedality, along with the associated family reproductive unit, played a pivotal role in shaping human evolutionary strategies and behaviours.

However, nakedness also caused many clear costs for the naked ape. The 'naked skin' also made humans more vulnerable to UV radiation, resulting in cancer and aging changes [14].

What, however, deserves an explanation is the persistence of hairs in certain areas such as under the arms, around the genitals, and on the head. Darwin suggests a plausible theory that elaborates that, as hairlessness has no direct advantage and therefore cannot have evolved through natural selection, human hairlessness may have evolved through sexual selection, where males came to see the nakedness of the female skin as sexually attractive [15]. Wyatt suggests this selective persistence of hair causes different signals with at least three functions: individual recognition, priming effects of various kinds, and potential mate selection [16]. All of these indicate that the primary function of scalp hair may also be sexual. The fact that male pattern hair loss is related to androgens also supports this hypothesis. These facts explain why the little hair prevalent amongst relative nakedness is so precious to the nude ape, and its loss causes so much concern.

But why is occipital hair not lost to baldness? The occipital scalp has less androgen receptors; hence it can tolerate and withstand androgen better, surviving longer in both men and women. While this persistence is useful as the donor in hair transplantation, it is not easily explained. There is a hypothesis that the occipital and rest of the scalp may be derived from a different embryological source. This may have been necessitated by the larger size of the head due to increased size of the frontal brain in humans.

The notion that male pattern baldness (MPL) extends beyond cosmetic concerns to potentially serve as a risk factor for cardiovascular disease has been proposed by Cotton et al. and other researchers [17–22]. Severe and early onset of MPL in individuals before the age of 30 may be linked to a higher risk of ischemic heart disease, elevated serum cholesterol levels, and increased blood pressure when compared to men of similar age without hair loss [23, 24]. Additionally, there is evidence suggesting an increased incidence of benign prostatic hyperplasia associated with male androgenetic alopecia (MAA), although this has been a topic of dispute in some studies [25–27]. Prostate cancer has also been found to be positively associated with MAA in various research findings [28, 29]. A meta-analysis has indicated that an elevated risk of prostate cancer is linked to vertex baldness, though other baldness patterns may also be seen [30].

Male androgenetic alopecia (MAA) exhibits a familial tendency, and there are recognized racial variations in its prevalence [31, 32]. Twin studies have indicated that heredity accounts for nearly 80% of the predisposition to baldness [33]. It is believed that the baldness gene follows an autosomal dominant pattern in men and an autosomal recessive pattern in women [34]. Polygenic inheritance is also suggested by an Australian study that found a high correlation between balding sons and fathers with significant balding [35].

Moreover, an association between male pattern baldness and a polymorphism of the androgen receptor gene on the X chromosome has been identified [35, 36]. Shorter triplets repeat haplotypes (RFLP) associated with a functional variant of the androgen receptor (AR) gene are found in higher frequency in bald men compared to normal controls. A gene test has recently been developed to assess an individual's response to finasteride therapy based on specific variations in the AR gene [37]. This test provides the patient's CAG repeat length score in the AR gene, with a shorter CAG repeat length (<22) being associated with a higher likelihood of benefiting from finasteride administration.

AGA has three key pathophysiological features: alteration (shortening of anagen and prolongation of telogen) in hair cycle development, follicular miniaturization and inflammation. The key event is the detachment of the arrector pili muscle from its follicular attachment and its replacement by fat, making hair loss irreversible. Prolongation of the kenogen phase (or the lag phase) leads to the delayed replacement of telogen hair, leaving a higher percentage of empty hair follicles contributing to balding [38, 39].

The 5-alpha reductase enzyme plays a pivotal role in miniaturization by converting testosterone to the more active metabolite, dihydrotestosterone (DHT), within hair follicles [40]. DHT has a significantly higher binding affinity to the androgen receptor compared to testosterone [41]. Two isoforms of the 5-α reductase enzyme have been identified: Type 1 is present in sebaceous glands, epidermis, eccrine sweat glands, apocrine sweat glands, and hair follicles, while Type 2 is found in the dermal papilla, the inner layer of the outer root sheath, sebaceous ducts, proximal inner root sheath of scalp hair follicles, as well as in the prostate, testes, and liver [42, 43]. Type 2 enzyme accounts for approximately 80% of circulating DHT [44]. Several other enzymes contribute to the pathogenesis of androgenetic hair loss, including 17β- and 3β-hydroxysteroid dehydrogenases (HSD) [45]. Major steroidogenic enzymes involved in the formation of potent androgens include steroid sulfatase, 3β-HSD1, 17β-HSD3, and type 1 5α reductase. On the other hand, 17β-HSD2, 3α-HSD, and aromatase are believed to deactivate excess androgens locally to maintain androgen homeostasis in the hair follicles [45].

It is indeed intriguing to observe that androgens can have paradoxically different effects on human hair follicles in various body sites. While androgens stimulate hair growth in certain areas like the beard, axillary (armpit), and pubic regions, they concurrently suppress the growth of frontal scalp hair in individuals genetically predisposed to hair loss. This dual action of androgens on hair follicles in different body locations may be linked to the second messenger system, highlighting the complex and context-dependent nature of androgenic effects on hair growth [46]. Beard dermal papilla cells (DPC) are known to secrete growth-inducing autocrine growth factors such as IGF-1 in response to testosterone, leading to an increase in dermal papilla size and enlargement of the hair follicle and hair cortex.

The dermal papilla, derived from mesenchyme and situated at the center of the hair bulb in the follicle base, plays a crucial role in regulating various aspects of the epithelial follicle. It serves as the target for androgen-mediated events that lead to miniaturization and changes in the hair cycle [47–49]. The size of the dermal papilla directly influences the size of the hair bulb and, consequently, the hair shaft produced [50, 51]. The mechanism of cell death in this context can take various forms, including apoptotic cell death, decreased proliferation of keratinocytes, cell displacement with a loss of cellular adhesion resulting in dermal papilla fibroblasts dropping into the dermis, or migration of dermal papilla cells into the dermal sheath associated with the outer root sheath of the hair follicle [51–53]. Balding dermal papilla cells may release inhibitory factors, such as Insulin-like growth factor binding protein 3 (IGFBP3), which contribute to the formation of smaller dermal papillae and subsequently smaller hairs in male androgenetic alopecia (MAA). This leads to a reduction in the caliber of hair shafts from 0.08 mm to less than 0.06 mm [53–56].

Traditionally, follicular miniaturization has been thought to occur in a stepwise fashion. Still, evidence suggests that the transition from terminal to vellus hair may happen abruptly as a single large-step process [55]. This could explain the rapid progression of miniaturization observed in some patients. Additionally, follicular miniaturization occurs between anagen cycles rather than within the anagen phase, explaining the delay in response seen after the initiation of therapy [56].

Arrectores play a fascinating and pivotal role in these events. Arrectores are responsible for the architecture of the follicular unit. Each follicular unit is comprised of 1–4 terminal hair follicles, 1–2 vellus hair follicles, a sebaceous gland, arrector pili muscle and surrounding collagen. It is pyramidal in shape, being narrow at the top and splaying at the bottom. This architecture, first described by Headington, marks a landmark discovery in the pathology and surgical management of hair loss.

The arrector pili muscle forms an obtuse angle with the skin surface and covers the sebaceous glands around the sebaceous lobules. The hair follicle bulge area is a contiguous portion of the outer root sheath at the level of insertion of the arrector pili muscle, also called trochanter. The bulge cells are composed of stem cells, which are multipotent and possess high proliferative capacity [57]. The arrector pili muscle and its bulge connection persists throughout the hair growth cycle and has a role in the renewal as well as morphogenesis of hair. The level of arrectores attachment is variable, and this, along with the hold of perifollicular collagen, is responsible for the challenges encountered in extraction by the follicular unit extraction process.

The follicular basement membrane is responsible for anchoring of the arrector pili muscle to the bulge. Genes of tendons like SCX (scleraxis), Mitf (microphthalmia-associated transcription factor), Fbln1 (fibulin 1), Postn (periostin) and Tnc (Tenascin-c) are expressed by bulge stem cells. The bulge cells express periostin, which is a major component of the tendon extracellular matrix; hence, it is postulated that the bulge stem cells serve as tendon cells for the arrector pili muscle [58]. The nephronectin and $\alpha 8\beta 1$ integrin play a significant role in determining the proximal attachment site of the arrector pili muscle [59]. It has been seen that fibroblasts positive for $\alpha 8$ integrin are the progenitor cells for arrector pili muscle, which attach to nephronectin in bulge area and differentiate into α-smooth muscle actin (SMA)-expressing arrector pili muscle cells.

There are some proposed hypotheses for the role of arrectores. One of these, the *bulge hypothesis*, comprises of four important elements; the slow-cycling bulge cells are activated by dermal papillae to undergo transient proliferation during early anagen, the bulge cells undergo transient proliferation in response to matrix signals; the matrix cells derived from bulge stem cells are transient amplifying cells and thus have limited proliferative potential; and during late catagen the dermal papilla moves upward which allows interaction of resting bulge cells and dermal papilla essential to start new hair cycle [60].

A critical event recognized recently is the degeneration of arrectores, with a decrease in muscle volume and fat infiltration around the arrector pili muscle of hair follicles in androgenetic alopecia. This fat deposition occurs due to a disrupted cholesterol synthesis pathway, which leads to the accumulation of proinflammatory lipids. This is somewhat similar to the ectopic fat deposits in mesenchymal progenitor cell conditions like obesity, Duchenne muscular dystrophy and aging-related sarcopenia [61]. This loss of mesenchymal progenitor cells in androgenetic alopecia leads to loss of arrector pili muscle and dermal papilla interaction, which finally leads to miniaturization [62].

Most hair loss disorders can be attributed to changes in the normal dynamic behavior of the hair follicle. Therefore, any treatment would have to cut-short telogen, prolong anagen or hasten entry into anagen. However, all the key molecules of the hair loss cycling have not been identified, resulting in management gaps. In most types of hair loss, even in the so-called permanent hair loss, the AGA, there is no destruction in contrast to the scarring alopecia (which is indeed the true permanent hair loss), and it should therefore be possible to find a key to unlock the reverse transition of vellus-like hair back to terminal hair.

Since their fortuitous and serendipitous discoveries, minoxidil and finasteride have remained the only FDA-approved medications for decades. A number of other agents such as cyclosporin A (CsA), topical immunophilin ligands, prostaglandin, ezetimibe and simvastatin, minoxidil, retinoids, estrogen, adenosine, calcitriol, estradiol, prednisolone, zinc, and candida antigen have all flattered to deceive [63–74]. Biologics and small molecules such as JAK inhibitors offer hope in alopecia areata treatment [75–78]. The role of prolactin receptor antagonists and the regulators of thyroid hormones and vitamin-D receptor modulators are yet to be fully established [79].

In the absence of substantial breakthroughs in pharmacological options, surgical options have caught the imagination of patients, and many significant advances have occurred in this field, which are discussed below. Regenerative treatments such as autologous platelet-rich plasma (PRP) and stem cells from different sources, including fat, have attracted attention.

Hair is a complicated organ with multiple modes of keratinization, multiple types of cells of different origins, a unique cycling phenomenon, and most importantly, a largely cosmetic function. It is therefore not surprising that efforts at cloning and culture have remained largely experimental [80].

Finasteride is a selective inhibitor of the intracellular enzyme 5-α reductase type 2, responsible for converting the androgen testosterone (T) into 5α-dihydrotestosterone (DHT). On the other hand, dutasteride is a synthetic 4-azasteroid that acts as a competitive inhibitor of the type-1, type-2, and type-3 isoenzymes of 5-α reductase, significantly reducing DHT levels to 6% of normal [81]. In addition to catalyzing the rate-limiting step in the conversion of T into DHT, finasteride also limits the conversion of progesterone and deoxycortisone to dihydroprogesterone and dihydrocortisone, respectively. This process, facilitated by the enzyme 3-α-hydroxysteroid oxidoreductase (3αHSOR), leads to the formation of neurosteroids like tetrahydroprogesterone and isopregnanolone. These neurosteroids enhance GABAergic transmission, exerting anticonvulsant, antidepressant, and anxiolytic effects. Changes in the levels of these neurosteroids have been suggested as a possible reason for depression, anxiety, mood disturbances, and suicidal thoughts in patients using finasteride [82].

While the efficacy of the drugs has never been questioned, finasteride has been linked to impaired spermatogenesis and poor motility, which reverses after cessation of the drug, in a limited number of studies [83]. However, some studies conclude that the use of finasteride does not increase the risk of sexual dysfunction compared to placebo [84–87]. There are some explanations for these conflicting data, such as the nocebo effect, poor body image associated with AGA, and psychological comorbidities associated with AGA, such as depression and sexual dysfunction [88–90].

Several psychiatric side effects have been attributed to finasteride: depression, anxiety, panic attacks, insomnia and fatigue through a reduction in levels of neurosteroids, which also may be the cause for sexual side effects. Recently, studies have also shown that individuals with a preexisting history of psychiatric illness or neurotic personality traits are at a higher risk of developing these side effects, thereby also underlining the importance of screening [91].

These symptoms have caused much debate and have been given the controversial name of the post-finasteride syndrome, although the criteria for the same are ill-defined. The relation to sexual selection, hormones and hair has already been alluded to. This plays out in the way finasteride is perceived. These side-effects and the aggressive propaganda against the drug have made drug authorities in several countries issue advisories cautioning against the use of finasteride and advocating informing patients about the risks [92].

Topical minoxidil, as 2% and 5% formulations, is the only other medication to receive FDA approval for AGA treatment and is the only topical medication with this approval. Minoxidil solution is as such a prodrug. The enzyme sulfotransferases convert it into its active form minoxidil sulphate in the outer root sheath [93].

Minoxidil sulfation varies among individuals. Individuals with higher enzyme activity have better results compared to individuals with lower enzyme activity. Minoxidil causes prolongation of the latent period of the hair cycle while moving to the G1 phase of the cell cycle, opens the potassium channels, thus opposing the effect of calcium-mediated EGF-induced inhibition of the hair follicle, and also causes vasodilation by inhibition of phosphodiesterase.

While minoxidil is relatively safe and side effects are minor, these side effects are common enough to affect compliance with the drug [94]. Recently, low-dose oral minoxidil has been reported to be effective. While its efficacy is not in doubt, its safety profile, which can include potentially serious cardiovascular side effects, remains a question mark.

Regenerative medicine, particularly the role of stem cells, has become a focal point of study across various medical disciplines. Unsurprisingly, this approach has also been explored in hair loss treatment, considering the limitations of traditional medical management options. The conventional methods of obtaining stem cells were complex multi-stage procedures, often involving cultivation, making them costly. However, recent advances in the field have sparked increased interest. Simplified techniques for isolating regenerative elements and stem cells have evolved, facilitating easy outpatient procedures with immediate injection. These procedures are typically single sessions involving harvest with minimal manipulation, usually of a physical nature. This not only reduces costs but also eliminates regulatory concerns associated with the use of stem cells [95]. The simplicity and effectiveness of these techniques, along with the rise of social media, have contributed to heightened awareness and publicity. As a result, there has been a growing demand from patients, leading to the clinical use of these approaches and, in some cases, premature commercial exploitation.

The management of alopecia involves modifications to two types of stem cells: hair follicle stem cells (HFSCs) and dermal papilla cells (DPCs). In scarring alopecia, there is irreversible loss of these stem cells. However, in androgenetic alopecia (AGA) and other non-scarring alopecias, these cells are preserved until the late stages, allowing for potential reversal [96, 97]. In the balding scalp, the number of hair follicle stem cells (HFSCs) remains intact, but the number of actively proliferating CD34 and CD200-positive progenitor cells decreases significantly. This suggests that the balding scalp may either lack an activator or has an inhibitor of hair follicle growth [98].

HFSCs express markers including CD34, K15, K19, CD200, PHLDA1, EpCAM/Ber-EP4, while DPCs express alkaline phosphatase, alphaSMA, laminin, fibronectin, and CD133 [99, 100]. These markers can be modified in disease states, with CK15 and CD34 being lower, especially in the frontal scalp in AGA. Stem cells in the bulge of the hair follicle remain in the resting phase for the majority of their lives and are influenced by the mesenchymal cells of the dermal papilla. They play a key role in transmitting signals for hair growth. Early techniques of stem cell treatment for AGA involve isolating these stem cells, culturing them, and then reinjecting them. The main sources for stem cells include the bone marrow, adipose tissue, scalp tissue, blood, and other tissues such as Wharton's jelly.

Based on physiological considerations, there appears to be a reasonable hypothesis for the use of adipocyte-derived stem cells (ADSCs) for androgenetic alopecia (AGA). The technique involves a simple and safe outpatient procedure and is well-established in various other medical indications. Different methods of harvesting and using adipose-derived cells, such as autologous whole fat, a stromal vascular fraction (SVF), and nano fat, have been described and tested in various types of alopecias, including traumatic scars, alopecia areata, scarring alopecias like scleroderma, and AGA [101–109].

However, it's important to note that most studies on this topic have had small sample sizes, variable control groups, different durations, methodologies, and outcome measures. Currently, no large controlled studies exist, and the level of evidence is considered low. Therefore, while adipose tissue (AT) and ADSCs may represent a potential therapy for hair regeneration, the modality cannot be recommended as a routine option for the management of AGA at this stage. Further research with robust study designs is needed to establish the efficacy and safety of this approach in treating hair loss.

Follicle-derived stem cells have shown promise in stimulating hair regrowth. Ruiz et al. developed a novel method to isolate human adult stem cells by mechanically centrifuging punch biopsies from human hair follicles. Using the Rigenera® technology, scalp biopsy samples were mechanically disaggregated to obtain an extract [110]. This extract was then directly infiltrated into patients' scalps, resulting in increased hair density and hair count during a two-month follow-up period [111, 112]. However, it's important to note that there are only two published studies on this topic, and it is too premature to make any recommendations based on this limited data.

Platelet-rich plasma (PRP) treatment has gained popularity as a treatment option for hair loss, particularly androgenetic alopecia (AGA), in both men and women. PRP is autologous plasma with a platelet concentration 2–7 times higher than the baseline after centrifugation [112–114]. The activation of platelet α-granules releases more than 20 different growth factors and cytokines, promoting cell proliferation and differentiation [115, 116]. These include platelet-derived growth factor (PDGF), insulin-like growth factor-1 (IGF-1), transforming growth factor (TGF), endothelial growth factor (EGF), basic fibroblast growth factor (bFGF), granulocyte-macrophage colony-stimulating factor (GM-CSF), and hepatocyte growth factor (HGF).

However, it's important to recognize that the actions of different growth factors can be conflicting in various situations, requiring careful interpretation. Published data on the use of platelet-rich plasma (PRP) in androgenetic alopecia (AGA) has been expanding over the years, with several studies reporting varying results in terms of improvement in hair count, hair diameter, and patient satisfaction [117, 118]. A critical analysis of these studies reveals a significant issue: the lack of standardization and wide variability in every aspect of PRP preparation, administration, and assessment of results. Variations exist in blood volume, type of spin, duration of spin, assessment criteria, type of kit and activator used, frequency, duration, and follow-up period. Despite PRP being available for nearly 5 years in the field of hair loss and even earlier in other specialties, the debate about its role in management has persisted. It's noteworthy that European guidelines for AGA classified the evidence available as Level 3 (Studies grade B evidence or studies with mainly consistent results grade C evidence), stating that efficacy to improve or prevent hair loss is doubtful. The guidelines concluded, "There is no standardized technique for performing PRP to permit objective evaluation of its effects on AGA. We cannot make a recommendation for or against treatment of AGA with platelet-rich plasma at the present time" [119]. The impact of PRP treatment on the quality of life of patients should be further investigated, and high-quality controlled studies are needed to accurately predict its long-term efficacy.

The origins of modern hair transplantation as we know it today can be traced back to the early twentieth century. The New York dermatologist Norman Orentreich is heralded as the father of modern hair transplantation due to his pioneering work in the 1950s [120].

Hair transplantation, as much else in hair loss management, suffered from a checkered history with forgotten discoveries that are rediscovered decades later. All the major advances in hair transplantation, such as the use of small punches, adoption of follicular unit transplantation, extraction technique, and use of body hair, suffered from delay in application for years and decades after their initial discovery. After decades of Orentreich's 4 mm punch grafting technique affecting a generation of patients with a doll look and the resulting disrepute, single strip dissection and microscopic dissection led to the concept of 'Follicular Unit Transplantation' and mega sessions by Bernstein and Rassman in 1995 [121]. After a spate of initial advancements such as trichophytic closure, video microscopic dissection, the technique came to be questioned by patients as aggressive harvesting lead to unacceptably wide donor scars. Patients demanded not just a natural looking aesthetic result in the recipient area, but also a similar outcome in the donor!

This led to the return of the prodigal—the ubiquitous punch but in its minimal form. The technique had a delightfully simple concept: Release the hold of the arrectores with a very small punch so that the unit will just pop up. The Follicular Unit Extraction (FUE) technique is credited to Bernstein and Rassman for their paper in 2002 [122]. This technique of FUE shows that the technique of Hair Transplantation has come full circle in a sense, back to the days of individual graft harvest (albeit micrografts instead of punches). The outcome for the donor was very pleasant, with downtime reduced to a day. The technique saw several advances in motorization and in the types of punches. Principles of physics, such as torque and speed, were applied and studied to enhance both safety, accuracy and extraction speed. The final outcome of this technique was the discovery of a robotic machine for extraction. Now the technique has become the primary method of donor harvesting worldwide.

However, one fundamental problem remained—using a small area of donor hair in the occipital scalp to cover a much larger recipient site. This seemingly imbalanced equation underscores the possibilities and limitations of this procedure. The discovery of recipient influence by Tommy Hwang in a series of interesting hair transplants using hairs from different areas of his own body showed body hair could grow longer and thicker [123]. FUE provided an apt technique to extract body hair. These discoveries have made it possible to give satisfactory results to almost every patient with any extent of baldness.

So now hair transplantation has become simple, safe and effective. FUE technique revolutionized the approach to surgery by removing the fear of surgery from the minds of the patients. But here was the real danger: It removed fear from the minds of everyone, with the result that every caregiver thought this was a simple surgery and could be done by anyone anywhere. Hence, we have seen quackery resulting in its fullest and most abusive form: crass commercialism, exaggeration and hype, and many unethical practices. As part of medical tourism, HT soon grew to be an industry, particularly in certain places such as Turkey. ISHRS and other societies such as AHRS has, therefore, had to initiate campaigns such as FIGHT THE FIGHT, SAY NO TO BLACK MARKETING AND SAY NO TO GHOST SURGERY. We had the unedifying news of deaths from hair transplantation. This has led to the formulation of guidelines and calls for regulations to tackle quackery. However, in the absence of significant medical advancements in recent types, hair transplantation remains a popular option for most patients.

In conclusion, the field of hair loss and androgenetic alopecia is pregnant with possibilities, particularly in the application of regenerative treatments. Amidst all this cacophony of different treatments, one more advance has caught the attention—the possibility of printing hairs—by 3D printing. While the introduction of synthetic hairs in the late 1970s ended in a disastrous ban by the FDA, 3D printing offers yet another hope to meet the endless and limitless demand for hairs. Whether it meets the hope or will only flatter to deceive remains to be seen.

References

1. Weitz R. Rapunzel's daughters: what women's hair tells us about women's lives. New York: Farrar, Straus and Giroux; 2004.
2. Gan DC, Sinclair RD. Prevalence of male and female pattern hair loss in Maryborough. J Investig Dermatol Symp Proc. 2005;10:184–9.
3. DeMuro-Mercon C, Rhodes T, Girman CJ, Vatten L. Male-pattern hair loss in Norwegian men: a community-based study. Dermatology. 2000;200:219–22.

4. Norwood OT. Male pattern baldness: classification and incidence. South Med J. 1975;68:1359–65.
5. Severi G, Sinclair R, Hopper JL, et al. Androgenetic alopecia in men aged 40-69 years: prevalence and risk factors. Br J Dermatol. 2003;149:1207–13.
6. Bakry OA, Moneim Shoeib MA, El Shafiee MK, Hassan A. Androgenetic alopecia, metabolic syndrome, and insulin resistance: is there any association? A case–control study. Indian Dermatol Online J. 2014;5:276–81.
7. González-González JG, Mancillas-Adame LG, Fernández-Reyes M, et al. Androgenetic alopecia and insulin resistance in young men. Clin Endocrinol (Oxf). 2009;71:494–9.
8. Mumcuoglu C, Ekmekci TR, Ucak S. The investigation of insulin resistance and metabolic syndrome in male patients with early-onset androgenetic alopecia. Eur J Dermatol. 2011;21:79–82.
9. Cannarella R, Condorelli RA, Mongioì LM, La Vignera S, Calogero AE. Does a male polycystic ovarian syndrome equivalent exist? J Endocrinol Invest. 2018;41:49–57.
10. Hunt N, McHale S. Clinical review: the psychological impact of alopecia. Br Med J. 2005;331:951–3.
11. Hunt N, McHale S. Reported experiences of persons with alopecia areata. J Loss Trauma. 2005;10:33–50.
12. Hunt N, McHale S. Understanding alopecia. London: Sheldon; 2004.
13. Practice census results, International Society of Hair Restoration Surgery, Relevant Research, Inc., Chicago; 2017.
14. do Amaral LQ. Loss of body hair, bipedality and thermoregulation. Comments on recent papers in the Journal of Human Evolution. J Hum Evol. 1996;30:357–66.
15. Darwin C. The descent of man, and selection in relation to sex. London: John Murray; 1871.
16. Wyatt TD. Pheromones and animal behaviour: communication by smell and taste. Cambridge: Cambridge University Press; 2003.
17. Tabolli S, Sampogna F, di Pietro C, Mannooranparampil TJ, Ribuffo M, Albeni D. Health status, coping strategies, and alexithymia in subjects with androgenetic alopecia. A questionnaire study. Am J Clin Dermatol. 2013;14:139–45.
18. Cotton SG, Nixon JM, Carpenter RG, Evans DW. Factors discriminating men with coronary heart disease from healthy controls. Br Heart J. 1972;34:458–64.
19. Herrera CR, D'Agostino RB, Gerstman BB, Bosco LA, Belanger AJ. Baldness and coronary heart disease rates in men from the Framingham study. Am J Epidemiol. 1995;142:828–33.
20. Ford ES, Freedman DS, Byers T. Baldness and ischemic heart disease in a national sample of men. Am J Epidemiol. 1996;143:651–7.
21. Lesko SM, Rosenberg L, Shapiro S. A case-control study of baldness in relation to myocardial infarction in men. JAMA. 1993;269:998–1003.
22. Schnohr P, Lange P, Nyboe J, Appleyard M, Jensen G. Gray hair, baldness, and wrinkles in relation to myocardial infarction: the Copenhagen City heart study. Am Heart J. 1995;130:1003–10.
23. Agac MT, Bektas H, Korkmaz L, Cetin M, Erkan H, Gurbak I, Hatem E, Celik S. Androgenetic alopecia is associated with increased arterial stiffness in asymptomatic young adults. Eur Acad Dermatol Venereol. 2015;29:26–30.
24. Ahouansou S, Le Toumelin P, Crickx B, Descamps V. Association of androgenetic alopecia and hypertension. Eur J Dermatol. 2007;17:220–2.
25. Oh BR, Kim SJ, Moon JD, Kim HN, Kwon DD, Won YH, Ryu SB, Park YI. Association of benign prostatic hyperplasia with male pattern baldness. Urology. 1998;51:744–8.
26. Arias-Santiago S, Arrabal-Polo MA, Buendia-Eisman A, Arrabal-Martin M, Gutierrez-Salmeron MT, Giron-Prieto MS, Jimenez-Pacheco A, Calonje JE, Naranjo-Sintes R, Zuluaga-Gomez A, Serrano OS. Androgenetic alopecia as an early marker of benign prostatic hyperplasia. J Am Acad Dermatol. 2012;66:401–8.
27. Chen W, Yang CC, Chen GY, Wu MC, Sheu HM, Tzai TS. Patients with a large prostate show a higher prevalence of androgenetic alopecia. Arch Dermatol Res. 2004;296:245–9.

28. Dastheib L, Shirazi M, Moezzi I, Deghan S, Sadati M. Is there a relationship between androgenic alopecia and benign prostatic hyperplasia? Acta Med Iran. 2015;53:30–2.
29. Hawk E, Breslow RA, Graubard BI. Male pattern baldness and clinical prostate cancer in the epidemiologic follow-up of the first National Health and Nutrition Examination Survey. Cancer Epidemiol Biomarkers Prev. 2000;9:523–7.
30. Muller DC, Giles GG, Sinclair R, Hopper JL, English DR, Severi G. Age-dependent associations between androgenetic alopecia and prostate cancer risk. Cancer Epidemiol Biomarkers Prev. 2013;22:209–15.
31. Setty LR. Hair patterns of scalp of white and Negro males. Am J Phys Anthropol. 1970;33:49–55.
32. Denmark-Wahnefried W, Schildkraut JM, Thompson D, Lesko SM, McIntyre L, Schwingl P, Paulson DF, Robertson CN, Anderson EE, Walther PJ. Early onset baldness and prostate cancer risk. Cancer Epidemiol Biomarkers Prev. 2000;9:325–8.
33. Ellis JA, Sinclair R, Harrap SB. Androgenetic alopecia: pathogenesis and potential for therapy. Expert Rev Mol Med. 2002;4:1–11.
34. Ellis JA, Harrap SB. The genetics of androgenetic alopecia. Clin Dermatol. 2001;19:149–54.
35. Kuster W, Happle R. The inheritance of common baldness: two B or not two B? J Am Acad Dermatol. 1984;11:921–6.
36. Ellis JA, Stebbing M, Harrap SB. Genetic analysis of male pattern baldness and the 5alpha-reductase genes. J Invest Dermatol. 1998;110:849–53.
37. Brockschmidt FF, Heilmann S, Ellis JA, Eigelshoven S, Hanneken S, Herold C, Moebus S, Alblas MA, Lippke B, Kluck N, Priebe L, Degenhardt FA, Jamra RA, Meesters C, Jockel KH, Erbel R, Harrap S, Schumacher J, Frohlich H, Kruse R, Hillmer AM, Becker T, Nothen MM. Susceptibility variants on chromosome 7p21.1 suggest HDAC9 as a new candidate gene for male-pattern baldness. Br J Dermatol. 2011;165:1293–302.
38. Olsen EA. Female pattern hair loss: clinical features and potential hormonal factors. J Am Acad Dermatol. 2001;45:S70–80.
39. Kligman AM. The human hair cycle. J Invest Dermatol. 1959;33:307–16.
40. Schweikert HU, Wilson JD. Regulation of human hair growth by steroid hormones. II. Androstenedione metabolism in isolated hairs. J Clin Endocrinol Metab. 1974;39:1012–9.
41. Randall VA, Thornton MJ, Hamada K, Messenger AG. Androgen action in cultured dermal papilla cells from human hair follicles. Skin Pharmacol. 1994;7:20–6.
42. Kaufman KD. Androgen metabolism as it affects hair growth in androgenetic alopecia. Dermatol Clin. 1996;14:697–711.
43. Itami S, Kurata S, Sonoda T, Takayasu S. Characterization of 5 alpha-reductase in cultured human dermal papilla cells from beard and occipital scalp hair. J Invest Dermatol. 1991;96:57–60.
44. Chen W, Thiboutot D, Zouboulis CC. Cutaneous androgen metabolism: basic research and clinical perspectives. J Invest Dermatol. 2002;119:992–1007.
45. Bayne EK, Flanagan J, Einstein M, Ayala J, Chang B, Azzolina B, Whiting DA, Mumford RA, Thiboutot D, Singer II, Harris G. Immunohistochemical localization of types 1 and 2 5alpha-reductase in human scalp. Br J Dermatol. 1999;141:481–91.
46. Hoffmann R, Happle R. Current understanding of androgenetic alopecia. Part I: etiopathogenesis. Eur J Dermatol. 2000;10:319–27.
47. Sinclair R, Torkamani N, Jones L. Androgenetic alopecia: new insights into the pathogenesis and mechanism of hair loss [version 1; referees: 4 approved]. F1000Res. 2015;4(F1000 Faculty Rev):585.
48. Jahoda CA, Horne KA, Oliver RF. Induction of hair growth by implantation of cultured dermal papilla cells. Nature. 1984;311:560–2.
49. Jahoda CA, Reynolds AJ. Dermal-epidermal interactions. Adult follicle-derived cell populations and hair growth. Dermatol Clin. 1996;14:573–83.
50. Obana NJ, Uno H. Dermal papilla cells in macaque alopecia trigger a testosterone-dependent inhibition of follicular cell proliferation. In: van Neste D, Randall VA, editors. Hair research in the next millenium. Amsterdam: Elsevier; 1996. p. 307–10.

51. Randall VA. The use of dermal papilla cells in studies of normal and abnormal hair follicle biology. Dermatol Clin. 1996;14:585–94.
52. Van Scott EJ, Ekel TM. Geometric relationships between the matrix of the hair bulb and its dermal papilla in normal and alopecic scalp. J Invest Dermatol. 1958;31:281–7.
53. Elliott K, Stephenson TJ, Messenger AG. Differences in hair follicle dermal papilla volume are due to extracellular matrix volume and cell number: implications for the control of hair follicle size and androgen responses. J Invest Dermatol. 1999;113:873–7.
54. Jahoda CA. Cellular and developmental aspects of androgenetic alopecia. Exp Dermatol. 1998;7:235–48.
55. Sinclair R. Male pattern androgenetic alopecia. Br Med J. 1998;317:865–9.
56. Prieto VG, Sadick NS, Shea CR. Androgenetic alopecia: analysis of proliferation and apoptosis. Arch Dermatol. 2002;138:1101–2.
57. Ohyama M, Vogel JC, Amagai M. Gene ontology analysis of human hair follicle bulge molecular signature. J Dermatol Sci. 2007;45:147–50.
58. Fujiwara H, Ferreira M, Donati G, Marciano DK, Linton JM, Sato Y, et al. The basement membrane of hair follicle stem cells is a muscle cell niche. Cell. 2011;144:577–89.
59. Zargham R, Touyz RM, Thibault G. Alpha 8 integrin overexpression in de-differentiated vascular smooth muscle cells attenuates migratory activity and restores the characteristics of the differentiated phenotype. Atherosclerosis. 2007;195:303–12.
60. Sun TT, Cotsarelis G, Lavker RM. Hair follicular stem cells: the bulge-activation hypothesis. J Invest Dermatol. 1991;96:77S–8S.
61. Uezumi A, Fukada S, Yamamoto N, Takeda S, Tsuchida K. Mesenchymal progenitors distinct from satellite cells contribute to ectopic fat cell formation in skeletal muscle. Nat Cell Biol. 2010;12:143–52.
62. Lowell S, Jones P, Le Roux I, Dunne J, Watt FM. Stimulation of human epidermal differentiation by delta-notch signalling at the boundaries of stem-cell clusters. Curr Biol. 2000;10:491–500.
63. Yamamoto S, Kato R. Hair growth-stimulating effects of cyclosporin A and FK506, potent immunosuppressants. J Dermatol Sci. 1994;7 Suppl:S47–54.
64. Maurer M, Handjiski B, Paus R. Hair growth modulation by topical immunophilin ligands: induction of anagen, inhibition of massive catagen development, and relative protection from chemotherapy-induced alopecia. Am J Pathol. 1997;150:1433–41.
65. Johnstone MA, Albert DM. Prostaglandin-induced hair growth. Surv Ophthalmol. 2002;47(Suppl 1):S185–202.
66. Ali A, Martin JM 4th. Hair growth in patients with alopecia areata totalis after treatment with simvastatin and ezetimibe. J Drugs Dermatol. 2010;9:62–4.
67. Ramelet AA. Minoxidil induces selective regrowth of androgenetic dependent hair. Dermatologica. 1986;173:301–2.
68. Foitzik K, Spexard T, Nakamura M, Halsner U, Paus R. Towards dissecting the pathogenesis of retinoid-induced hair loss: all-trans retinoic acid induces premature hair follicle regression (catagen) by upregulation of transforming growth factor-beta2 in the dermal papilla. J Invest Dermatol. 2005;124:1119–26.
69. Ohnemus U, Unalan M, Handjiski B, Paus R. Topical estrogen accelerates hair regrowth in mice after chemotherapy-induced alopecia by favoring the dystrophic catagen response pathway to damage. J Invest Dermatol. 2004;122:7–13.
70. Oura H, Iino M, Nakazawa Y, et al. Adenosine increases anagen hair growth and thick hairs in Japanese women with female pattern hair loss: a pilot, double-blind, randomized, placebo-controlled trial. J Dermatol. 2008;35:763–7.
71. Paus R, Schilli MB, Handjiski B, Menrad A, Henz BM, et al. Topical calcitriol enhances normal hair regrowth but does not prevent chemotherapy-induced alopecia in mice. Cancer Res. 1996;56:4438–43.
72. Bodó E, van Beek N, Naumann V, Ohnemus U, Brzoska T, et al. Modulation of chemotherapy-induced human hair follicle damage by 17-beta estradiol and prednisolone: potential stim-

ulators of normal hair regrowth by "dystrophic catagen" promotion? J Invest Dermatol. 2009;129:506–9.
73. Park H, Kim CW, Kim SS, Park CW. The therapeutic effect and the changed serum zinc level after zinc supplementation in alopecia areata patients who had a low serum zinc level. Ann Dermatol. 2009;21:142–6.
74. Rosenberg EW, Skinner RB Jr. Immunotherapy of alopecia areata with intralesional Candida antigen. Pediatr Dermatol. 2006;23:299.
75. Garcia Bartels N, Lee HH, Worm M, Burmester GR, Sterry W, et al. Development of alopecia areata universalis in a patient receiving adalimumab. Arch Dermatol. 2006;142:1654–5.
76. Pelivani N, Hassan AS, Braathen LR, Hunger RE, Yawalkar N. Alopecia areata universalis elicited during treatment with adalimumab. Dermatology. 2008;216:320–3.
77. Ettefagh L, Nedorost S, Mirmirani P. Alopecia areata in a patient using infliximab: new insights into the role of tumor necrosis factor on human hair follicles. Arch Dermatol. 2004;140:1012.
78. Posten W, Swan J. Recurrence of alopecia areata in a patient receiving etanercept injections. Arch Dermatol. 2005;141:759–60.
79. Amor KT, Rashid RM, Mirmirani P. Does D matter? The role of vitamin D in hair disorders and hair follicle cycling. Dermatol Online J. 2010;16:3.
80. Yoshida R, Tanaka K, Amagai M, Ohyama M. Involvement of the bulge region with decreased expression of hair follicle stem cell markers in senile female cases of alopecia areata. J Eur Acad Dermatol Venereol. 2011;25:1346–50.
81. Olsen EA, Hordinsky M, Whiting D, Stough D, Hobbs S, Ellis ML, Wilson T, Rittmaster RS, Dutasteride Alopecia Research Team. The importance of dual 5alpha-reductase inhibition in the treatment of male pattern hair loss: results of a randomized placebo-controlled study of dutasteride versus finasteride. J Am Acad Dermatol. 2006;55(6):1014–23.
82. Finn DA, Beadles-Bohling AS, Beckley EH, Ford MM, Gililland KR, Gorin-Meyer RE, et al. A new look at the 5alpha-reductase inhibitor finasteride. CNS Drug Rev. 2006;12(1):53–76.
83. Amory JK, Wang C, Swerdloff RS, Anawalt BD, Matsumoto AM, Bremner WJ, et al. The effect of 5alpha-reductase inhibition with dutasteride and finasteride on semen parameters and serum hormones in healthy men. J Clin Endocrinol Metab. 2007;92(5):1659–65.
84. Clark RV, Hermann DJ, Cunningham GR, Wilson TH, Morrill BB, Hobbs S. Marked suppression of dihydrotestosterone in men with benign prostatic hyperplasia by dutasteride, a dual 5alpha-reductase inhibitor. J Clin Endocrinol Metab. 2004;89(5):2179–84.
85. Erdemir F, Harbin A, Hellstrom WJ. 5-alpha reductase inhibitors and erectile dysfunction: the connection. J Sex Med. 2008;5(12):2917–24.
86. Hagberg KW, Divan HA, Persson R, Nickel JC, Jick SS. Risk of erectile dysfunction associated with use of 5-α reductase inhibitors for benign prostatic hyperplasia or alopecia: population based studies using the clinical practice research datalink. BMJ. 2016;354:i4823.
87. Haber RS, Gupta AK, Epstein E, Carviel JL, Foley KA. Finasteride for androgenetic alopecia is not associated with sexual dysfunction: a survey-based, single-center, controlled study. J Eur Acad Dermatol Venereol. 2019;33(7):1393–7.
88. Mondaini N, Gontero P, Giubilei G, Lombardi G, Cai T, Gavazzi A, et al. Finasteride 5 mg and sexual side effects: how many of these are related to a nocebo phenomenon? J Sex Med. 2007;4:1708–12.
89. Cash TF. The psychosocial consequences of androgenetic alopecia: a review of the research literature. Br J Dermatol. 1999;141(3):398–405.
90. Samplaski MK, Lo K, Grober E, Jarvi K. Finasteride use in the male infertility population: effects on semen and hormone parameters. Fertil Steril. 2013;100(6):1542–6.
91. Ganzer CA, Jacobs AR. Emotional consequences of finasteride: fool's gold. Am J Mens Health. 2018;12(1):90–5.
92. Mysore V, Shashikumar BM. Guidelines on the use of finasteride in androgenetic alopecia. Indian J Dermatol Venereol Leprol. 2016;82(2):128–34.
93. Goren A, Mccoy J, Kovacevic M, Situm M, Chitalia J, Dhurat R. The effect of topical minoxidil treatment on follicular sulfotransferase enzymatic activity. J Biol Regul Homeost Agents. 2018;32(4):937–40.

94. Rundegren J. A one-year observational study with minoxidil 5% solution in Germany: results of independent efficacy evaluation by physicians and patients. J Am Acad Dermatol. 2004;50(3):91.
95. Coelho MB, Cabral JM, Karp JM. Intraoperative stem cell therapy. Annu Rev Biomed Eng. 2012;14:325–49.
96. Ohyama M, Terunuma A, Tock CL, Radonovich MF, Pise-Masison CA, Hopping SB, Brady JN, Udey MC, Vogel JC. Characterization and isolation of stem cell-enriched human hair follicle bulge cells. J Clin Invest. 2006;116:249–60.
97. Mohammadi P, Youssef KK, Abbasalizadeh S, Baharvand H, Aghdami N. Human hair reconstruction: close, but yet so far. Stem Cells Dev. 2016;25:1767–79.
98. Garza LA, Yang CC, Zhao T, et al. Bald scalp in men with androgenetic alopecia retains hair follicle stem cells but lacks CD200-rich and CD34-positive hair follicle progenitor cells. J Clin Invest. 2011;121:613–22.
99. Purba TS, Haslam IS, Poblet E, Jiménez F, Gandarillas A, Izeta A, Paus R. Human epithelial hair follicle stem cells and their progeny: current state of knowledge, the widening gap in translational research and future challenges. Bioessays. 2014;36:513–25.
100. Inoue K, Aoi N, Sato T, Yamauchi Y, Suga H, Eto H, Kato H, Araki J, Yoshimura K. Differential expression of stem-cell-associated markers in human hair follicle epithelial cells. Lab Invest. 2009;89:844–56.
101. Banyard DA, Sarantopoulos CN, Borovikova AA, et al. Phenotypic analysis of stromal vascular fraction after mechanical shear reveals stress-induced progenitor populations. Plast Reconstr Surg. 2016;138:237e–47e.
102. Oberbauer E, Steffenhagen C, Wurzer C, et al. Enzymatic and nonenzymatic isolation systems for adipose tissue-derived cells: current state of the art. Cell Regen. 2015;4:7.
103. van Dongen JA, Stevens HP, Harmsen MC, et al. Mechanical micronization of lipoaspirates: squeeze and emulsification techniques. Plast Reconstr Surg. 2017;139:1369e–70e.
104. Nilforoushzadeh MA, Lotfi E, Heidari-Kharaji M, Torkamaniha E, Hanifnia AR. Autologous whole fat injection stimulates hair growth in resistant androgenetic.
105. Tedesco M. Adipose tissue transplant in recurrent folliculitis decalvans. Int J Immunopathol Pharmacol. 2018;32:1–4.
106. Dini M, Mori A, Quattrini LA. Eyebrow regrowth in patient with atrophic scarring alopecia treated with an autologous fat graft. Dermatol Surg. 2014;40:926–8.
107. Zanzottera F, Lavezzari E, Trovato L, Icardi A, Graziano A. Adipose derived stem cells and growth factors applied on hair transplantation follow-up of clinical outcome. J Cosmet Dermatol Sci Appl. 2014;4:268–74.
108. Lee YI, Kim J, Kim J, Park S, Lee JH. The effect of conditioned media from human adipocyte-derived mesenchymal stem cells on androgenetic alopecia after nonablative fractional laser treatment. Dermatol Surg. 2020;46:1698–704.
109. Narita K, Fukuoka H, Sekiyama T, Suga H, Harii K. Sequential scalp assessment in hair regeneration therapy using an adipose-derived stem cell-conditioned medium. Dermatol Surg. 2020;46:819–25.
110. Ruiz RG, Rosell JMC, Ceccarelli G, De Sio C, De Angelis GC, Pinto H, Astarita C, Graziano A. Progenitor-cell-enriched micrografts as a novel option for the management of androgenetic alopecia. J Cell Physiol. 2019;235:4587–93.
111. Gentile P, Scioli MG, Bielli A, Orlandi A, Cervelli V. Stem cells from human hair follicles: first mechanical isolation for immediate autologous clinical use in androgenetic alopecia and hair loss. Stem Cell Investig. 2017;4:58.
112. Wu PI, Diaz R, Borg-Stein J. Platelet-rich plasma. Phys Med Rehabil Clin N Am. 2016;27(4):825–53.
113. Stevens J, Khetarpal S. Platelet-rich plasma for androgenetic alopecia: a review of the literature and proposed treatment protocol. Int J Womens Dermatol. 2018;5(1):46–51.
114. Marx RE. Platelet-rich plasma (PRP): what is PRP and what is not PRP? Implant Dent. 2001;10(4):225–8.

115. Amable PR, Carias RB, Teixeira MV, da Cruz PI, Corrêa do Amaral RJ, Granjeiro JM, Borojevic R. Platelet-rich plasma preparation for regenerative medicine: optimization and quantification of cytokines and growth factors. Stem Cell Res Ther. 2013;4(3):67.
116. Trink A, Sorbellini E, Bezzola P, et al. A randomized, double-blind, placebo- and active-controlled, half-head study to evaluate the effects of platelet-rich plasma on alopecia areata. Br J Dermatol. 2013;169(3):690–4.
117. Almohanna HM, Ahmed AA, Griggs JW, Tosti A. Platelet-rich plasma in the treatment of alopecia Areata: a review. J Investig Dermatol Symp Proc. 2020;20(1):S45–9.
118. Kahn RA, Cossette I, Friedman LI. Optimum centrifugation conditions for the preparation of platelet and plasma products. Transfusion. 1976;16(2):162–5.
119. Kanti V, Messenger A, Dobos G, Reygagne P, Finner A, Blumeyer A, Trakatelli M, Tosti A, Del Marmol V, Piraccini BM, Nast A, Blume-Peytavi U. Evidence-based (S3) guideline for the treatment of androgenetic alopecia in women and in men—short version. J Eur Acad Dermatol Venereol. 2018;32:11–22.
120. Orentreich N. Autografts in alopecias and other selected dermatological conditions. Ann N Y Acad Sci. 1959;83:463–79.
121. Bernstein RM, Rassman WR, Szaniawski W, Halperin A. Follicular transplantation. Int J Aesthet Restorative Surg. 1995;3:119–32.
122. Rassman WR, Bernstein RM, McClellan R, Jones R, Worton E, Uyttendaele H. Follicular unit extraction: minimally invasive surgery for hair transplantation. Dermatol Surg. 2002;28(8):720–8.
123. Hwang ST, Kim HY, Lee SJ, Lee WJ, Kim DW, Kim JC. Recipient-site influence in hair transplantation: a confirmative study. Dermatol Surg. 2009;35(6):1011–4.

Functional, Aesthetic, and Procedural Significance of the Nail Unit

7

Eckart Haneke

The nail is a cutaneous appendage poorly understood by many physicians and even some dermatologists. However, recent basic and clinical research has broadened our knowledge of this important, though often underestimated, part of our body. In-depth knowledge of the nail's biology, development, anatomy, and pathology is essential to manage ungual alterations.

This short essay is not meant to substitute a textbook on nails nor to be an update; it is intended to give some ideas about a few common nail conditions and problems related to nails.

The nail is the hardest and least abundant skin appendage [1, 2]. Because of its intimate functional relationship to the underlying bone, the distal interphalangeal joint, its capsule, ligaments, aponeuroses, and tendons, it is also called a musculoskeletal appendage [3].

The nail develops from gestation weeks 7–8 onwards, with the fingernails first, then the toenails, in parallel with the later embryonal development of the toes compared to the fingers. For nail development, virtually all growth factors and signaling proteins known for hair development are necessary, but correct nail development requires the anlage of the distal phalanx bone to be formed first; in the condition called atelephalangia where the distal digital bone is absent, no nail is formed as the nail unit-inducing factors are also lacking [4]. Further, signaling proteins for anterior-posterior orientation must act in a timely manner; otherwise, the nail may remain at the tip of the digital pulp and not move to its dorsal aspect. Probably the same factors differentially expressed in folliculogenesis to ensure that each hair

E. Haneke (✉)
Dermatology Practice Dermaticum, Freiburg, Germany

Department of Dermatology, Inselspital, University of Bern, Bern, Switzerland

Centro de Dermatología Epidermis, Insituto CUF, Matosinhos, Porto, Portugal

Department of Dermatology, University of Ghent, Ghent, Belgium

S. Gupta et al. (eds.), *Critical Thinking in Contemporary Dermatology: Cognitive Essays*, https://doi.org/10.1007/978-981-97-0411-8_7

follicle has its characteristic angle are also responsible for the fact that the nail lies flat, i.e., grows out and not up [5].

Nail development starts with the formation of a cellular densification at the tip of the digit called the placode. Under the influence of β-catenin, this placode proliferates to a peg, which then gets an orientation to grow proximally so that first a nail field is seen, from which all components of the nail organ develop. Its most proximal portion grows under the skin of the dorsal distal digit, forming the matrix and the nail pocket. From here, the nail plate, which usually reaches the tip of the digital pulp at the term of birth, is formed.

The primate nail developed from the claw. The shape of the bone of the distal phalanx is the decisive factor. In claw formation, the distal phalanx is conical; in the flat primate nail, its tip is wider, making the nail more than a tool for defense and attack but allowing it to pick up fine and soft objects without piercing them. The nail also enhances the sensory function of the fingertip and improves the grip.

The nail plate consists of keratins, which are fibrous sulfur-rich proteins embedded in an amorphous ground substance even richer in sulfur. Hair and nail proteins are highly similar in their physico-chemical composition; this has many clinical implications. Mutations in keratins present in hair and nails may have similar clinical effects, with thin fragile hair being analogous to thin and soft nails. However, as the hair grows about 10 times faster than nails, any real deficiency of amino acids, sulfur, zinc, various vitamins, and many more substances is usually seen on hair first before the nails are visibly affected. Like hair, nail keratin is birefringent, and polarization microscopy can give valuable information on the nail keratin and its fibrillar structure. Nail keratin, in contrast to hair, readily takes up water, making the nail softer and allowing it to be trimmed without major mechanical trauma. Immersing the digit tips in water for 5–10 min also makes the nails softer and facilitates certain types of nail surgery [6].

Correct nail formation is also associated with the cellular immune system. In the human analog of the nu-nu mouse, which is characterized by thymus aplasia, FOXN1 family signal proteins are mutated, and the nails are extremely soft and white [7].

The nail serves many purposes, with the protection of the dorsal aspect of the distal finger phalanx and support of the toe pulp during gait probably being the most important biological functions in the human being. Further, as a hard keratin plate, the nail is a powerful weapon for attack and defense, although not to the same degree as in big felines or bears. The nail plate gives counterpressure to the fingertips and thus enhances the sensory palpatory function of the finger pulp. For the toes, particularly the big toes, a sufficiently long nail slightly overlapping the toe tip is indispensable to avoid the soft tissue of the pulp becoming dislocated dorsally, forming a wrong distal bulge, which in turn impedes the outgrowth of the short nail or correct regrowth of the great toenail. However, the distal bulge formation is also often seen when the thumbnail is too short after avulsion, too short trimming of the nail, and onychophagia. This gives strong evidence of the forces the finger and toe tips have to withstand in daily life. Further, the nail is an exceedingly versatile tool for many everyday activities [8]. Individuals with no thumbnails have great difficulty buttoning a shirt, and the nails are critical to picking up fine objects from a plane surface [9].

The aesthetic importance of the nails cannot be overestimated. Nail adornment dates back to 5000 BC when nails were stained with henna in India, Egypt, and China [10]. More than 5000 years ago, rich Chinese would adorn their fingertips with golden thimbles. Having clean and well-groomed nails is a must for a cultivated appearance. Further, nail cosmetics are used more and more frequently, and the money spent on nail lacquers, hardeners, artificial nails, nail care products, and food additives hoped to improve nail quality is beyond US$ 20 billion annually. In addition, billions are spent on nail salons. The problem is that nail stylists, manicurists, beauticians, and other people involved in nail care are often not trained, as the designation of manicurist/pedicurist is not protected. Whereas most nail care products are not harmful, many procedures such as cuticle removal with high-concentration potassium hydroxide, cleaning the nail with sharp instruments, application of long gel nails which exert a lever action on the free edge of the nail and thus further worsen the tendency to onycholysis with consequent microbial colonization and infection, removal of gel nails with abrading devices that are very harmful to the nail, ultraviolet cure of cyanoacrylate nails with the theoretical potential of carcinoma induction, hazards of infection with atypical mycobacteria in nail salons, etc. are the real risks. Allergies, however, are surprisingly infrequent considering the number of daily nail varnish applications worldwide [11]. Most reactions are primary irritant contact dermatitides. Allergy to toluene sulphonamide-formaldehyde resin may occur, and then buffing is a valuable alternative to nail varnish. Some nail file kits specifically use the dust from filing the nail margin as a buffing and polishing powder to get a marvelous nail sheen. Nail beauty and function cannot be divided. A healthy nail is usually beautiful and can exert its full functions.

Hair and nails are often called siblings or even twins; however, this is certainly not true as they have different functions, macro- and micro-anatomy, and physiology. In contrast to hair, nails grow continuously and life-long with no cyclical growth; they are not hormone-dependent; thus, there is no equivalent to androgenetic alopecia in nails; they do not grey but rather tend to become more pigmented with age in dark-skinned individuals [12]. Alopecia areata often affects the nails but does not cause nail shedding [13].

Toenail changes are often associated with orthopedic abnormalities that are already evident at birth or in early infancy. The parents usually consult a pediatrician who is rarely knowledgeable about nails and often tells them to wait for puberty; however, puberty is no magical event to cure nails and associated orthopedic problems [14]. Newborns may present with lateral deviation of the big toenail, sometimes with an upward-growing nail or even a congenital pincer nail. Radiographs usually show an asymmetric epiphysis of the distal phalanx in case of a hallux valgus interphalangeus, of the proximal phalanx in case of hallux valgus, in the latter condition also an oblique plane of the joint between the os cuneiforme I—os metatarsale I with a medial deviation of the first metatarsal bone. X-rays taken in congenital malalignment of the great toenail almost invariably show a hallux valgus interphalangeus with an asymmetric cuneiform epiphysis of the distal phalanx. The treatment of nail abnormalities in newborns and infants is difficult as it is often simple: correction of the hallux valgus and hallux valgus interphalangeus is effective with taping: an adhesive tape is applied around the great toe commencing at its lateral side in the first webspace, leading over the tip and pulling it forcefully to the medial aspect of the toe and foot till about the mid-foot. As bone grows more rapidly when there is constant pull and is slowly reduced on continuous pressure, the asymmetric epiphysis and distal phalanx asymmetry can be corrected; this is the same principle used for orthodontic correction of malpositioned teeth [14].

Another relatively frequent though less known anomaly is the double little toenail [15]. It is apparently autosomal dominant and occurs in males, females, and all races. It can already be seen in newborns but is rarely noted in children because it remains asymptomatic until the patient develops an outward rotation of the little toe; then it causes pain similar to a Lister's corn [16]. Good radiographs exhibit a tiny lateral bone spike of the tip of the distal phalanx that apparently induces an extra rudimentary nail anlage. Treatment consists of segmental excision of the accessory nail matrix [17].

Although onychomycoses are commonly held to be the most common nail diseases a careful examination of the feet often reveals that there are very frequently orthopedic abnormalities: flat and splay foot, hallux valgus, hallux valgus interphalangeus, hallux erectus, and pincer nails with widening of the base of the distal phalanx, which often lead to onycholysis and nail bed hyperkeratosis that are confused with fungal infection in many cases. This complex condition is called the asymmetric gait (toe)nail unit syndrome (AGNUS) [18]. Another problem is determining whether the nails' non-dermatophyte mold infections exist [19]. It is even postulated that AGNUS is the most common toenail condition in the world [20]. The niche under the onycholytic nail with hyperkeratosis of the nailbed causes alterations clinically identical to distal-lateral subungual onychomycosis; however, it is primarily fungus-free and may secondarily be colonized by environmental molds that are not able to actively invade corneocytes [21]. Non-dermatophyte molds, though unable to directly digest keratin, may invade the nail plate by using the intercellular cement substance to cause a real infection [22]. Further, some fungi have acid proteases that are able to split up keratin. Histopathology of *Fusarium* onychomycoses definitely shows fungal elements in the nail plate [23]; however, their exact localization whether between or within the onychocytes cannot definitely be defined by light microscopy. The treatment of onychomycoses has become more complex and difficult in recent years as some dermatophytes have developed resistance and non-dermatophyte molds have low sensitivity to common antifungals [24]. Recently, compounded amphotericin B was proposed for the treatment of mold nail infections [25].

Procedural onychology comprises virtually all treatments of nails beyond drugs, starting with grooming the nails for cosmetic reasons and reaching from simple to highly advanced nail surgery. Grooming includes cleansing and all cosmetic measures described in detail in many articles and chapters [26].

Nail surgery is a classical example of procedural nail therapy. It is still not widely performed by dermatologists and dermatosurgeons although they are the ones that ought to do it as they are the only medical specialists with in-depth knowledge of the nail organ. In principle, nail surgery is not difficult though sometimes delicate. Surgical skills, atraumatic surgery and instruments, and an intimate knowledge of the anatomy, physiology, biology, and growth characteristics as well as basic pathology are necessary for a good result. A dermatosurgeon who knows how the nail grows, where the various nail alterations come from, and what might happen post-operatively does not need to be afraid of performing a surgical intervention on the nail organ [8]. Unfortunately, the intervention most frequently performed on nails is their avulsion. This is very often done "just in order to do something" because the surgeon cannot make a diagnosis or is otherwise helpless.

The prerequisite of any nail procedure is good and long-lasting anesthesia. The first-choice anesthetic is ropivacaine, which has a rapid onset like lidocaine and a long action like bupivacaine, which outweighs its slightly higher price.

Nail avulsion is rarely a treatment per se, except severe retronychia [27]. Otherwise, it is the most severe iatrogenic nail trauma that can be done to the patient and often makes the nail susceptible to infection and post-avulsion nail dystrophy [28].

Ingrown toenails are very frequent. They occur in all age groups with different clinical characteristics [29]. Neonatal and infantile ingrown nails are not treated surgically. In neonates, the distal and sometimes distal-lateral nail fold is gently moved away from the nail margin by cautious massage of the hypertrophic nail wall in a warm bath. In infants, the cause of ingrowing may be a so-called hypertrophic lip, i.e., a hyperplastic medial, rarely lateral, nail fold that lies on the nail and forms a deep fold in which debris of keratin and foreign substances may accumulate and degrade and thus cause inflammation. If the hypertrophic lip cannot be successfully corrected by massage it is easily removed with the electric loop. Another cause of infantile ingrown nails is congenital malalignment [30]. This complex anomaly should usually be treated according to the underlying orthopedic abnormality. We have seen considerable improvement by correcting the malpositioned metatarsal and toe bones with consistent taping [14]. Surgery consists of dissecting the entire nail unit from the underlying terminal phalanx bone, rotating it into an orthograde position, and suturing it back. The results are best—though still not really satisfying in many cases—when this surgery is done before the age of 2 years [31].

The most common type of ingrown toenail is seen in school children, adolescents, and young adults. Usually the distal-lateral or distal-medial or both sides of the nail pierce into the depth of the distal portion of the nail sulcus. There is almost always an over-curvature of the nail; ungues incarnati are extremely rarely observed in flat nails! There are many claims as to the etiology and pathogenesis of this condition, but in the end, there is a disbalance between too wide a nail and too narrow the (distal) nail bed. Hyperhidrosis, being overweight, wrong nail clipping, and many more factors may aggravate or precipitate an ingrown nail. This is a painful condition interfering with daily activities and sports at an age when the children are physically most active. Treatment is taking the offending nail margin away from the injured soft tissue, either by conservative means or surgery [29]. Non-invasive therapy requires high patient compliance and is very effective in Japanese patients. There are many different modalities: Packing of cotton between the offending nail edge and the soft tissue, pulling the nail fold away from the nail by consistent taping, protecting the nail sulcus by inserting a gutter over the lateral nail margin or thickening it by building an artificial nail that would not cut into the soft tissue; these methods may be combined to enhance their efficacy [32, 33]. However, it has to be stressed that the result of treatment cannot be better than its execution!

When conservative therapy is not an option for whatever reason surgery is indicated. There are two fundamentally different approaches that are even reflected by the different terminologies of ingrown nails and onychocryptosis. If you believe the nail is too wide, it should be narrowed by selective lateral matrix horn removal, either by surgical extirpation or by chemocautery with liquefied phenol, 10–20% sodium hydroxide or 85–100% trichloroacetic acid; healing time and success rates are comparable [34]. If you assume that the primary event is a hypertrophy of the nail folds, their reduction or removal would be logical. This may be done by excision of a fusiform wedge of soft tissue from the lateral aspect of the distal phalanx to radical extirpation of both lateral nail folds according to Vandenbos or an even bigger resection of the super-U technique [29, 35]. It is imperative to note that as early as 150 years ago, the Swiss surgeon Emmert stressed that either the nail matrix and nail bed or the lateral nail folds should be operated on, not both, as is unfortunately done by most surgeons worldwide with the many different variations of wedge excisions. Unfairly, these wedge excisions that in most cases are wrong from their design and have an unacceptably high recurrence rate of 25% to greater than 70%, are incorrectly named in many countries after Emmert or even after Kocher, his successor on the chair of surgery in Berne, who had never published anything about nails [29].

There are many misconceptions concerning nail melanoma. It is certainly the most serious nail condition. It is still claimed that it is a rare neoplasm, and this would be the reason for its late diagnosis, insufficient treatment, and poor prognosis. However, this is not true. Nail melanoma makes up about 2% of all melanomas in light-skinned Caucasians. The surface of all nails taken together is much less than 1% of the body surface. Most ungual melanomas arise from the matrix, which is about one-quarter of the nail field, and within the matrix, the apical portion is most commonly the site of origin of nail melanomas in contrast to benign functional and lentigo- or nevus-associated melanonychia. Thus, the nail matrix is rather a hotspot of melanoma development, and ungual melanoma is not rare, particularly not when considering the high percentage of ungual melanomas in dark-skinned individuals in whom cutaneous melanomas are rare or even exceptional [36]. However, this makes the proportion of ungual melanomas in relation to all melanomas in dark-skinned individuals much higher, although it is roughly equal in absolute numbers. Nail melanoma is not a particularly aggressive form of melanoma, as many have a history of many years or even decades before being correctly diagnosed and treated. It is not really challenging to make the diagnosis as two-thirds to three-quarters of nail melanomas are pigmented and arise in the matrix causing longitudinal melanonychia. If this develops in a person over 30 years, it is suspicious and requires an exact diagnosis. The nature of the pigment is easy to determine. Melanin is in the nail plate and thus reaches into the free margin of the nail, which is virtually never the case with blood; exogenous pigment can be scraped off the surface of the nail plate, and blood never forms as regular a longitudinal band as melanin. A nail clipping stained with Fontana's argentaffin reaction shows finely granular pigment in the nail plate cells. Blood is seen as clumps and lakes of a brown to reddish-brown substance under the nail by dermatoscopy, completely different from melanin. Neither the color's width nor intensity is proof of, or rules out, nail melanoma [37]. Melanoma treatment is primarily surgical. For decades, amputation was the treatment dogma. As many publications evidence, the prognosis was very poor and is still poor. It was shown that the extent of amputation had no influence on the cure rates, it was the time of treatment: early treatment by complete local excision guarantees the best therapeutic results and long-term prognosis [36, 38, 39]. Amputation was shown to have no survival benefit and is evidently associated with a poorer quality of life. The surgery is performed under digital block anesthesia; we recommend 0.5–1% ropivacaine as the anesthetic of choice as it has a long action. The excision margins are generally 5 mm around the anatomical borders of the nail unit; however, as so-called field cells were demonstrated in the epidermis up to 9 mm around acral melanoma [40], we recommend a 10 mm safety margin in the case of Hutchinson's sign. The crucial point is the nail unit's total extirpation, including the lateral matrix horns, which often extend far distal and volar; from here, recurrences may develop. They can be re-excised without worsening the patient's prognosis. The wound may be left for second-intention healing, repaired with a free full-thickness skin graft, or with various flaps [41].

In contrast to just 40–50 years ago, many nail conditions can nowadays be treated with drugs or surgery. Understanding the nail as a special organ is the essential point.

References

1. Heller J. Die Krankheiten der Nägel. Berlin: Hirschwald; 1900.
2. Pinkus F. Anatomie des Nagels. In: Jadassohn J, editor. Handbuch der Haut- und Geschlechtskrankheiten, vol. I/1. Berlin: Springer; 1927.
3. McGonagle D, Tan AL, Benjamin M. The nail as a musculo-skeletal appendage—implications for an improved understanding of the link between psoriasis and arthritis. Dermatology. 2009;218:97–102.
4. Cooks RG, Hertz M, Katznelson MB, Goodman RM. A new nail dysplasia syndrome with anonychia and absence and/or hypoplasia of distal phalanges. Clin Genet. 1985;27:85–91.
5. Haneke E. Histopathology of the nail. Boca Raton: CRC Press; 2017.
6. Richert B, Di Chiacchio N, Haneke E. Nail surgery. New York: Informa Healthcare; 2011.
7. Pignata C, Fusco A, Amorosi S. Human clinical phenotype associated with FOXN1 mutations. Adv Exp Med Biol. 2009;665:196–206.
8. Saito M, Ohyama M, Amagai M. Exploring the biology of the nail: an intriguing but less-investigated skin appendage. J Dermatol Sci. 2015;79:187–93.
9. Padda I. What are the functions of nails? Queios ID: HMT8LH. https://doi.org/10.32388/HMT8LH.

10. Shafer L. Nail care: from ancient times to new heights. nailsmag.com/392664.
11. Goossens A, Beck M, Haneke E, McFadden JP, Nolting S. Cutaneous reactions to cosmetic products, a retrospective survey in 5 European dermatological centres. Contact Derm. 1999;40:112–3.
12. Baran R, Dawber RP, Haneke E. Hair and nail relationship. Skinmed. 2005;4:18–23.
13. Haneke E. Chapter 91. Nail disorders. In: Kang et al., editors. Fitzpatrick's dermatology, 9th ed. 2020.
14. Haneke E. Toenails: where orthopedics and onychology meet. In: Baran R, editor. Advances in nail disease and management. Springer Nature Switzerland. 2021. pp. 71–85.
15. Hundeiker M. Hereditäre Nageldysplasie der 5. Zehe [Hereditary nail dysplasia of the 5th toe]. Hautarzt. 1969;20:281–282.
16. Haneke E. Double nail of the little toe. Skin Appendage Disord. 2016;1:163–7.
17. Haneke E. Therapie von Nagelfehlbildungen. In: Landthaler M, Hohenleutner U, editors. Fortschritte der operativen Dermatologie, vol. 12. Berlin: Blackwell Wissenschafts-Verlag; 1997. p. 180–7.
18. Zaias N, Rebell G, Casal G, Appel J. The asymmetric gait toenail unit sign. Skinmed. 2012;10:213–7.
19. Zaias N, Escovar SX, Rebell G. Opportunistic toenail onychomycosis. The fungal colonization of an available nail unit space by non-dermatophytes is produced by the trauma of the closed shoe by an asymmetric gait or another trauma. A plausible theory. J Eur Acad Dermatol Venereol. 2014;28:1002–6.
20. Zaias N, Rebell G, Escovar S. Asymmetric gait nail unit syndrome: the most common worldwide toenail abnormality and onychomycosis. Skinmed. 2014;12:217–23.
21. Zaias N, Escovar SX, Zaiac MN, et al. Onychomycosis, the active invasion of a normal nail unit by a dermatophytic versus the colonization of an existing abnormal nail unit by environmental fungus. Skinmed. 2020;18:18–22.
22. Summerbell RC. Epidemiology and ecology of onychomycosis. Dermatology. 1997;194(Suppl 1):32–6.
23. Rammlmair A, Mühlethaler K, Haneke E. Fusarium onychomycoses in Switzerland—a mycological and histopathological study. Mycoses. 2019;62:928–31.
24. Gupta AK, Summerbell RC, Venkataraman M, Quinlan EM. Nondermatophyte mould onychomycosis. J Eur Acad Dermatol Venereol. 2021;35:1628–41.
25. Monod M, Lurati M, Baudraz-Rosselet F. Diagnostic des onychomycoses à moisissures et importance pour le traitement. Rev Med Suisse. 2013;9(380):730–3.
26. Richert B, Scheers C, André J. Nail care, nail modification techniques and camouflage strategies. In: André P, Haneke E, Marini L, Rowland Payne C, editors. Cosmetic medicine & surgery. Boca Raton: CRC Press; 2016. p. 139–53.
27. Baumgartner M, Haneke E. Retronychia: diagnosis and treatment. Dermatol Surg. 2010;36:1610–3.
28. Haneke E. Nail surgery: indications and outcome. Expert Rev Dermatol. 2006;1:93–104.
29. Haneke E. Controversies in the treatment of ingrown nails. Dermatol Res Pract. 2012;2012:783924. https://doi.org/10.1155/2012/783924.
30. Baran R, Haneke E. Etiology and treatment of nail malalignment. Dermatol Surg. 1998;24:719–21.
31. Haneke E. Pathogenese-orientierte Behandlung eingewachsener Zehennägel und des angeborenen Nagelschiefstandes bei Kindern. In: Burg G, Hartmann AA, Konz B, editors. Fortschritte der operativen Dermatologie 7: Onkologische Dermatologie, neue Aspekte, altersbedingte Besonderheiten. Springer: Berlin; 1992. p. 243–5.
32. Arai H, Arai T, Nakajima H, Haneke E. Formable acrylic treatment for ingrowing nail with gutter splint and sculptured nail. Int J Dermatol. 2004;43:759–65.
33. Arai H, Arai T, Haneke E. Simple and effective non-invasive treatment methods for ingrown and pincer nail including acrylic affixed gutter splint, anchor taping, sculptured nails, shape memory alloy nail clip and plastic nail braces as well as 40% urea paste. J Kochi Med Ass. 2011;16:37–56.

34. André MS, Caucanas M, André J, Richert B. Treatment of ingrowing toenails with phenol 88% or trichloroacetic acid 100%: a comparative, prospective, randomized, double-blind study. Dermatol Surg. 2018;44:645–50.
35. Thakur V, Vinay K, Haneke E. Onychocryptosis—decrypting the controversies. Int J Dermatol. 2020;59:656–69.
36. Haneke E. Ungual melanoma—controversies in diagnosis and treatment. Dermatol Ther. 2012;25:510–24.
37. Haneke E. Eleven myths on nail melanoma. EMJ Dermatol. 2021;9(1):83–6.
38. Haneke E, Binder D. Subunguales Melanom mit streifiger Nagelpigmentierung [Subungual melanoma with streaky nail pigmentation]. Hautarzt. 1978;29:389–391.
39. Moehrle M, Metzger S, Schippert W, Garbe C, Rassner G, Breuninger H. "Functional" surgery in subungual melanoma. Dermatol Surg. 2003;29:366–74.
40. North JP, Kageshita T, Pinkel D, LeBoit PE, Bastian BC. Distribution and significance of occult intraepidermal tumor cells surrounding primary melanoma. J Invest Dermatol. 2008;128:2024–30.
41. Haneke E. Advanced nail surgery. J Cutan Aesthet Surg. 2011;4:167–75.

Dermatoscopy: What Does It Add?

8

Deepak Jakhar and Ishmeet Kaur

8.1 Introduction

A dermatoscope is an optical device that uses visible light (polarizing and non-polarizing) to inspect suspicious skin lesions. Currently, dermatoscopes are either available as handheld devices (used individually or connected to a camera) or videodermatoscopes [1]. Dermatoscope for a dermatologist is like a stethoscope for a physician. Dermatoscopy (epiluminescence microscopy) is a noninvasive modality (using a dermatoscope) that enables the visualization of submacroscopic structures invisible to the naked eye. It acts as a link between naked-eye examination and histopathology. Though initially utilized only for pigmented melanocytic lesions, dermatoscopy has now become an essential tool to assist dermatologists in diagnosing and prognosis various skin, hair, nail, and mucosal disorders. This chapter allows us to elaborate on various aspects of dermatoscopy and its applications in everyday clinical practice (diagnosis, biopsy site selection, prognosis, and procedural dermatology). We have focused on studies with high evidence; however, weaker evidence with significant future potential has also been mentioned. Since 'dermatoscopy' and 'dermoscopy' are both accepted terminologies, we have used them interchangeably.

D. Jakhar (✉)
Dermosphere Clinic, New Delhi, India

I. Kaur
Department of Dermatology, NDMC Medical College and Hindu Rao Hospital, New Delhi, India

S. Gupta et al. (eds.), *Critical Thinking in Contemporary Dermatology: Cognitive Essays*, https://doi.org/10.1007/978-981-97-0411-8_8

8.2 Evolving Dermatoscopes

The popularity of dermatoscopy can partially be attributed to the advancement in the dermatoscope. Better designs, ease of handling, improved illuminations, and magnification has increased its acceptability amongst dermatologists. Dermoscopes come in two main types: handheld dermatoscopes and video-dermatoscopes. The handheld dermatoscope typically offers a magnification range of 10×–20×, while video-dermatoscopes have a broader range of 10×–220×, and some newer models may exceed this magnification. Optical resolution is generally quite good for handheld dermatoscopes, whereas video-dermatoscopes vary in resolution, with higher-cost versions matching the quality of handheld devices. Both types of dermatoscopes offer polarized and non-polarized modes. Handheld dermatoscopes are usually contact devices, but some newer models allow for non-contact use with a disposable faceplate. Video-dermatoscopes, on the other hand, are typically non-contact and use a sterilizable spacer to maintain a distance between the lens and the skin, enabling a rim of material to come into contact with the skin. When it comes to sharing and teaching, handheld dermatoscopes have limitations, as images can only be seen by the operator, and capturing images is relatively cumbersome. In contrast, video-dermatoscopes display images on a screen (laptop/desktop/phone), facilitating live viewing by multiple people, including the patient. Furthermore, these images can be easily shared, printed, or stored. Handheld dermatoscopes come with a rechargeable battery lasting 0.5–8 hours. Video-dermatoscopes usually require a direct cord connection to a laptop, but newer models feature rechargeable batteries with Bluetooth connectivity to phones or laptops. Accessories required are different as well: handheld dermatoscopes may have magnetic connectors for smartphones and digital cameras to ease image capture, while video-dermatoscopes typically require no additional accessories apart from the device being used with them to view the image. In terms of compatibility, handheld dermatoscopes are primarily compatible with smartphones, while video-dermatoscopes can connect to laptops, desktops, and smartphones. Older video-dermatoscope models may need a USB port or converter for connection. Regarding ease of use and specific dermatoscopic evaluations, handheld dermatoscopes excel in pigment evaluation, perform well in vascular evaluation, and are also suitable for trichoscopy, while video-dermatoscopes are superior in vascular evaluation, and they excel in onychoscopy, nail-fold capillaroscopy, trichoscopy, entomo-dermoscopy, oculoscopy, hidroscopy, and can be used over mucous membranes. Additionally, the latter offer the advantage of being non-contact, making certain vascular evaluations easier [1].

Any dermatoscope has the following basic parts: lighting or illumination system, magnification, and power supply [2]. Lighting system usually consists of light-emitting diode (LED) lights. The initial dermatoscopes used to have non-polarized light, which limited their ability to scope sub-surface structures. In most incidents, non-polarized light is reflected from the skin's surface. The use of immersion fluids aided the non-polarizing dermatoscopes to some extent, but the breakthrough came with incorporating polarized light in the devices [3]. Similarly, contact dermatoscopes have evolved into non-contact dermatoscopes due to better visualization of vascular structures and decreased chances of nosocomial infection spreading with the latter [1]. Another important development in the device is the incorporation of WiFi. This enables the device to connect with multiple devices simultaneously and may be better suited for teaching and discussion amongst dermatology residents [4].

8.3 Technique

Before starting dermatoscopy, cleaning the skin surface or using alcohol-containing immersion fluid as an interface medium is always advisable. Dermatoscopy is performed using either contact or non-contact techniques. In contact dermatoscopy, the glass plate of the dermatoscope comes in direct contact with the skin lesion. On the other hand, in non-contact dermatoscopy, only the rim of the contact faceplate meets the skin. This reduces the chances of cross-infection and avoids blanching of the vasculature [5]. Both polarized and non-polarized light dermoscopy should be done while evaluating the skin lesion as they complement each other. Non-polarized dermoscopy provides details about surface changes (Like scales, comedo-like openings, etc.), while polarizing dermatoscopy provides details about sub-surface changes (like pigmentary changes, vascular changes, etc.). After doing dermatoscopy at 10× magnification, if the device allows, a higher magnification (50–200×) should also be performed for a detailed evaluation of features.

8.4 Clinical Evaluation with Dermoscopy

Dermatoscope should be considered and used as an essential part of clinical evaluation. It shouldn't be considered a second-level examination tool restricted to selected cases. Even when the diagnosis is confirmed on clinical examination, dermoscopy can be used to support the diagnosis. There are concerns that dermoscopy use in routine clinical practice is time-consuming; however, in experienced hands, it only adds a little time to the whole process of examination [6]. It is important to understand that dermoscopy should be viewed as an integral part of patient management, and information provided by dermoscopy should be correlated with the patient's history, inspection, or palpation.

In vivo direct skin microscopy was first applied to detect cutaneous filariae [7]. Leon Goldman later also provided the first description of clinically invisible morphologic structures of skin tumors with skin microscopy [8]. Later, Rona Mackie described microscopic features of nevi, melanoma, angioma, and basal cell carcinoma [9]. Some of the most popular and accepted dermoscopic methods, like the ABCD rule of dermoscopy, the 7-point checklist, and the Menzies method, came into light between 1994 and 1998 [10–12]. Initial literature was primarily focused on the use of dermoscopy for the evaluation of melanocytic skin tumors (mainly nevi and melanoma) [13]. With time, dermatologists started describing the dermoscopic features of several non-melanocytic pigmented and non-pigmented tumors [14, 15]. Reports about its utility in the assessment of infectious and inflammatory dermatoses are more recent [16–23].

8.5 Melanocytic Tumors

Dermoscopy of pigmented skin lesions follows a two-step procedure [24]. The first step is to distinguish melanocytic tumors from nonmelanocytic ones based on several defined dermoscopic features: pigment network (reticular pattern), globules (globular pattern), streaks (starburst pattern), homogeneous blue pigmentation (homogeneous pattern), parallel pattern (for acral lesions). Once the melanocytic nature of the tumors is established, the next step is to distinguish nevi from melanoma. This is achieved by following pattern analysis or algorithms such as the ABCD rule (Table 8.1), Menzies' scoring method (Table 8.2), the 7-point and the revised 7-point checklist (Table 8.3), and the 3-point checklist (Table 8.4) [10–12].

The pattern analysis includes the lesional symmetry, the presence of one or more colors, the local features of the lesions, and the global dermoscopic appearance. The global dermoscopic appearance includes reticular (pigment network), globular (multiple globules), homogenous (structureless pigmentation), starburst (peripheral streaks or pseudopods), and multi-component (resulting from the combination of

Table 8.1 ABCD rule of melanoma detection

1. **A**symmetry in 0, 1 and 2 axes, regarding contour, color and structures—*Score 0–2*
2. **B**order abruptly interrupted at the periphery in 0–8 segments—*Score 0–8*
3. Color: Presence of up to 6 colors (white, red, light brown, dark brown, blue-gray, black)—*Score 1–6*
4. Dermoscopic structures: presence of pigment network, dots, globules, streaks, structureless homogeneous areas—*Score 1–5*
Total dermoscopic score (TDS): (A score × 1.3) + (B score × 0.1) + (C score × 0.5) + (D score × 0.5) = TDS
Interpretation of TDS: <4.75 Benign melanocytic lesion, 4.75–5.45 suspicious lesion, >5.45 Melanoma

Table 8.2 Menzies method for melanoma detection

Negative features	Positive features
1. Symmetry of dermoscopic structures	1. Blue-white veil
2. The presence of a single color	2. Multiple brown dots
	3. Pseudopods
	4. Radial streaks
	5. Scar like depigmentation
	6. Peripheral dots/globules
	7. Multiple (5 or 6) colors
	8. Multiple blue-gray dots
	9. Broadened network
Interpretation: Melanoma is diagnosed when both negative features are absent, and 1 or more of the 9 positive features are present	

Table 8.3 7-point checklist algorithm for melanoma detection

Dermoscopic features	Score
Major criteria	
1. Atypical pigment network	2
2. Blue-white veil	2
3. Atypical vascular pattern	2
Minor criteria	
4. Irregular streaks	1
5. Irregular dots and globules	1
6. Irregular blotches	1
7. Regression structures	1
Interpretation: Total score ≥ 3: melanoma, total score < 3: nonmelanoma	

Table 8.4 3-point checklist for suspicious lesions

1. Asymmetry of colors and/ or structures 2. Atypical pigment network 3. Blue-white structures	Excision should be planned if more than one criterion is present

Table 8.5 Dermoscopic features suggestive of melanoma

Atypical pigment network	Brown-black network with irregular meshes and irregularly distributed lines of different thicknesses (high specificity for the diagnosis of melanoma)
Irregular dots and/or globules	Brown-black or gray dots and globules of different sizes, irregularly distributed within the lesion
Irregular blotches	Black, brown, or gray areas with irregular shape and/or distribution
Irregular steaks and pseudopods	Radial lines irregularly distributed at the periphery of the lesion (streaks), sometimes with a bulbous projection at their peripheral ending (pseudopods)
Regressional structures	White scarlike areas corresponding to fibrosis or blue-gray areas (peppering) corresponding to melanophages
Blue-white veil	Blue-gray or blue-white, diffuse, irregular pigmentation
Irregular vascular structures	Polymorphous vessels, the coexistence of dotted, linear, or hairpin vessels in the same lesion

more than two of the above patterns). The presence of a multi-component pattern is directly suggestive of melanoma. On dermoscopy, nevi generally shows symmetry of structures and displays one or two colors. Melanoma-specific dermoscopic features are summarized in Table 8.5. The location of lesions may influence the dermoscopic features, like facial lesions may show a pseudo reticular network (because of the appendageal openings) [25]. Similarly, lesions of palms and soles show specific dermoscopic features (Table 8.6). It is to be remembered that dermoscopy for melanocytic lesions is still an adjunctive tool, and histopathology remains the gold standard for all suspicious lesions.

Table 8.6 Dermoscopic features of melanocytic lesions on palms and soles

Benign dermoscopic features	Malignant dermoscopic features
• Parallel furrow pattern: pigmentation along the furrows of the skin markings (most common dermoscopic pattern) • Fibrillar pattern: fine fibrillar pigmentation perpendicular to the furrows • Lattice-like pattern: pigmentation along and across the furrows • Homogeneous pattern, Reticular pattern, Globular pattern	• Parallel ridge pattern: pigmentation located on the ridges of the skin markings (acral melanoma in situ or early invasive melanoma) • Multicomponent pattern • Diffuse pigmentation

8.6 Common Benign Nonmelanocytic Tumors

Dermatoscopy has been described for several nonmelanocytic tumors and shows certain pathognomonic features in some of them [26]. Classic dermoscopic features of seborrheic keratosis include comedo-like openings (roundish-to-ovoid, or irregularly shaped, sharply defined structures with brown-yellow to brown-black color corresponding to keratin plugs in dilated follicular openings) and milia-like cysts (round, white-yellow colored structures corresponding to intraepidermal horn globules). Other features include cerebriform appearance (ridges and fissures), fingerprint and fat finger signs, and a "moth-eaten" border [27]. Dermatofibroma may show a range of patterns involving classical dermoscopic features like a white scar-like patch and a fine pigment network [28]. Zaballos et al. described ten different dermoscopic features for dermatofibroma [29]. Vascular tumors like hemangioma show lacunae (red-blue-black, well-circumscribed, round or ovoid structures) and red-blue-black homogenous areas [30]. Homogenous blue appearance is the characteristic dermoscopic feature of a venous lake [31]. Pyogenic granuloma shows red homogeneous areas, the white collaret, "white rail lines" intersecting the lesion, and ulceration [32]. Angiokeratoma shows 3 dermoscopic patterns: dark lacunae and a whitish veil; dark lacunae, whitish veil, and peripheral erythema; dark lacunae, whitish veil, and presence of hemorrhagic crusts [31, 33].

8.7 Common Malignant Nonmelanocytic Tumors

One of the important utilities of dermatoscopy has been in the differentiation of malignant nonmelanocytic lesions from benign lesions. Some of these tumors might show characteristic clinical features, and dermatoscopy has served as a collaborative tool in these cases. Other cases have benefited from biopsy site selection, early prognosis, and treatment initiation. Basal cell carcinoma (BCC) dermoscopy is predominantly based on vascular and pigmentary structures. Dermoscopic features may depend on clinicopathological subtype, location, gender, age, etc. BCC is one of the prototypic skin lesions where dermoscopic features convincingly correlate with histopathological features (Table 8.7) [34–38].

Table 8.7 Common dermatoscopic features of basal cell carcinoma and their histopathology correlation

Dermatoscopic feature	Histopathological correlation
Arborizing vessels	Vessels located on the surface of the tumor (just below the epidermis)
Blue-gray ovoid nests	Large, well-defined tumor nests with pigment aggregates, invading the dermis
Blue-gray dots and globules	Small, roundish tumor nests with central pigmentation, localized to the papillary or reticular dermis
Maple leaf-like areas	Multifocal tumor nests containing pigment aggregates connected to each other by lobular extensions (in the epidermis or upper dermis)
Spoke-wheel areas	Tumor nests arising and connected to the epidermis, characterized by fingerlike projections and centrally located pigmentation
In-focus dots	Melanophages or free pigment deposition in the papillary and reticular dermis
Chrysalis structures or short white streaks	Presence of collagenous stroma and fibrosis in the dermis

The role of regular or sequential dermoscopy is very important in actinic keratosis (AK). The 5-year cumulative probability of developing SCC in patients with multiple AKs is 14%, highlighting the need for regular dermoscopic examination [39]. This is especially important since dermoscopy's diagnostic sensitivity and specificity in the diagnosis of non-pigmented AK reaches 98% and 95%, respectively [40]. Dermoscopic features of AK depend on the grade of AK, signifying that dermatoscopy may not show consistent features even with the same disease. Grade I shows white scales and red pseudo-network, grade II shows the "strawberry" pattern (erythematous background interrupted by white to yellow enlarged follicular openings with or without keratin plugs). In contrast, grade III shows a white-yellow structureless area [15].

Dermatoscopy of Bowen's disease (BD) consists of a red-yellow background color, white-yellow surface scales, and dotted and/or glomerular vessels [41]. The closest differential based on dermatoscopy is psoriasis, which is sometimes very difficult to differentiate. Here comes the role of detailed analysis of dermatoscopy features [42]. The vessels (diameter larger in BD than psoriasis) in BD are usually clustered, while those of psoriasis are regularly distributed [43]. Pigmented BD shows, in addition to vascular structures, brown structureless areas, a mixed pattern of hypopigmented structureless eccentric areas, and small brown/black dots [44]. Dermatoscopy of squamous cell carcinoma depends on the histological differentiation of the tumor. A well-differentiated tumor shows white structureless areas, white halos (surrounding vessels), white circles (surrounding the follicular openings), and white amorphous masses of keratin, out of which white circles represent the most specific feature of SCC [45]. A poorly differentiated tumor shows a predominantly red color, dense vascularity, and the presence of bleeding. The presence of vessels, their distribution and morphology can give valuable clues regarding the differentiation of the tumor [46]. Lesions where vessels cover more than 50% of the lesion surface are more likely to be poorly differentiated [46]. In addition, a small vessel caliber is associated with poor differentiation.

8.8 Pigmentary Dermatoses (Other than Tumors)

Dermatoscopy, in general dermatology, has been described for both hypo- and hyper-pigmentary disorders. Frequently, dermatoscopy of pigmentary disorders is described under the following headings: pigment color/pattern, pigment distribution, surface changes like scaling, vascular morphology and distribution, appendageal features, and other specific features. With these dermatoscopy clues, it is possible to rule out close differentials. Large-scale studies, however, are still lacking in most of these diseases.

Hypopigmentary disorders: The salient dermatoscopic features of various hypopigmentary disorders are described in Table 8.8 [47–55]. Although the level of evidence is still low, dermoscopy can also be used in assessing the disease activity. Certain dermatoscopy features of vitiligo point towards active disease: reduced

Table 8.8 Common dermoscopic features of hypopigmentary disorders

Disease	Dermatoscopic features
Vitiligo	Diffuse white glow; distorted pigment network in the form of absent, broken, or reverse pigment network; perifollicular changes (perifollicular depigmentation, perifollicular re-pigmentation), follicular changes (leukotrichia), micro-Koebnerisation (visible as small areas of depigmentation/hypopigmentation in surrounding areas), starburst appearance, and tapioca sago appearance [47, 48]
Idiopathic guttate hypomelanosis	Loss of pigmentary network, diffuse white glow, margins are described as amoeboid, petaloid, feathery and nebuloid
Lichen sclerosus et atrophicus	Background erythema, follicular keratinous plugs, and linear telangiectatic vessels, linear fibrotic strands, peppering of brown and blue-gray pigment dots and globules
Pityriasis alba	Focal white areas, broken pigmentary network and diffuse fine scaling
Pityriasis versicolor	Faint pigment network, white scales, halo sign
Nevus depigmentosus	White area with faint uniform pigment network and feathery margins
Nevus anemicus	Preserved pigment network, paucity of vessels in the lesional skin
Leprosy	Yellow-orange areas, white chrysalis structures with broken pigmentary network, and loss/diminution of hair follicle and appendages
Progressive macular hypomelanosis	Focal white areas, broken pigmentary network, widened skin lines and focal white scales

Table 8.9 Common dermoscopic features of hyperpigmentary disorders

Disease	Dermatoscopic features
Melasma	Exaggerated pseudo network, brown colored dots and globules, annular and arcuate structures, and telangiectasia
Exogenous ochronosis	Blue-gray pigment globules in arciform or annular patterns, obliterated appendageal openings
Pigment demarcation lines	Exaggerated pseudo network
Acquired dermal maturational hyperpigmentation	Pigment dots, globules, and blotches (in various patterns like dotted pattern, arcuate/Chinese letter pattern, hem-like pattern, reticular pattern, and diffuse)
Nevus of ota	Blue structureless area and scattered brown-grey dots
Acanthosis nigricans	Multiple cristae and sulci, pigment dots & globules
Fixed drug eruption	Pigment dots and globules with various shades

pigment network, peripheral white globules, micro-Koebnerisation, and starburst/feathery pattern [47].

Hyperpigmented disorders: The salient dermatoscopy features of various hyperpigmented disorders are described in Table 8.9 [56–59].

8.9 Inflammatory Dermatoses

For dermoscopy of inflammatory dermatoses, the following parameters are generally evaluated: background color, morphology and arrangement of vascular patterns, scales (color and distribution), follicular abnormalities, and other specific features (clues). While some diseases like psoriasis show consistent features, certain dermatoses like dermatitis and lichen planus might show varied dermatoscopy features based on the site and chronicity of the lesions. Nail involvement in psoriasis can also be differentiated from onychomycosis using dermoscopic features as clues, especially when there is no skin involvement beyond nails and distal onycholysis is the only feature observable by the naked eye [60]. The salient dermatoscopy features for common cutaneous conditions are summarized in Table 8.10 [61–65].

In the context of connective tissue diseases, Nail-fold Capillaroscopy (NFC) in patients with isolated Raynaud's phenomenon has been shown to be effective in identifying patients at-risk for developing scleroderma-spectrum disorders later. A significant prognostic value was found for the presence of giant loops and microhemorrhages [66].

Table 8.10 Salient dermatoscopic features of inflammatory diseases

Diseases	Dermatoscopic feature
Psoriasis	Dotted vessels with regular distribution, white scales
Lichen planus	Wickham striae, peripheral dotted/linear vessels
Dermatitis	Dotted vessels with patchy distribution, yellow crusts/scales
Discoid lupus erythematosus	Early lesions: perifollicular whitish halo, follicular plugging, and white scales Late lesions: telangiectasias, pigmentation structures, and whitish structureless areas
Pityriasis rosea	Yellowish background, peripheral white scales, dotted vessels with patchy distribution
Pityriasis rubra pilaris	Yellowish areas, dotted and linear vessels with patchy or peripheral distribution
Sarcoidosis	Orange-yellowish globules or areas, linear vessels
Granuloma annulare	Dotted, linear, or dotted/linear vessels; white, red, or yellow background
Rosacea	Erythematotelangiectatic type: polygonal vessels Papulopustular type: follicular plugs, follicular pustules, polygonal vessels
Porokeratosis	White-yellowish or brownish peripheral annular structure; in the center, brownish pigmentation, dotted/ linear vessels, or structureless whitish areas
Granuloma faciale	Dilated follicular openings, perifollicular whitish haloes, pigmentation structures, follicular keratotic plugs, elongated or linear branching vessels
Pigmented purpuric dermatosis	Purpuric dots or globules, orange-brown background
Morphea	Whitish fibrotic beams, linear vessels
Urticarial vasculitis	Purpuric dots or globules, orange-brown background
Urticaria	Network of linear vessels surrounding avascular areas
Mycosis fungoides	Short linear vessels, orange-yellowish areas, spermatozoa-like structures
Mastocytosis	Light-brown blot, pigment network, reticular vascular pattern, or yellow-orange blot

8.10 Infectious Diseases

Dermatoscopic features have been described for several parasitic, viral and fungal diseases. The important thing while doing dermatoscopy of infectious diseases is to minimize the risk of cross-infection. Several measures have been proposed to limit the risk of cross-infection [67, 68]. The salient dermatoscopy features are summarized in Table 8.11 [68–72].

Table 8.11 Salient dermatoscopic features of infectious diseases

Disease	Dermatoscopic feature
Scabies	"Jet with contrail" structure
Pediculosis	The lice itself, ovoid brownish structures (nits with vital nymphs), ovoid translucent structures (empty nits)
Molluscum contagiosum	Central pore or umbilication, white to yellow amorphous structures, peripheral linear or branching vessels ("red corona")
Human papilloma virus infection	Common warts: multiple densely packed papillae with a central red dot or loop, surrounded by a whitish halo; hemorrhages (small red to black dots or streaks) may also be present Plantar warts: prominent hemorrhages within a well-defined, yellowish papilliform surface in which skin lines are interrupted Plane warts: regularly distributed red dots, light brown to yellow background Genital warts: mosaic pattern (early/flat lesions), fingerlike and knoblike pattern (raised/ papillomatous lesions), unspecific pattern
Lupus vulgaris	Orange-yellowish globules or areas, linear vessels
Leishmaniasis	Orange-yellowish globules or areas, linear vessels, erythema, follicular plugs, hyperkeratosis, central ulceration

8.11 Nail Disorders

Onychoscopy is dermatoscopic examination of the nail unit and its components, namely, the proximal nail fold, lateral nail fold, hyponychium, nail plate, and bed. The nail matrix can ordinarily be visualized only in larger nails (that too partly) or can be seen intraoperatively. Onychoscopy enables easier and closer observation of nail features not visible to the naked eye. Just as dermoscopy is skin surface microscopy, onychoscopy is surface microscopy of nails (Table 8.12) [73].

Table 8.12 Onychoscopic diagnoses and features with level of evidence (where available) [73]

Disease	Level of evidence	Common signs
Melanonychia	Level-2	• Subungual hemorrhages • Benign melanonychia • Nail pigment origin
Onychomycosis	Level-3	• Jagged proximal edge with spikes of onycholytic edge • Longitudinal striae/Aurora borealis pattern • Ruin pattern
Nail psoriasis	Level-3	Nail pitting, onycholysis, splinter hemorrhages, salmon patch
Nail lichen planus	Level-5	• Nail matrix changes: trachyonychia, pitting, pterygium and red lunula • Nail bed changes: Chromonychia, nail fragmentation, splinter hemorrhages, onycholysis and subungual keratosis • Other features: paronychia, longitudinal streaks and anonychia
Onychomatricoma	Level-5	Longitudinal parallel white bands, parallel lateral edges, splinter hemorrhages, dark dots, nail pitting and thickening of the free edge
Onychopapilloma	Level-5	• Red bands originating from lunula along with splinter hemorrhages • The distal edge has keratotic subungual mass corresponding to streaks
Subungual glomus tumor	Level-5	• Ramified telangiectasiae over a blue background at the site of tumor • Tumor margin can be considered corresponding to the abrupt loss of telangiectasiae at the periphery of the mass • The homogeneous white area of the nail plate and the disappearance of the lunula • Onychoschizia
Digital myxoid cyst	Level-5	• Onychoscopic features depend on the pressure applied to lesion • No pressure: vascular patterns in the form of linear, branched, or serpentine vessels • Pressure: vascular pattern diminishes, and lesion shows translucent bright white areas
Periungual pyogenic granuloma	Level-5	Reddish homogenous area with white rail lines
Periungual warts	Level-5	Multiple red-black dots corresponding to thrombosed vessels in the keratotic lesions
Periungual Bowen's disease	Level-5	Islands of whitish scale and numerous, diffusely distributed red-dotted vessels
Leukonychia	Level-5	White transverse bands in a deep plate with a normal smooth nail plate surface

8.12 Hair and Scalp Disorders

Trichoscopic analysis involves the assessment of the hair shaft, follicular openings, and inter-follicular skin. Table 8.13 summarizes the findings and their associated diseases [74].

Table 8.13 Trichoscopic diagnosis of hair disorders [74]

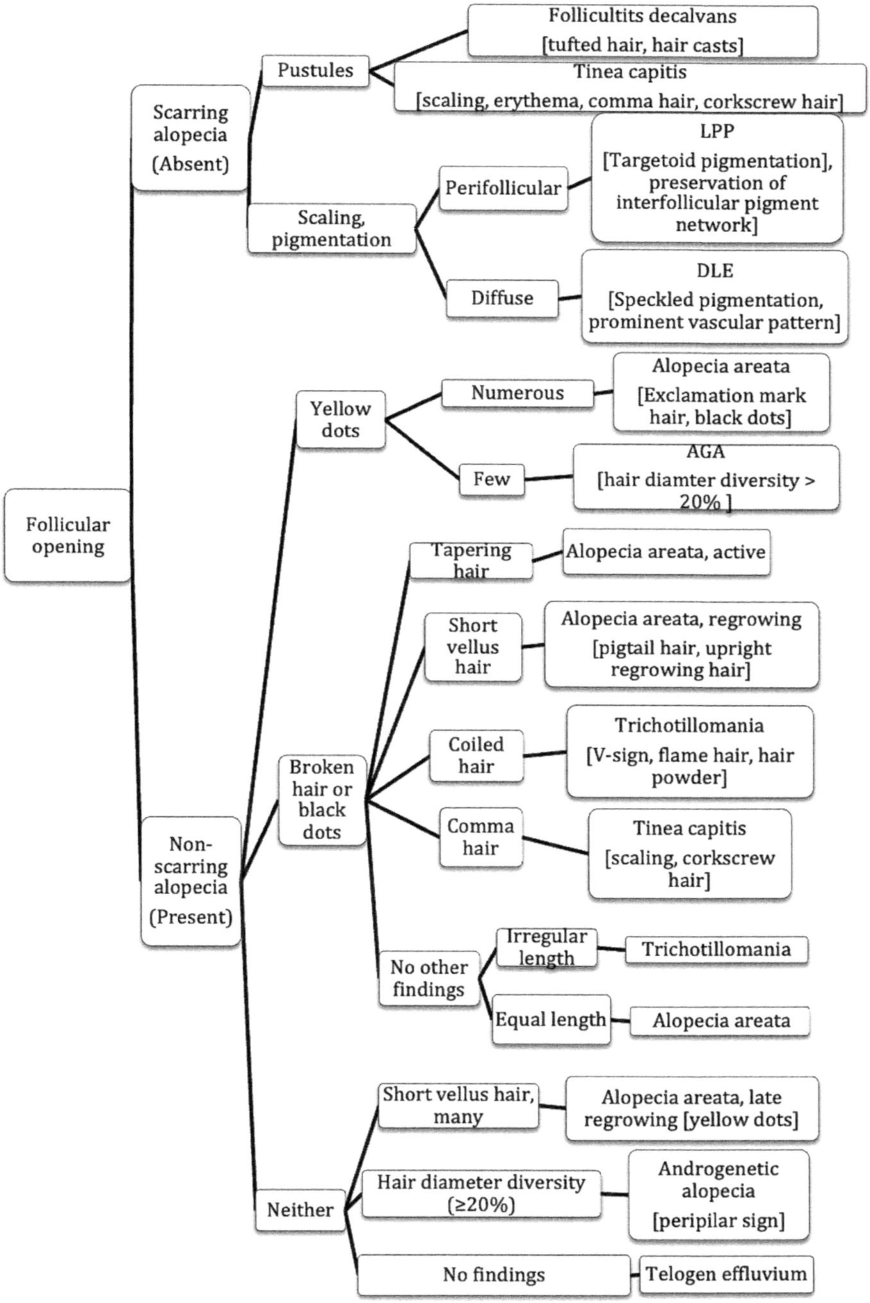

8.13 Dermatoscopy Beyond Diagnosis

The uses of dermoscopy beyond diagnosis include:

(a) Reducing the need for biopsy: In suspected melanoma lesions, dermoscopy was seen to reduce the need for biopsy by 76.5% [75].
(b) Biopsy site selection: Several reports suggest that dermoscopy-guided biopsy of various cutaneous and scalp lesions can improve the outcomes of histopathology reports [76]. For this, all lesions are dermoscopically scanned, and the lesion showing the most specific dermatoscopy feature is selected for biopsy.
(c) Disease activity evaluation: Dermoscopy can be used for the evaluation of disease activity in vitiligo (as described above). Similarly, it has been used for alopecia areata where features like black dots, yellow dots, 'exclamation-mark' hairs, broken hairs, and clustered short vellus hairs are associated with disease activity [77]. Activity in lichen planopilaris and discoid lupus erythematosus of the scalp is also identified and localized using dermoscopy.
(d) Ensuring complete excision of tumor: Dermatoscopy can be used as a tool to ensure complete excision of a tumor. A post-excision dermatoscopy can give valuable clues towards a residual tumor [78].
(e) Intra-operative dermatoscopy: This is a relatively newer application of dermatoscopy where a dermatoscope is used intra-operatively. The advantages include guiding to the most appropriate site for biopsy, confirming the diagnosis, ascertaining tumor margins, and completing surgical excision [79].
(f) Ex-vivo dermatoscopy: Ex-vivo dermatoscopy means performing dermatoscopy on the lesions after removal. It has been successfully utilized for eruptive vellus hair cysts, trichostasis spinulosa, keratosis pilaris, molluscum contagiosum, and lesions of milia [80, 81].
(g) Dermoscopy for aesthetic procedures: The outcomes of laser hair reduction can be monitored with dermatoscopy. Evaluation of the density and thickness of hair follicles and image documentation is possible with dermatoscope [82].

8.14 Teledermatoscopy

Teledermatoscopy can become a novel diagnostic tool for the prevention, diagnosis, and treatment of skin disease, especially when face-to-face (FTF) consultations are not possible [83]. The inclusion of clinical and dermoscopic images in teledermatology clinics has shown improvement in the diagnostic accuracy of clinicians. It further reduces healthcare costs as it reduces the number of patient visits, simultaneously reducing the burden on the healthcare provider. Teledermoscopy can become an indispensable tool for monitoring chronic conditions requiring frequent follow-up and treatment modifications. With the emergence of inexpensive mobile-based dermatoscopes, teledermoscopy may become a more feasible and viable option. With the integration of artificial intelligence in teledermoscopy, diagnostic accuracy is also expected to improve [84].

8.15 Conclusion

Dermatoscopy is probably the most-studied diagnostic modality in dermatology in the past two decades. It has fast become an essential tool for a dermatologist. The diagnostic potential of dermatoscope has improved and is expected to improve with more large-scale studies. With the incorporation of teledermatoscopy, improvement of devices, and utilization of artificial intelligence, the scope of dermatoscopy is expected to increase immensely.

References

1. Grover C, Jakhar D. Handheld dermatoscope or videodermatoscope: which one to buy? Indian J Dermatol Venereol Leprol. 2021;87(5):739–41. https://doi.org/10.25259/IJDVL_802_19. PMID 33666053.
2. Nischal KC, Khopkar U. Dermoscope. Indian J Dermatol Venereol Leprol. 2005;71(4):300–3. https://doi.org/10.4103/0378-6323.16633. PMID 16394450.
3. Micali G, Lacarrubba F. Dermatoscopy: instrumental update. Dermatol Clin. 2018;36(4):345–8. https://doi.org/10.1016/j.det.2018.05.001. PMID 30201143.
4. Jakhar D, Kaul S, Kaur I, Kumar S. Wifi-enabled dermoscopy: what is the potential in clinical practice and education? Clin Exp Dermatol. 2021;46(7):1317–9. https://doi.org/10.1111/ced.14692. PMID 33872396.
5. Jakhar D, Grover C, Kaur I. Polyethylene tube as an attachment to universal serial bus (USB) dermatoscope for preventing cross-infection. Indian J Dermatol Venereol Leprol. 2020;86(4):459–60. https://doi.org/10.4103/ijdvl.IJDVL_376_19. PMID 32235100.
6. Zalaudek I, Kittler H, Marghoob AA, Balato A, Blum A, Dalle S, et al. Time required for a complete skin examination with and without dermoscopy: a prospective, randomized multicenter study. Arch Dermatol. 2008;144(4):509–13. https://doi.org/10.1001/archderm.144.4.509. PMID 18427045.
7. Goldman L, Figueroa Ortiz LF. Types of dermatitis in American onchocerciasis. Arch Dermatol Syphilol. 1946;53:79–93. https://doi.org/10.1001/archderm.1946.01510310003001. PMID 21015824.
8. Goldman L. Some investigative studies of pigmented nevi with cutaneous microscopy. J Invest Dermatol. 1951;16(6):407–27. https://doi.org/10.1038/jid.1951.48. PMID 14841402.
9. MacKie RM. An aid to the preoperative assessment of pigmented lesions of the skin. Br J Dermatol. 1971;85(3):232–8. https://doi.org/10.1111/j.1365-2133.1971.tb07221.x. PMID 5111687.
10. Argenziano G, Fabbrocini G, Carli P, De Giorgi V, Sammarco E, Delfino M. Epiluminescence microscopy for the diagnosis of doubtful melanocytic skin lesions. Comparison of the ABCD rule of dermatoscopy and a new 7-point checklist based on pattern analysis. Arch Dermatol. 1998;134(12):1563–70. https://doi.org/10.1001/archderm.134.12.1563. PMID 9875194.
11. Menzies SW, Ingvar C, Crotty KA, McCarthy WH. Frequency and morphologic characteristics of invasive melanomas lacking specific surface microscopic features. Arch Dermatol. 1996;132(10):1178–82. PMID 8859028.
12. Stolz W, Riemann A, Cognetta AB, et al. ABCD rule of dermatoscopy: a new practical method for early recognition of malignant melanoma. Eur J Dermatol. 1994;4:521–7.
13. Kittler H, Pehamberger H, Wolff K, Binder M. Diagnostic accuracy of dermoscopy. Lancet Oncol. 2002;3(3):159–65. https://doi.org/10.1016/s1470-2045(02)00679-4. PMID 11902502.
14. Menzies SW, Westerhoff K, Rabinovitz H, Kopf AW, McCarthy WH, Katz B. Surface microscopy of pigmented basal cell carcinoma. Arch Dermatol. 2000;136(8):1012–6. https://doi.org/10.1001/archderm.136.8.1012. PMID 10926737.

15. Zalaudek I, Giacomel J, Schmid K, Bondino S, Rosendahl C, Cavicchini S, et al. Dermatoscopy of facial actinic keratosis, intraepidermal carcinoma, and invasive squamous cell carcinoma: a progression model. J Am Acad Dermatol. 2012;66(4):589–97. https://doi.org/10.1016/j.jaad.2011.02.011. PMID 21839538.
16. Lallas A, Giacomel J, Argenziano G, García-García B, González-Fernández D, Zalaudek I, et al. Dermoscopy in general dermatology: practical tips for the clinician. Br J Dermatol. 2014;170(3):514–26. https://doi.org/10.1111/bjd.12685. PMID 24266695.
17. Nwako-Mohamadi MK, Masenga JE, Mavura D, Jahanpour OF, Mbwilo E, Blum A. Dermoscopic features of psoriasis, Lichen planus, and Pityriasis rosea in patients with skin type IV and darker attending the regional dermatology training centre in northern Tanzania. Dermatol Pract Concept. 2019;9(1):44–51. https://doi.org/10.5826/dpc.0901a11. PMID 30775148.
18. Bhat YJ, Jha AK. Dermatoscopy of inflammatory diseases in skin of color. Indian Dermatol Online J. 2021;12(1):45–57. https://doi.org/10.4103/idoj.IDOJ_613_20. PMID 33768022.
19. Jha AK, Lallas A, Sonthalia S, Jhakar D, Udayan UK, Chaudhary RKP. Differentiation of Pityriasis rubra pilaris from plaque psoriasis by dermoscopy. Dermatol Pract Concept. 2018;8(4):299–302. https://doi.org/10.5826/dpc.0804a10. PMID 30479860.
20. Jakhar D, Kaur I, Sonthalia S. Dermoscopy of Tinea manuum. Indian Dermatol Online J. 2019;10(2):210–1. https://doi.org/10.4103/idoj.IDOJ_95_18. PMID 30984609.
21. Jakhar D, Kaur I, Chaudhary R. Dermoscopy of pityrosporum folliculitis. J Am Acad Dermatol. 2019;80(2):e43–4. https://doi.org/10.1016/j.jaad.2018.08.057. PMID 30244060.
22. Conforti C, Dri A, Toffoli L, Zelin E, Zalaudek I, Di Meo N. Entodermoscopy: a useful tool for the diagnosis of cutaneous larva migrans. Dermatol Pract Concept. 2021;11(2):e2021014. https://doi.org/10.5826/dpc.1102a14. PMID 33747627.
23. Jakhar D, Misra A, Dabas S. Myiasis under dermatoscope: the hidden story. Indian Dermatol Online J. 2018;9(3):220–1. https://doi.org/10.4103/idoj.IDOJ_258_17. PMID 29854656.
24. Braun RP, Rabinovitz HS, Oliviero M, Kopf AW, Saurat JH. Pattern analysis: a two-step procedure for the dermoscopic diagnosis of melanoma. Clin Dermatol. 2002;20(3):236–9. https://doi.org/10.1016/s0738-081x(02)00216-x. PMID 12074858.
25. Lallas A, Argenziano G, Moscarella E, Longo C, Simonetti V, Zalaudek I. Diagnosis and management of facial pigmented macules. Clin Dermatol. 2014;32(1):94–100. https://doi.org/10.1016/j.clindermatol.2013.05.030. PMID 24314382.
26. Marghoob AA, Usatine RP, Jaimes N. Dermoscopy for the family physician. Am Fam Physician. 2013;88(7):441–50. PMID 24134084.
27. Braun RP, Rabinovitz HS, Krischer J, Kreusch J, Oliviero M, Naldi L, et al. Dermoscopy of pigmented seborrheic keratosis: a morphological study. Arch Dermatol. 2002;138(12):1556–60. https://doi.org/10.1001/archderm.138.12.1556. PMID 12472342.
28. Espasandín-Arias M, Moscarella E, Mota-Buçard A, Moreno-Moreno C, Lallas A, Longo C, et al. The dermoscopic variability of dermatofibromas. J Am Acad Dermatol. 2015;72(1 Suppl):S22–4. https://doi.org/10.1016/j.jaad.2014.04.048. PMID 25500030.
29. Zaballos P, Puig S, Llambrich A, Malvehy J. Dermoscopy of dermatofibromas: a prospective morphological study of 412 cases. Arch Dermatol. 2008;144(1):75–83. https://doi.org/10.1001/archdermatol.2007.8. PMID 18209171.
30. Oiso N, Kawada A. The dermoscopic features in infantile hemangioma. Pediatr Dermatol. 2011;28(5):591–3. https://doi.org/10.1111/j.1525-1470.2011.01385.x. PMID 21854412.
31. Zaballos P, Daufí C, Puig S, Argenziano G, Moreno-Ramírez D, Cabo H, et al. Dermoscopy of solitary angiokeratomas: a morphological study. Arch Dermatol. 2007;143(3):318–25. https://doi.org/10.1001/archderm.143.3.318. PMID: 17372096.
32. Zaballos P, Carulla M, Ozdemir F, Zalaudek I, Bañuls J, Llambrich A, et al. Dermoscopy of pyogenic granuloma: a morphological study. Br J Dermatol. 2010;163(6):1229–37. https://doi.org/10.1111/j.1365-2133.2010.10040.x. PMID 20846306.
33. Jha AK, Sonthalia S, Jakhar D. Dermoscopy of angiokeratoma. Indian Dermatol Online J. 2018;9(2):141–2. https://doi.org/10.4103/idoj.IDOJ_278_17. PMID 29644211.

34. Lallas A, Apalla Z, Argenziano G, Longo C, Moscarella E, Specchio F, et al. The dermatoscopic universe of basal cell carcinoma. Dermatol Pract Concept. 2014;4(3):11–24. https://doi.org/10.5826/dpc.0403a02. PMID 25126452.
35. Giacomel J, Zalaudek I. Dermoscopy of superficial basal cell carcinoma. Dermatol Surg. 2005;31(12):1710–3. https://doi.org/10.2310/6350.2005.31314. PMID 16336893.
36. Lallas A, Argenziano G, Kyrgidis A, Apalla Z, Moscarella E, Longo C, et al. Dermoscopy uncovers clinically undetectable pigmentation in basal cell carcinoma. Br J Dermatol. 2014;170(1):192–5. https://doi.org/10.1111/bjd.12634. PMID 24117444.
37. Lallas A, Tzellos T, Kyrgidis A, Apalla Z, Zalaudek I, Karatolias A, et al. Accuracy of dermoscopic criteria for discriminating superficial from other subtypes of basal cell carcinoma. J Am Acad Dermatol. 2014;70(2):303–11. https://doi.org/10.1016/j.jaad.2013.10.003. PMID 24268311.
38. Balagula Y, Braun RP, Rabinovitz HS, Dusza SW, Scope A, Liebman TN, et al. The significance of crystalline/chrysalis structures in the diagnosis of melanocytic and nonmelanocytic lesions. J Am Acad Dermatol. 2012;67(2):194.e1–8. https://doi.org/10.1016/j.jaad.2011.04.039. PMID 22030020.
39. Glogau RG. The risk of progression to invasive disease. J Am Acad Dermatol. 2000;42(1 Pt 2):23–4. https://doi.org/10.1067/mjd.2000.103339. PMID 10607353.
40. Huerta-Brogeras M, Olmos O, Borbujo J, Hernández-Núñez A, Castaño E, Romero-Maté A, Martínez-Sánchez D, Martínez-Morán C. Validation of dermoscopy as a real-time noninvasive diagnostic imaging technique for actinic keratosis. Arch Dermatol. 2012;148(10):1159–64. https://doi.org/10.1001/archdermatol.2012.1060. PMID: 23069952.
41. Zalaudek I, Argenziano G, Leinweber B, Citarella L, Hofmann-Wellenhof R, Malvehy J, et al. Dermoscopy of Bowen's disease. Br J Dermatol. 2004;150(6):1112–6. https://doi.org/10.1111/j.1365-2133.2004.05924.x. PMID 15214896.
42. Pan Y, Chamberlain AJ, Bailey M, Chong AH, Haskett M, Kelly JW. Dermatoscopy aids in the diagnosis of the solitary red scaly patch or plaque-features distinguishing superficial basal cell carcinoma, intraepidermal carcinoma, and psoriasis. J Am Acad Dermatol. 2008;59(2):268–74. https://doi.org/10.1016/j.jaad.2008.05.013. PMID 18550207.
43. Lallas A, Kyrgidis A, Tzellos TG, Apalla Z, Karakyriou E, Karatolias A, et al. Accuracy of dermoscopic criteria for the diagnosis of psoriasis, dermatitis, lichen planus and Pityriasis rosea. Br J Dermatol. 2012;166(6):1198–205. https://doi.org/10.1111/j.1365-2133.2012.10868.x. PMID 22296226.
44. Cameron A, Rosendahl C, Tschandl P, Riedl E, Kittler H. Dermatoscopy of pigmented Bowen's disease. J Am Acad Dermatol. 2010;62(4):597–604. https://doi.org/10.1016/j.jaad.2009.06.008, PMID 20079953.
45. Rosendahl C, Cameron A, Argenziano G, Zalaudek I, Tschandl P, Kittler H. Dermoscopy of squamous cell carcinoma and keratoacanthoma. Arch Dermatol. 2012;148(12):1386–92. https://doi.org/10.1001/archdermatol.2012.2974, PMID 22986634.
46. Lallas A, Pyne J, Kyrgidis A, Andreani S, Argenziano G, Cavaller A, et al. The clinical and dermoscopic features of invasive cutaneous squamous cell carcinoma depend on the histopathological grade of differentiation. Br J Dermatol. 2015;172(5):1308–15. https://doi.org/10.1111/bjd.13510, PMID 25363081.
47. Jha AK, Sonthalia S, Lallas A. Dermoscopy as an evolving tool to assess vitiligo activity. J Am Acad Dermatol. 2018;78(5):1017–9. https://doi.org/10.1016/j.jaad.2017.12.009, PMID 29229577.
48. Kumar Jha A, Sonthalia S, Lallas A, Chaudhary RKP. Dermoscopy in vitiligo: diagnosis and beyond. Int J Dermatol. 2018;57(1):50–4. https://doi.org/10.1111/ijd.13795. PMID 29076154.
49. Oiso N, Kawada A. The diagnostic usefulness of dermoscopy for nevus depigmentosus. Eur J Dermatol. 2011;21(4):639–40. https://doi.org/10.1684/ejd.2011.1414. PMID 21697055.
50. Ankad BS, Beergouder SL. Dermoscopic evaluation of idiopathic guttate hypomelanosis: a preliminary observation. Indian Dermatol Online J. 2015;6(3):164–7. https://doi.org/10.4103/2229-5178.156383. PMID 26009709.

51. Larre Borges A, Tiodorovic-Zivkovic D, Lallas A, Moscarella E, Gurgitano S, Capurro M, et al. Clinical, dermoscopic and histopathologic features of genital and extragenital lichen sclerosus. J Eur Acad Dermatol Venereol. 2013;27(11):1433–9. https://doi.org/10.1111/j.1468-3083.2012.04595.x. PMID 22646723.
52. Errichetti E, Lallas A, Apalla Z, Di Stefani A, Stinco G. Dermoscopy of morphea and cutaneous lichen sclerosus: clinicopathological correlation study and comparative analysis. Dermatology. 2017;233(6):462–70. https://doi.org/10.1159/000484947. PMID 29237158.
53. Kaur I, Jakhar D, Singal A. Dermoscopy in the evaluation of pityriasis versicolor: a cross sectional study. Indian Dermatol Online J. 2019;10(6):682–5. https://doi.org/10.4103/idoj.IDOJ_502_18. PMID 31807448.
54. Vinay K, Kamat D, Chatterjee D, Narang T, Dogra S. Dermatoscopy in leprosy and its correlation with clinical spectrum and histopathology: a prospective observational study. J Eur Acad Dermatol Venereol. 2019;33(10):1947–51. https://doi.org/10.1111/jdv.15635. PMID 31004456.
55. Lallas A, Apalla Z, Lefaki I, Tzellos T, Karatolias A, Sotiriou E, et al. Dermoscopy of early stage mycosis fungoides. J Eur Acad Dermatol Venereol. 2013;27(5):617–21. https://doi.org/10.1111/j.1468-3083.2012.04499.x. PMID 22404051.
56. Gil I, Segura S, Martínez-Escala E, Lloreta J, Puig S, Vélez M, et al. Dermoscopic and reflectance confocal microscopic features of exogenous ochronosis. Arch Dermatol. 2010;146(9):1021–5. https://doi.org/10.1001/archdermatol.2010.205. PMID 20855704.
57. Vinay K, Bishnoi A, Parsad D, Saikia UN, Sendhil Kumaran M. Dermatoscopic evaluation and histopathological correlation of acquired dermal macular hyperpigmentation. Int J Dermatol. 2017;56(12):1395–9. https://doi.org/10.1111/ijd.13782. PMID 28971471.
58. Sharma V, Gupta V, Pahadiya P, Vedi K, Arava S, Ramam M. Dermoscopy and patch testing in patients with lichen planus pigmentosus on face: a cross-sectional observational study in fifty Indian patients. Indian J Dermatol Venereol Leprol. 2017;83(6):656–62. https://doi.org/10.4103/ijdvl.IJDVL_469_16.
59. Russo F, Flori ML, Taddeucci P, Rubegni P, Cinotti E. Pigmentary demarcation lines of Voigt-Futcher: dermoscopic and reflectance confocal microscopy features. Skin Res Technol. 2020;26(3):440–2. https://doi.org/10.1111/srt.12795. PMID 31562651.
60. Rigopoulos D, Papanagiotou V, Daniel R III, Piraccini BM. Onychomycosis in patients with nail psoriasis: a point to point discussion. Mycoses. 2017;60(1):6–10. https://doi.org/10.1111/myc.12542. PMID 27523738.
61. Vázquez-López F, Manjón-Haces JA, Maldonado-Seral C, Raya-Aguado C, Pérez-Oliva N, Marghoob AA. Dermoscopic features of plaque psoriasis and lichen planus: new observations. Dermatology. 2003;207(2):151–6. https://doi.org/10.1159/000071785. PMID: 12920364.
62. Lallas A, Argenziano G, Apalla Z, Gourhant JY, Zaballos P, Di Lernia V, et al. Dermoscopic patterns of common facial inflammatory skin diseases. J Eur Acad Dermatol Venereol. 2014;28(5):609–14. https://doi.org/10.1111/jdv.12146. PMID 23489377.
63. Lallas A, Apalla Z, Lefaki I, Sotiriou E, Lazaridou E, Ioannides D, et al. Dermoscopy of discoid lupus erythematosus. Br J Dermatol. 2013;168(2):284–8. https://doi.org/10.1111/bjd.12044. PMID 22985425.
64. Vázquez-López F, Maldonado-Seral C, Soler-Sánchez T, Perez-Oliva N, Marghoob AA. Surface microscopy for discriminating between common urticaria and urticarial vasculitis. Rheumatology (Oxf Engl). 2003;42(9):1079–82. https://doi.org/10.1093/rheumatology/keg301, PMID 12730524.
65. Zaballos P, Puig S, Malvehy J. Dermoscopy of pigmented purpuric dermatoses (lichen aureus): a useful tool for clinical diagnosis. Arch Dermatol. 2004;140(10):1290–1. https://doi.org/10.1001/archderm.140.10.1290, PMID 15492206.
66. Ingegnoli F, Boracchi P, Gualtierotti R, Lubatti C, Meani L, Zahalkova L, Zeni S, Fantini F. Prognostic model based on nailfold capillaroscopy for identifying Raynaud's phenomenon patients at high risk for the development of a scleroderma spectrum disorder: PRINCE (prognostic index for nailfold capillaroscopic examination). Arthritis Rheum. 2008;58(7):2174–82. https://doi.org/10.1002/art.23555. PMID: 18576359.

67. Jakhar D, Bhat YJ, Chatterjee M, Keshavmurthy V, Ankad BS, Jha AK, et al. Dermoscopy practice during COVID-19 pandemic: recommendations by SIG dermoscopy (IADVL academy). Indian Dermatol Online J. 2020;11(3):343–4. https://doi.org/10.4103/idoj.IDOJ_231_20, PMID 32695690.
68. Jakhar D, Kaur I, Kaul S. Art of performing dermoscopy during the times of coronavirus disease (COVID-19): simple change in approach can save the day! J Eur Acad Dermatol Venereol. 2020;34(6):e242–4. https://doi.org/10.1111/jdv.16412, PMID 32223004.
69. Zalaudek I, Giacomel J, Cabo H, Di Stefani A, Ferrara G, Hofmann-Wellenhof R, et al. Entodermoscopy: a new tool for diagnosing skin infections and infestations. Dermatology. 2008;216(1):14–23. https://doi.org/10.1159/000109353, PMID 18032894.
70. Zaballos P, Ara M, Puig S, Malvehy J. Dermoscopy of molluscum contagiosum: a useful tool for clinical diagnosis in adulthood. J Eur Acad Dermatol Venereol. 2006;20(4):482–3. https://doi.org/10.1111/j.1468-3083.2006.01480.x, PMID 16643165.
71. Di Stefani A, Hofmann-Wellenhof R, Zalaudek I. Dermoscopy for diagnosis and treatment monitoring of pediculosis capitis. J Am Acad Dermatol. 2006;54(5):909–11. https://doi.org/10.1016/j.jaad.2005.11.1083, PMID 16635683.
72. Zalaudek I, Argenziano G. Images in clinical medicine. Dermoscopy of nits and pseudonits. N Engl J Med. 2012;367(18):1741. https://doi.org/10.1056/NEJMicm1103059. PMID 23113485.
73. Grover C, Jakhar D. Onychoscopy: a practical guide. Indian J Dermatol Venereol Leprol. 2017;83(5):536–49. https://doi.org/10.4103/ijdvl.IJDVL_242_16. PMID: 28485306.
74. Kinoshita-Ise M, Sachdeva M. Update on trichoscopy: integration of the terminology by systematic approach and a proposal of a diagnostic flowchart. J Dermatol. 2022;49(1):4–18. https://doi.org/10.1111/1346-8138.16233. Epub 2021 Nov 22. PMID: 34806223.
75. Grimaldi L, Silvestri A, Brandi C, Nisi G, Brafa A, Calabrò M, et al. Digital epiluminescence dermoscopy for pigmented cutaneous lesions, primary care physicians, and telediagnosis: a useful tool? J Plast Reconstr Aesthet Surg. 2009;62(8):1054–8. https://doi.org/10.1016/j.bjps.2008.01.011. PMID 18547883.
76. Jakhar D, Kaur I. IA muselet and USB dermatoscope: a precise way to mark a site for biopsy. Pediatr Dermatol. 2020;37(4):774–5. https://doi.org/10.1111/pde.14182. PMID 32333609.
77. Kibar M, Aktan Ş, Lebe B, Bilgin M. Trichoscopic findings in alopecia areata and their relation to disease activity, severity and clinical subtype in Turkish patients. Australas J Dermatol. 2015;56(1):e1–6. https://doi.org/10.1111/ajd.12102. PMID 23991834.
78. Apalla Z, Lallas A, Tzellos T, Sidiropoulos T, Lefaki I, Trakatelli M, et al. Applicability of dermoscopy for evaluation of patients' response to nonablative therapies for the treatment of superficial basal cell carcinoma. Br J Dermatol. 2014;170(4):809–15. https://doi.org/10.1111/bjd.12749. PMID 24283541.
79. Kaur I, Chowdhry S, D'Souza P, Jakhar D, Yadav MK, Kaur O. Intra-operative dermoscopy in assessment of melanonychia and as a guide for biopsy. Indian Dermatol Online J. 2020;11(2):171–6. https://doi.org/10.4103/idoj.IDOJ_94_19. PMID 32477974.
80. Daruwalla SB, Dhurat RS, Agrawal S, Mahobia S, Naidu KS. 'Extraction dermoscopy': expanding the utility of epiluminescence microscopy. Skin Appendage Disord. 2020;6(4):220–3. https://doi.org/10.1159/000508518. PMID 32903886.
81. Daulatabad D, Grover C, Sharma S. 'Extraction dermoscopy' as a rapid and innovative diagnostic tool for eruptive vellus hair cyst. Clin Exp Dermatol. 2017;42(4):438–40. https://doi.org/10.1111/ced.13096. PMID 28429880.
82. Mohamed EE, Ahmed AM, Tawfik KM, Ibrahim SM. Trichoscopic changes in hair during treatment of hirsutism with 1064-nm neodymium:yttrium-aluminum-garnet laser. J Cosmet Dermatol. 2016;15(1):31–5. https://doi.org/10.1111/jocd.12164. PMID 26223429.
83. Uppal SK, Beer J, Hadeler E, Gitlow H, Nouri K. The clinical utility of teledermoscopy in the era of telemedicine. Dermatol Ther. 2021;34(2):e14766. https://doi.org/10.1111/dth.14766. PMID 33421232.
84. Veronese F, Branciforti F, Zavattaro E, Tarantino V, Romano V, Meiburger KM, et al. The role in teledermoscopy of an inexpensive and easy-to-use smartphone device for the classification of three types of skin lesions using convolutional neural networks. Diagnostics (Basel). 2021;11(3):451. https://doi.org/10.3390/diagnostics11030451. PMID 33807976.

9 Bedside, Real-Time Visualization and Diagnosis of Skin Lesions: A Myth or Reality?

Manu Jain

Diagnosis of skin lesions traditionally relies on clinical inspection followed by biopsy for histopathological confirmation. Although a skin biopsy seems like a trivial process compared to acquiring biopsies from other deep-seated organs, it remains an invasive procedure that can cause pain, bleeding, infection, and scarring. A biopsy is problematic for patients with multiple skin lesions, especially when they are located on the face (related to cosmetic concerns) [1, 2] or sensitive sites of genitalia. It may also be difficult in elderly or diabetic patients, who are prone to poor wound healing. Moreover, approximately 80% of biopsies for diagnosing skin cancers are benign, adding unnecessary trauma and cost [3–5]. A biopsy is also a terminal event, which makes it unsuitable for longitudinal monitoring of skin lesions during treatment. Likewise, even though histopathology is the gold standard for diagnosis, it is unable to render an immediate real-time diagnosis at the bedside due to necessary time-consuming tissue processing (tissue fixation, cutting, and staining) prior to evaluation by pathologists. Furthermore, only a fraction of the biopsied tissue is used for histopathological evaluation, which may miss early and focal changes in a given lesion.

Skin is a unique organ due to its visibility and accessibility, allowing it to be readily visualized and assessed by noninvasive surface microscopes. Dermoscopy, also called epiluminescence microscopy, is one of the earliest examples of surface imaging microscopes, which was described in 1920 by Johan Saphier [6]. Since then, it has been used extensively to diagnose skin lesions such as inflammatory and skin cancers. Diagnosis on dermoscopy relies only on pattern recognition

Supplementary Information The online version contains supplementary material available at https://doi.org/10.1007/978-981-97-0411-8_9.

M. Jain (✉)
Dermatology Service, Memorial Sloan Kettering Cancer Center, New York, NY, USA
e-mail: jainm@mskcc.org

S. Gupta et al. (eds.), *Critical Thinking in Contemporary Dermatology: Cognitive Essays*, https://doi.org/10.1007/978-981-97-0411-8_9

(pigmentary and vascular). Thus, it has improved the diagnosis of various skin cancers, especially melanoma, over visual inspection. However, lesions lacking pigment, i.e., lightly-colored or non-pigmented, are challenging to diagnose, leading to frequent biopsies for histopathology confirmation [7–9].

Several noninvasive imaging devices have been developed to overcome these limitations. These devices either use light as an imaging source ("optical imaging") or do not use light ("non-optical imaging") [10]. Optical imaging techniques that are not harmful to the patients use non-ionizing radiation, including visible and infrared light. Some well-known optical imaging techniques in dermatology include confocal microscopy [CM], optical coherence tomography [OCT], multiphoton microscopy (MPM), multi/hyperspectral imaging, Raman microscopy/spectroscopy, and photoacoustic tomography. Examples of non-optical imaging are ultrasound (US) and magnetic resonance imaging (MRI). Both optical and non-optical imaging devices are primarily used to acquire images in real time to render bedside diagnosis and aid in managing skin lesions. Thus, the field encompassing the use of these devices is referred to as in vivo *microscopy* (IVM). Not only can these devices image lesions in vivo, but some of them, including OCT and CM, can also image freshly excised tissues for rapid evaluation, avoiding the need for time-consuming tissue processing such as tissue cutting. Thus, these devices are also called ex vivo *microscopy* (EVM) devices.

This chapter will only focus on tools currently used or being integrated into clinics, including the US, OCT, RCM, and MPM. For each technique, we will briefly describe its principle, available commercial devices, as well as their applications, and limitations. We will also describe a combined optical coherence tomography (OCT) and reflectance confocal microscopy (RCM) device called the RCM-OCT device. Despite advances in noninvasive technologies, their use remains restricted to bigger academic institutes and some private clinics. Their limited use is related to the lack of expert readers, the high cost of the devices, and their bulky design. Lastly, we will discuss ongoing efforts aimed at overcoming these limitations.

9.1 In Vivo Microscopy in Dermatology (IVM)

9.1.1 Ultrasonography (US)

Principles: Ultrasound is one of the first noninvasive imaging techniques, first used in dermatology around the 1980s [11]. Since then, it has been the only non-optical imaging technique being extensively used in clinics. Unlike optical imaging techniques (OCT, RCM, MPM) that utilize light as a source of imaging, US imaging is based on the emission and reflection of sound waves. Images are formed with varying brightness intensities depending upon the ability of ultrasound waves to pass through the tissue. For example, bright or hyperechoic areas result from an abrupt increase in tissue density, dark or hypoechoic areas appear where tissue density decreases, and a black anechoic region appears in an area of tissue from which no waves are reflected.

Currently available commercial devices and their imaging capabilities: US devices for skin imaging are widely available in the market. These include high frequency or HFUS (20–30 MHz; GE, Canon, Toshiba, Esaote, Philips, Samsung, Mindray) and ultra-high frequency or UHFUS (30–70 MHz; VisualSonics) devices that generate an axial resolution of 100 μm–30 μm, respectively. Unlike optical imaging devices, which can image to a maximum depth of 2 mm, US images skin as deep as the deep fascia. Furthermore, several US devices include color Doppler analysis that provides vascular information, including blood flow (velocity, discriminating arterial from venous blood flow) and vascular morphology [12]. Figure 9.1 shows an image of normal skin with various layers acquired using a UHFUS.

Clinical applications: In dermatology, US is used to evaluate various cutaneous and nail lesions. This includes benign cystic lesions (epidermal cysts, trichilemmal cysts, pilonidal cysts) and solid tumors (lipoma, pilomatrixoma, and dermatofibromas) (Fig. 9.2). US also aids in the early diagnosis of nonmelanoma skin cancers (NMSC: basal cell and squamous cell carcinoma) and melanoma. In general, NMSCs appear as hypoechoic, heterogeneous lesions with irregular borders in a relatively hyperechoic epidermis and/or dermis [13]. Interestingly, hyperechoic spots have been described in some aggressive forms of BCCs [14] (Fig. 9.3). Melanoma appears as a fusiform hypoechoic lesion with hypervascularity and locoregional invasion. Increased and prominent vascularity is usually detected around or within the neoplasms. However, the main application of sonography is for pre-operative assessment of skin cancers, which is used to determine locoregional (including lymph nodes) spread. Other applications include the evaluation of inflammatory lesions (such as psoriasis, plantar warts, hidradenitis suppurativa, and atopic dermatitis), foreign bodies, and vascular lesions (hemangiomas, port-wine stains, and vascular malformations) [11] (Fig. 9.4). Cosmetic applications include but are

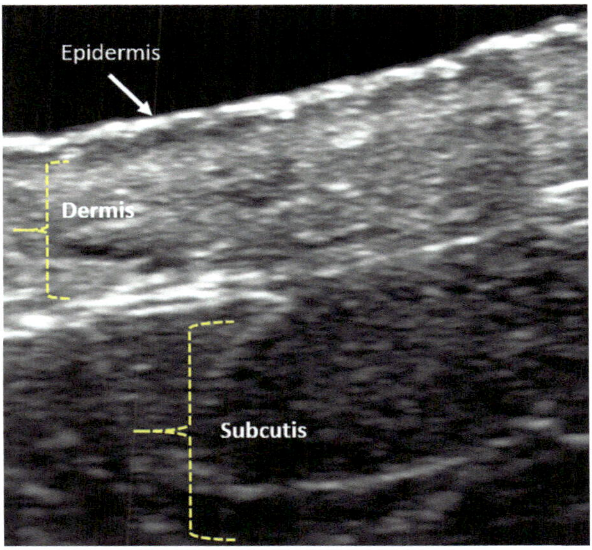

Fig. 9.1 Images of normal skin layers on ultrasound (grayscale; transverse view; 70 MHz). (*Courtesy:* Dr. Ximena Wortsman. Adjunct Professor, Dermatologic Ultrasound. Medical Director of IDIEP-Institute for Diagnostic Imaging and Research of the Skin and Soft Tissues. Departments of Dermatology. Universidad de Chile and/y Pontificia Universidad Católica de Chile. Santiago, Chile)

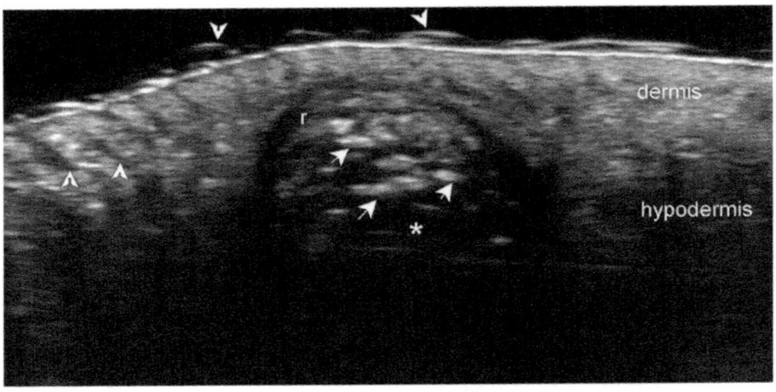

Fig. 9.2 Images of a pilomatrixoma on ultrasound (grayscale; frontal region; transverse view; 70 MHz). Round-shaped dermal and hypodermal structure with a hypoechoic rim (r) and heterogeneous center (*) presenting multiple hyperechoic deposits (arrows) that generate posterior acoustic shadowing artifacts suggestive of calcium. Notice the normal hair follicles (arrowheads pointing downward) and hair tracts (pointing upward) in the vicinity of the lesion. (*Courtesy:* Dr. Ximena Wortsman. Adjunct Professor, Dermatologic Ultrasound. Medical Director of IDIEP-Institute for Diagnostic Imaging and Research of the Skin and Soft Tissues. Departments of Dermatology. Universidad de Chile and/y Pontificia Universidad Católica de Chile. Santiago, Chile)

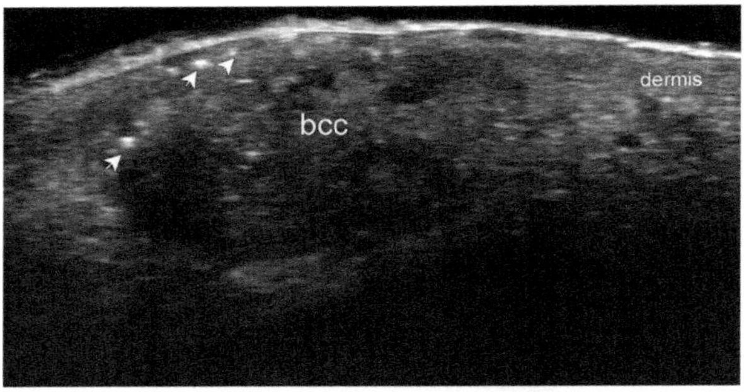

Fig. 9.3 Images of basal cell carcinoma (BCC) on ultrasound (grayscale; transverse view; 70 MHz) shows ill-defined hypoechoic dermal and a hypodermal lesion that contains multiple hyperechoic spots (arrows) in the superficial part. (*Courtesy*: Dr. Ximena Wortsman. Adjunct Professor, Dermatologic Ultrasound. Medical Director of IDIEP-Institute for Diagnostic Imaging and Research of the Skin and Soft Tissues. Departments of Dermatology. Universidad de Chile and/y Pontificia Universidad Católica de Chile. Santiago, Chile)

not limited to the visualization of fillers, monitoring botulinum toxin injections, and collagen response to topical vitamin C.

Status of approval: All the above-mentioned devices have FDA approval for clinical use.

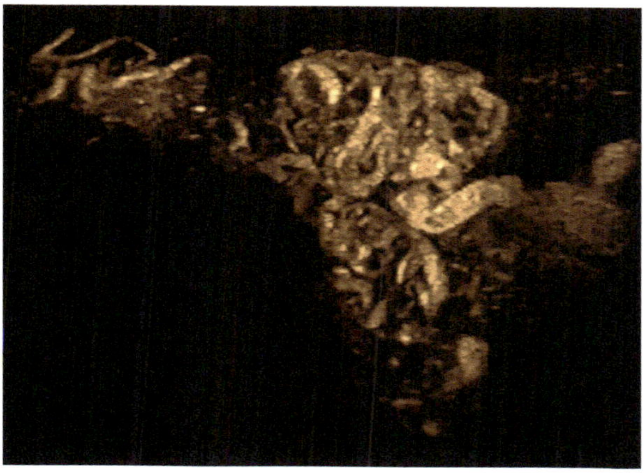

Fig. 9.4 Images of infantile hemangioma on ultrasound echoangio (longitudinal view; 24 MHz) demonstrates a hypervascular mass involving the medial part of the left intra-orbital extraconal lower fat pad. (*Courtesy:* Dr. Ximena Wortsman. Adjunct Professor, Dermatologic Ultrasound. Medical Director of IDIEP-Institute for Diagnostic Imaging and Research of the Skin and Soft Tissues. Departments of Dermatology. Universidad de Chile and/y Pontificia Universidad Católica de Chile. Santiago, Chile)

9.1.2 Optical Coherence Tomography (OCT)

Principles: Optical coherence tomography (OCT), an optical imaging technique, has been used in dermatology since the 1990s [15]. Fundamentally, OCT image generation relies on the principles of low-coherence interferometry. It detects the intensity of back-scattered infrared light (910–1305 nm wavelengths) from different layers within the skin and reconstructs the microstructure of the tissue [15].

Currently available commercial devices and their imaging capabilities: Typically, a standard or conventional frequency domain-based OCT device images skin in a B-mode or cross-section (similar to histopathology and US images) in vivo, in real-time [16]. Its imaging capabilities lie at a crossroads between US and RCM. Conventional OCT images skin up to a depth of 2 mm from the skin surface (deeper than RCM) and has a large field of view (FOV) measuring up to 6.0 × 6.0–10 mm. However, it cannot provide cellular details due to lateral resolution of approximately 15–20 μm [16]. Thus, the increase in the imaging depth comes at the cost of cellular resolution.

Newer OCT devices have improved the existing cellular resolution [16]. One such device is the Fourier-domain-based OCT (The VivoSight Dx; Michelson Diagnostics) (Figs. 9.5 and 9.6), which provides a lateral resolution of <7.5 microns and <5.0 microns axial resolution for better structural clarity. Its FOV (6 mm × 6 mm) and imaging depth (1–2 mm) remain similar to the conventional OCT.

With the advent of technology, the latest and the newest generation of OCT have dramatically improved lateral resolution from 20 μm to ~1–3 μm, thus called high-definition or HD-OCTs or ultrahigh-definition OCT [16]. However, this increase in resolution has come at the cost of decreased imaging depth to ~300–500 microns

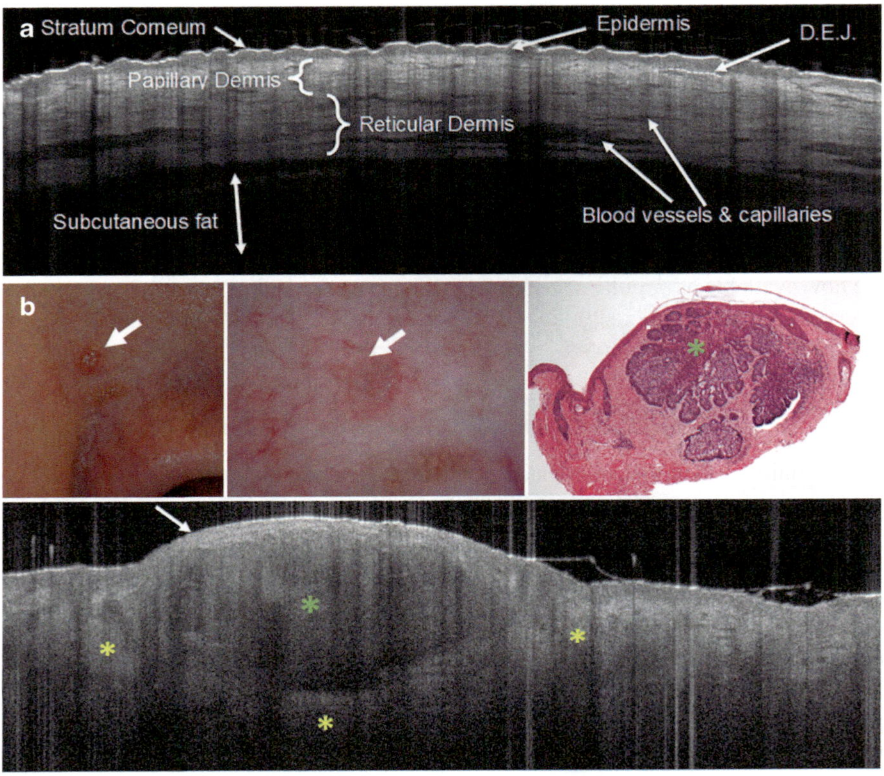

Fig. 9.5 Images of a normal skin and a basal cell carcinoma (BCC) on Fourier-domain-based OCT (VivoSight Dx; Michelson Diagnostics). (**a**) Layers of normal skin in a vertical section (from top to bottom) show *Epidermis:* grayish layer with bright, thin bright *stratum corneum* on the top; *Dermoepidermal junction*: border (dashed white line) between the grayish stratum spinosum and underlying bright papillary dermis; *Dermis:* white, thick layer containing linear, tubular, dark vessels; *Sub-cutis:* darkest layer below the dermis. (**b**) Nodular Basal cell carcinoma (BCC): *Top panel (left to right):* clinical, dermoscopy, and H&E images of a nodular BCC (green asterisk). *Bottom panel:* OCT image of the nodular BCC showing a well-defined round to oval grayish nodule (green asterisk) within a bright dermis (yellow asterisks). This nodule is pushing up the overlying epidermis (white arrow)

and a smaller FOV of ~1–2 mm to 500 × 500 μm. There are currently two such competing devices: Full-Field OCT or FF-OCT (ApolloVue®S100 Image System) [17] (Figs. 9.7 and 9.8) and Line-field confocal OCT or LC-OCT (Damae Medical) [18] (Figs. 9.9 and 9.10). These devices provide cellular-resolution images, similar to RCM. Additionally, they generate a cross-sectional and an *en face* view of skin lesions simultaneously. Both these devices have embedded dermatoscope to guide imaging within the lesion in real time. Similar to the US, dynamic OCT (D-OCT) can provide information about the vasculature of the lesions.

Clinical applications: The main application of OCT is for diagnosing keratinocyte carcinoma, especially basal cell carcinoma (Figs. 9.5, 9.8, and 9.10) [11, 19].

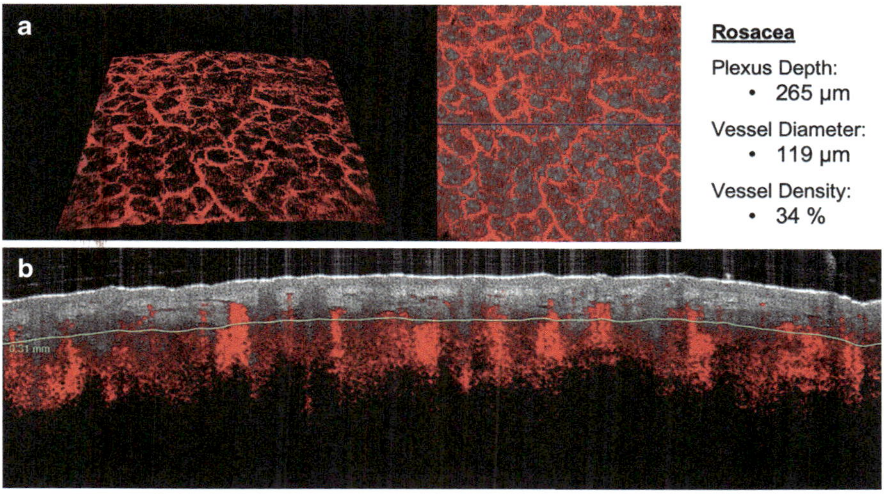

Fig. 9.6 Images of rosacea on Fourier-domain-based D-OCT (VivoSight Dx; Michelson Diagnostics). (**a**) *En face* views, and (**b**) Vertical view of skin with rosacea showing an increased number of dilated vessels in the dermis in the D-OCT images

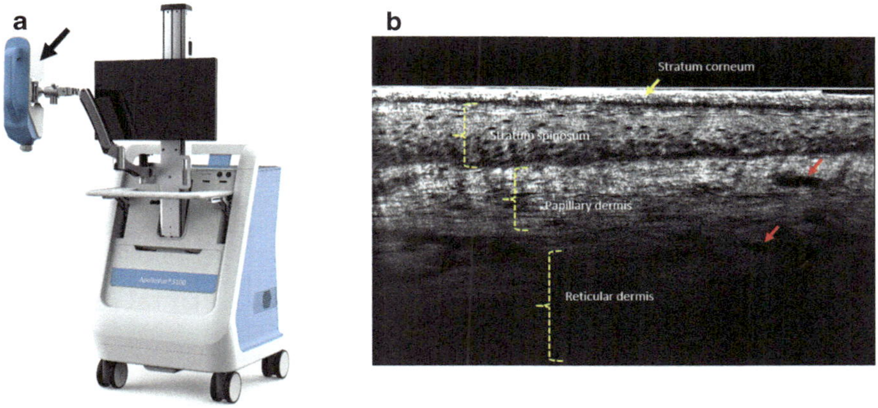

Fig. 9.7 Images of a normal skin on ultra-high-resolution FF-OCT (ApolloVue®S100 Image System). (**a**) Portable FF-OCT device with an imaging probe (arrow). (**b**) Normal skin layers (from top to bottom): *Stratum corneum*: bright and acellular; *Stratum spinosum*: grayish-white layer with a multi-layered dark round to oval nuclei; *Papillary dermis:* bright, white collagenous layer with dark tubular vessels (red arrows); *Reticular dermis:* dark gray layer beneath the papillary dermis. (*Images courtesy*: Dr. Chih-Shan Jason Chen, MD, Ph.D., FAAD. Memorial Sloan Kettering Cancer Center. Hauppauge, NY, USA)

As OCT can image lesions in vertical mode, BCC tumor nodules can be readily identified as round-to-oval, well-defined grayish structures within a bright collagenous dermis and separated by a surrounding dark area of clefting (Fig. 9.5). Thus,

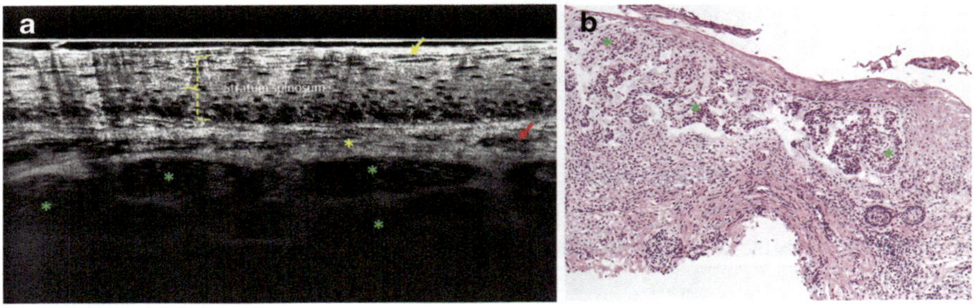

Fig. 9.8 Images of a nodular BCC on ultra-high-resolution FF-OCT (ApolloVue®S100 Image System). (**a**) BCC appears as dark to grayish nodules (green asterisks) within a bright dermis (yellow asterisk). There are dark tubular dilated vessels (red arrow) surrounding the BCC nodule, and (**b**) Corresponding H&E image of the BCC. (*Images courtesy:* Dr. Chih-Shan Jason Chen, MD, Ph.D., FAAD. Memorial Sloan Kettering Cancer Center. Hauppauge, NY, USA)

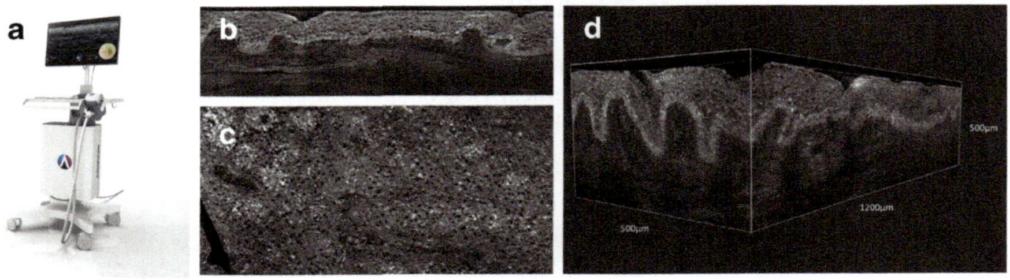

Fig. 9.9 Images of a normal skin on ultra-high-resolution LC-OCT (Damae Medical). (**a**) LC-OCT device on a wheelable trolley attached with a handheld imaging probe. (**b**) Vertical view of normal skin layers (from top to bottom): *Stratum corneum*: bright and acellular; *Stratum spinosum*: grayish-white layer with a multi-layered dark round to oval nuclei; *Dermoepidermal junction:* pigmented basal cells with bright cytoplasm (keratin and melanin) and dark nuclei; *Dermis:* grayish-dark collagenous layer with dark tubular vessels. (**c**) *En face* view of the normal skin site at DEJ shows bright rings of pigmented basal cells with central dark holes of the papillary dermis, surrounded by stratum spinosum with grayish cytoplasm and dark nuclei. (**d**) Three-dimensional visualization of the normal skin

OCT with dermoscopy has significantly improved the specificity (from 54.3 to 75.3%) [20, 21] of diagnosing BCC without any marked improvement in sensitivity (86–95%) [22]. Other subtypes of BCCs (micronodular and infiltrative) may not be evident on OCT. Furthermore, ultra-high-resolution OCT (FFOCT and LC-OCT) provides cellular details of BCC [23, 24] (Figs. 9.8 and 9.10), similar to the RCM device. Not only does OCT aid in diagnosing BCC, but it also aids in its management by providing information on the lesion's depth, location, and thickness. Based on this information, a dermatologist can opt for surgical or non-surgical treatment for BCC. It can also monitor the recurrence of BCC noninvasively following topical and photodynamic therapies and lasers. However, the role of OCT in detecting melanoma or SCC is not well-established. Ultra-high-resolution OCT devices [17, 18] are being explored to diagnose these lesions as well as lesions of acanthomas [17] and Paget's disease [17].

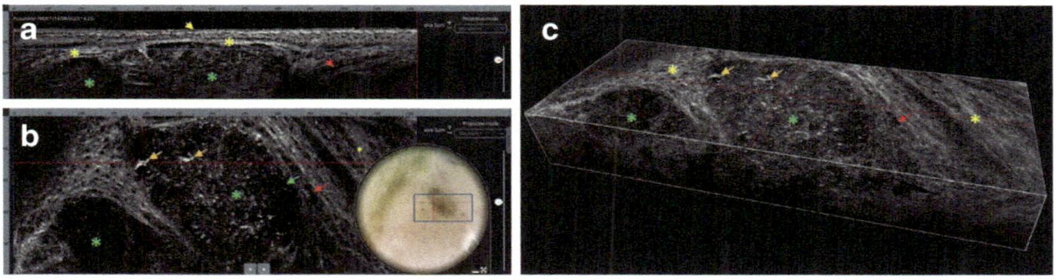

Fig. 9.10 Images of a nodular BCC on ultra-high-resolution LC-OCT (Damae Medical). (**a**) Vertical view of a nodular BCC showing epidermis (yellow arrow), beneath which a couple of hyporeflective ovoid BCC nodules (green asterisks) can be identified. These nodules are separated from the epidermis by bright collagen (yellow asterisks). Dark tubular vessels (red arrow) can be seen surrounding the BCC nodules. (**b**) *En face* view of the same nodular BCC at the level of superficial dermal level (dotted line in image **a**) shows cellular details (similar to RCM) of BCC nodules (green asterisks): increased nuclear: cytoplasmic (N:C) ratio and peripheral palisading (green arrow). Some bright dendritic cells (orange arrows) can be identified within the nodules, which are most likely melanocytes. The inset shows a dermoscopy image of the lesion, and the blue box indicates the site being imaged. (**c**) Three-dimensional visualization of the same nodular BCC (green asterisks). (*Image courtesy:* Prof. Jean-Luc Perrot. University Hospital of Saint-Etienne. Saint-Etienne, France)

The D-OCT can detect abnormal vasculature related to skin cancers. For example, early alteration in the vessel morphology can differentiate melanoma from dysplastic nevus [25].

Other applications of OCT include the evaluation and monitoring of inflammatory dermatosis [26] (Fig. 9.6) (e.g., contact dermatitis and psoriasis). Psoriasis shows characteristic features of hyperkeratosis, acanthosis, and dilated capillary loops on OCT [26]. Beyond its application in skin lesions, OCT is used to study skin aging, scars, wounds, burn assessments, and photodamage. It can image the nails and can diagnose onychomycosis [27].

Status of approval: All the OCT devices described have been accorded FDA approval in the United States and licensed for clinical use in Europe.

9.1.3 Reflectance Confocal Microscopy (RCM)

Principles: RCM imaging was demonstrated for in vivo human skin imaging for the first time in 1995 [28]. Since then, it has been the most promising noninvasive device for diagnosing skin cancers. The commercial RCM devices use a diode laser with a near-infrared wavelength (830 nm, laser power up to 35 mW). Unlike the US and conventional OCT, RCM images skin at cellular resolution (similar to histopathology). To achieve high-resolution images, in vivo, the RCM device has two pinholes in an optically conjugate plane (thus named 'confocal') that permit only selective transmission of the backscattered light from the illuminated point in the tissue while eliminating all the out-of-focus signals [29]. Various cells and organelles in the skin have different refractive indices, making them appear bright or dark on RCM. For example, cells with a high reflective index, such as melanin-containing cells (melanocytes and melanophages), collagen, and keratin, appear bright on RCM. On the other hand, the nucleus that has a low reflective index appears dark [30–32].

Currently available commercial devices and their imaging capabilities: RCM imaging provides optical sectioning of 2–5 μm and a lateral resolution of 1.0 μm. However, the imaging depth is limited to 250 microns (to the level of the papillary dermis) within the skin.

There are currently only two RCM devices available for clinical use: Vivascope 1500® (Vs 1500) and Vivascope 3000® (Vs 3000) (Caliber I.D. Inc. Rochester, NY, USA; MAVIG GmbH, Munich, Germany) (Fig. 9.11) [10]. Vs1500 is a bulkier skin contact device, also called a wide-probe RCM device, that needs to be attached to the skin to acquire images. This device is equipped with a dermatoscope or a "Vivacam® (Caliber I.D. Inc. Rochester, NY, USA; MAVIG GmbH, Munich, Germany)" to guide imaging within the lesion. One of the advantages of this device is the ability to image an entire lesion measuring up to 8 mm × 8 mm in size within a few minutes by creating mosaics (a large FOV image is obtained by stitching single frame images together at a given plane of depth within the skin). The mosaic enables a "bird's eye view" of the lesion (similar to 2× magnification images on

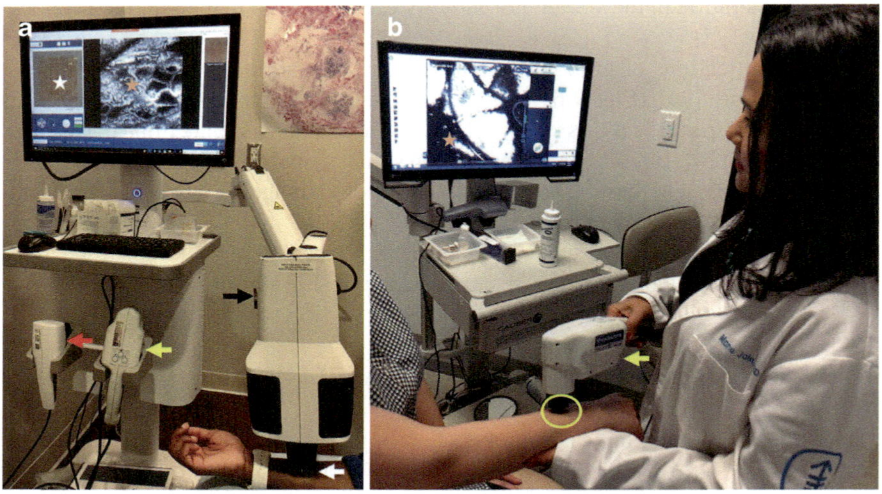

Fig. 9.11 Images of RCM devices (Vivascopes, Caliber I.D. Inc.). (**a**) A combined RCM device with an arm-mounted (Vivascope 1500; black arrow) and a handheld RCM (Vivascope 3000, also shown in **b**, yellow arrow) probe along with a digital dermatoscope (Vivacam; red arrow). The arm-mounted device (black arrow) is attached to the skin with a disposable plastic cone (white arrow). The device monitor shows a dermoscopy image (white asterisk) of the lesion acquired with the digital dermatoscope and the corresponding RCM image (pink asterisk). (**b**) Handheld RCM (Vivascope 3000; yellow arrow) probe pressed against the skin (yellow circle) with an RCM image shown on the monitor of the device (pink asterisk). There is no dermoscopy guidance while using the handheld device

histopathology) by providing architectural detail and identifying suspicious areas within the lesion. These areas can be digitally zoomed in to provide cellular-level information (similar to 20× magnification images on histopathology) that aids in diagnosis (Fig. 9.12).

RCM generates *en face* images. Thus, at least 3–4 mosaics are acquired at various depths in the skin: one at the stratum corneum, one at the stratum spinosum, one at the dermo-epidermal junction, and one at the dermis. Furthermore, to evaluate an area of interest within the mosaic, stacks (a collection of 0.5 mm × 0.5 mm images in consecutive depths) are acquired (Fig. 9.13 and Video 9.1). Contrary to the Vs 1500, the Vs 3000 is a handheld device that can be freely moved over the skin's surface. Therefore, it can evaluate lesions located in the anatomical sites of the nose, earlobes, eyelids, and genitalia where it is not possible to attach Vs1500. Although this device creates cellular-level images, it cannot provide architectural details of the lesions as only a small area of 0.5 mm × 0.5 mm within the lesion can be imaged. Ongoing efforts at 'video mosaicking' can mitigate this issue, where continuous videos can be captured by moving the device on the lesion and later stitched into a large FOV image.

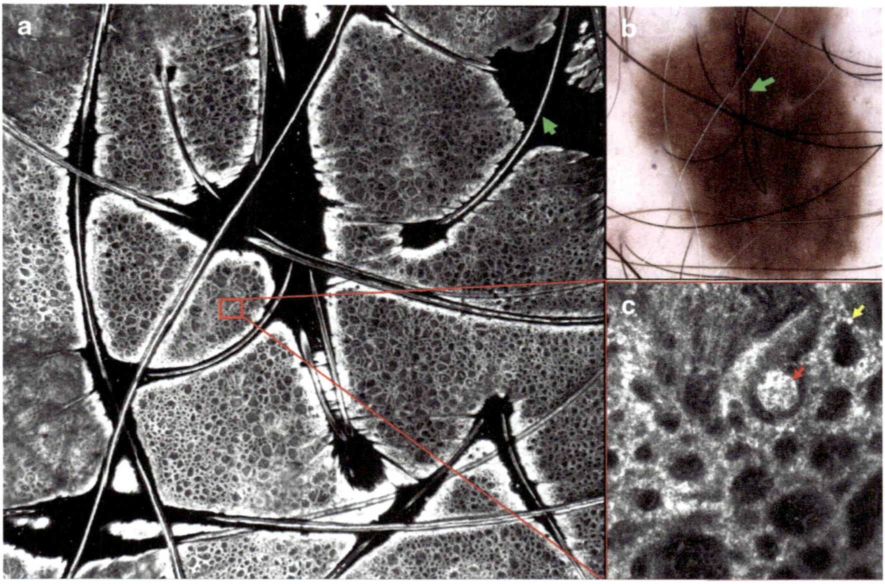

Fig. 9.12 Bedside image interpretation of a melanocytic lesion suspicious for melanoma using an arm-mounted (Vivascope 1500) RCM device. (**a**) Mosaic (~8 mm × 8 mm) acquired at the level of dermoepidermal junction (DEJ) covering the entire pigmented lesion seen in panel **b**. DEJ shows a "ringed pattern" and a few small dense dermal nests. Mosaic gives an overview of the architectural detail of the lesion (comparable with 2× magnification on H&E). (**c**) A digitally zoomed-in area from the mosaic (**a**) to evaluate an area of interest (red box on image **a**) within the mosaic shows a dermal nest (red arrow) and pigmented basal at the DEJ (yellow arrow). This magnification is similar to 30× on H&E. Green arrows indicate hair shafts in panels (**a**) and (**b**)

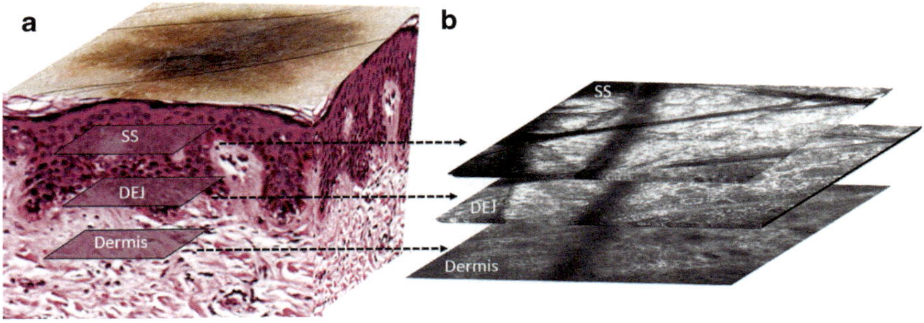

Fig. 9.13 Z-stack or Vivastack acquisition using RCM device. (**a**) Schematic diagram showing various skin layers, and (**b**) Several small fields of view (0.5 mm × 0.5 mm) RCM images were acquired in sequential depth from stratum spinosum to DEJ and then to the dermis. Vivastacks can be acquired using both the Vs1500 and Vs3000 RCM probes. See Video 9.1 for the movie

In addition to morphological details (Figs. 9.14, 9.15, 9.16, 9.17, and 9.18), RCM enables visualization of leukocyte trafficking within the vessels during live imaging sessions (Video 9.2).

Clinical applications: RCM's role as a noninvasive device has been well-established for diagnosing skin cancers, especially BCC and melanoma (Figs. 9.15 and 9.17) [33]. Features of skin cancers are well-defined on RCM and have their unique terminology [34, 35]. In clinics, it is primarily used in conjunction with clinical and dermoscopy. Its best application is to confirm lesions with high suspicion for BCC (clinically or on dermoscopy) to move directly to non-surgical treatment (lasers, PDT and Imiquimod) management by avoiding diagnostic biopsies. Overall, BCC has a sensitivity of 94% and a specificity of 85% with RCM. For melanoma, RCM is more accurate for diagnosis. It has improved the specificity of diagnosing melanoma over dermoscopy (from 42 to 82%) while maintaining a similar sensitivity (~90%) [36]. This improved specificity translates to a reduction of unnecessary surgical excisions by up to three-quarters compared to dermoscopy. Although RCM can identify features of SCCs, it cannot reliably differentiate between in situ SCC (SCCIS) and invasive SCC. A systematic review reported a sensitivity of 74% and specificity of 92% for diagnosing SCCs [37].

In addition, for diagnosing skin cancers, RCM is showing promise in monitoring treatment response noninvasively. Another excellent application of RCM is the margin mapping of large lesions with sub-clinical extensions such as lentigo maligna (LM). RCM also aids in procuring guided biopsies from these large lesions of LM [38] and EMPDs [39].

Other indications include the identification of superficial inflammatory skin diseases (psoriasiform, spongiotic, interface dermatitis) [40, 41], including features of graft-versus-host disease [42]. Additional applications are monitoring skin aging

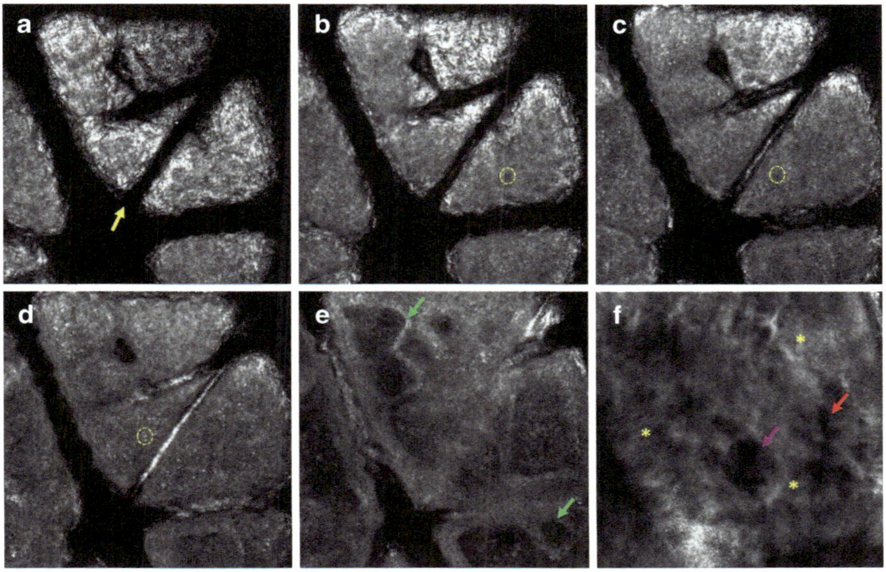

Fig. 9.14 Images of normal skin layers on RCM obtained from the left forearm of a 30-year-old female: (**a**) *Stratum corneum*: top-most brightest (keratin) anuclear layer of the epidermis. Dark linear structures are dermatoglyphics (yellow arrow). (**b**) *Stratum granulosum*: first nucleated layer composed of keratinocytes (yellow dotted-circle) that have bright cytoplasm (keratin) and dark nucleus forming a "regular honeycomb" pattern. (**c**) *Stratum spinosum*: similar in appearance to the granulosum but has smaller-sized keratinocytes. Dotted-circle shows three keratinocytes. (**d**) *Basal layer*: bright pigmented basal cells forming a "cobblestone pattern" (yellow dotted-circle). (**e**) *Dermoepidermal junction*: bright pigmented basal cells surrounding the central dark area of papillary dermis forming a "ringed pattern" (green arrows). (**f**) *Dermis*: mostly acellular composed of grayish to white collagen (yellow asterisks) with some dark, small, round-to-tubular vessels (red arrow) and bulb of a hair follicle (pink arrow). FOV of individual images = 500 μm × 500 μm

and hydration [43], assessing scar treatment [44], and skin pigmentation in melasma and vitiligo [45, 46].

RCM is not well-suited for imaging lesions with hyperkeratotic scales, ulceration or bleeding, and lesions located deeper than the papillary dermis [47].

Status of approval: RCM attained the current procedural terminology (CPT) code for 'billing' and 'image interpretation' in the United States for use as a routine diagnostic tool in dermatology [10].

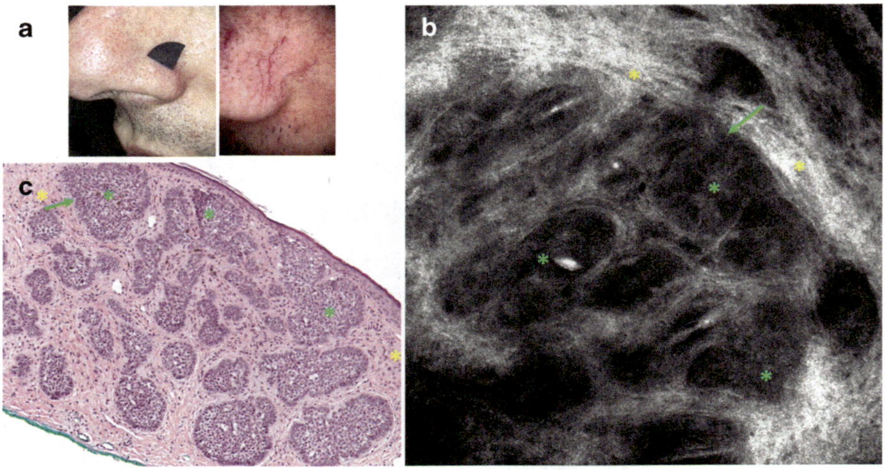

Fig. 9.15 Image of a nodular BCC on RCM obtained from a pink papule on the nose of a 50-year-old male: (**a**) Left: Clinical image of a pink papule, and right: dermoscopy image showing telangiectatic vessels. (**b**) RCM image shows multiple tumor nodules of BCC (green asterisks) along with palisading (green arrow) within the collagenous dermis (yellow asterisk). (**c**) The H&E revealed a nodular BCC (20× magnification)

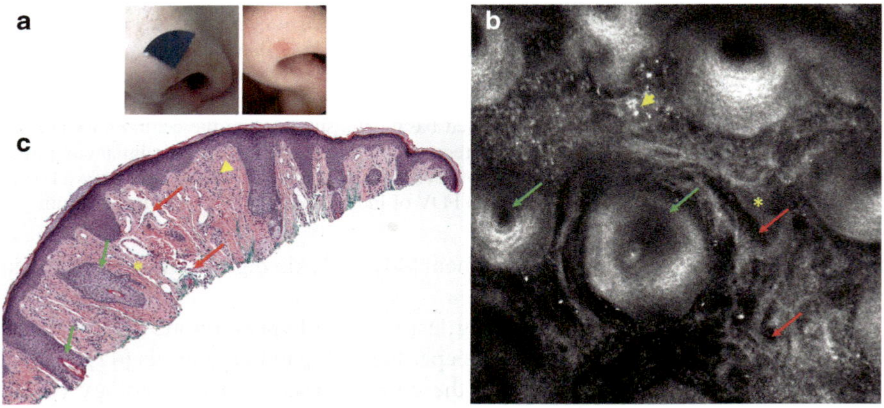

Fig. 9.16 Images of a fibrous papule on RCM obtained from a pink papule on the nose of a 30-year-old female: (**a**) On the left is a clinical image of a pink papule, and on the right is a dermoscopy image showing telangiectatic vessels. (**b**) The RCM image shows multiple hair follicles (green arrows) surrounded by a fibrous band (yellow asterisk), small bright inflammatory cells (yellow arrowheads), and prominent vessels (red arrows). BCC was not identified. (**c**) This lesion was diagnosed as a fibrous papule on H&E (20× magnification)

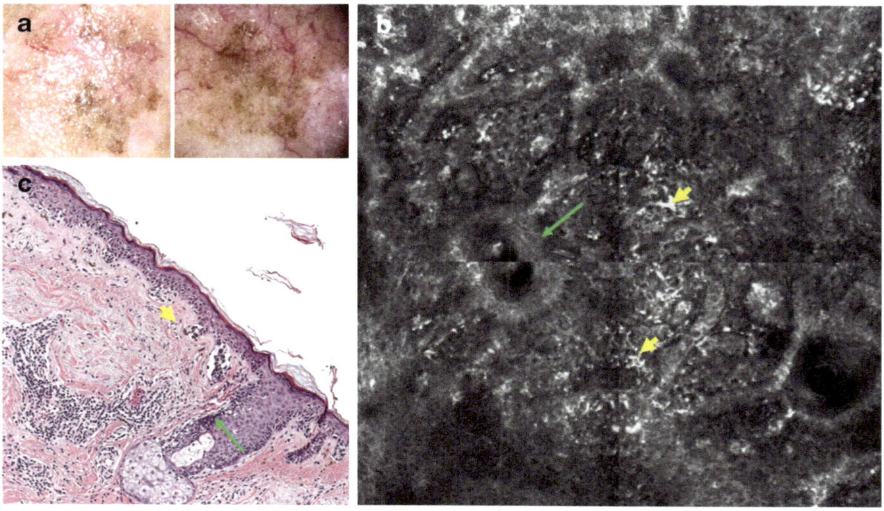

Fig. 9.17 Images of a lentigo maligna obtained from a brown macule on the cheek of a 65-year-old female: (**a**) On the left is a clinical image of a brown macule, and on the right is a dermoscopy image showing perifollicular pigmentation. (**b**) The RCM image shows big, round, and dendritic bright cells (pagetoid cells; yellow arrowheads) in the epidermis surrounding the hair follicles (green arrows). (**c**) This lesion was diagnosed as a lentigo maligna on H&E (20× magnification)

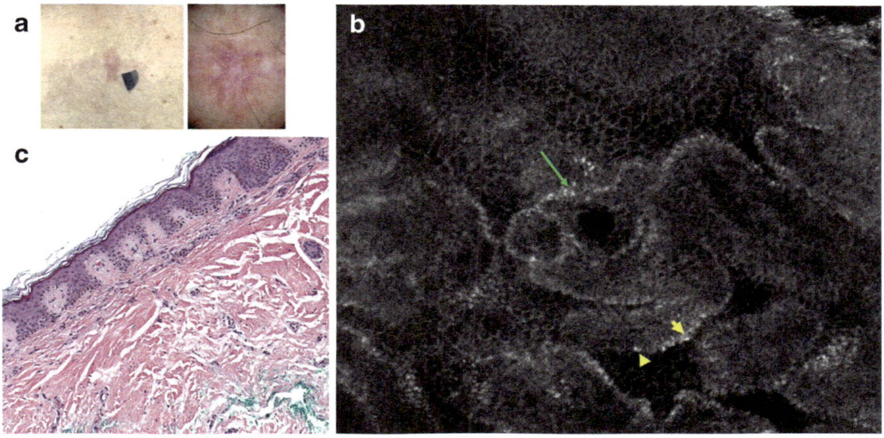

Fig. 9.18 Images of a solar lentigo (SL) obtained from a brown macule on the abdomen of a 50-year-old male: (**a**) On the left is a clinical image of a pigmented macule in a scar-like area, and on the right is a dermoscopy image showing shiny white structures and pigmentation. (**b**) The RCM image shows elongated rete-ridges (green arrows) lined by homogenous pigmented bright cells of the basal layer (yellow arrowheads). (**c**) The lesion was a lentigo-like lesion with hyperpigmentation overlying a dermal scar on H&E (20× magnification)

9.1.4 Multiphoton Microscopy (MPM)

Principles: MPM is a nonlinear optical imaging technique that provides unique molecular and cellular specificity based on the emission of endogenous signals from various tissue structures and cells within the skin. There are two distinct endogenous signals: two-photon excited fluorescence (TPEF) signal from reduced nicotinamide adenine dinucleotide phosphate (NADPH), flavin adenine dinucleotide (FAD), melanin, keratin, and elastin fibers, and second harmonic generation (SHG) signal from collagen [48–52]. These signals can be pseudo-color-coded to provide better and differential visualization of the tissue.

Currently available commercial devices and their imaging capabilities: MPTflex device (Jenlab, Germany) is the only MPM commercial device with promising results for imaging clinic skin lesions. It uses a tunable Ti:Sapphire femtosecond laser as a light source (laser power: 2–50 mW, wavelength: 710–920 nm). As compared to RCM and OCT, this device has a higher lateral and axial resolution of <0.5 μm and <2 μm; however, the FOV is relatively smaller ~350 μm × 350 μm. Like RCM, MPM images skin in an en face manner, and the imaging depth is limited to ~200 μm.

Clinical applications: The slow speed of image acquisition and a small field of view make MPM imaging in clinics challenging. MPM can potentially diagnose BCCs and melanoma [53–56] (Figs. 9.19 and 9.20). Their features have been

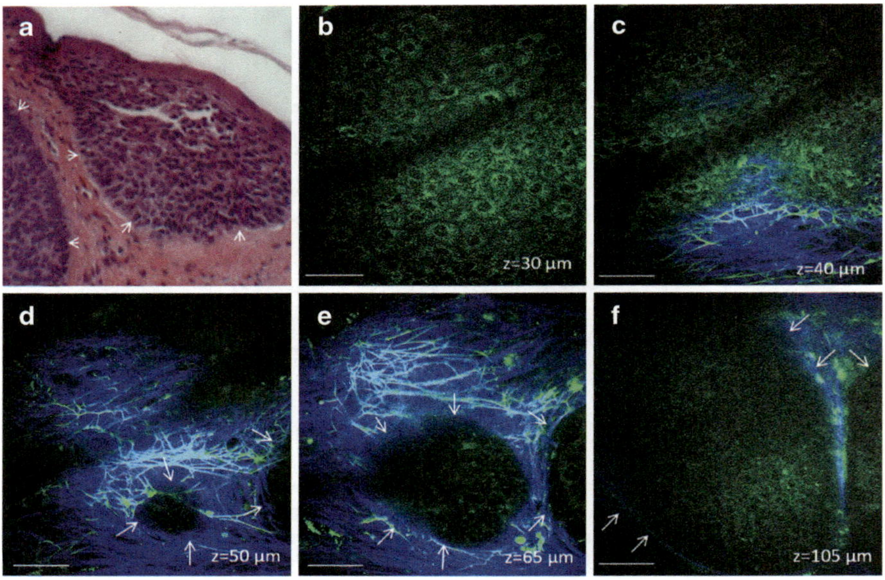

Fig. 9.19 Images of a basal cell carcinoma (BCC) on MPM. (**a**) H&E image showing BCC nests (arrows). (**b–f**) Horizontal MPM images (TPEF-green; SHG-blue) at different depths (z) showing the epidermal morphology of the lesion (**b**, **c**) and the BCC nests (**d–f**) (arrows) showing tumor cells surrounded by collagen (blue) and elastin (green) fibers. The scale bar is 40 μm. (*Courtesy:* Mihaela Balu, PhD, Associate Researcher. Nonlinear Optical Microscopy Lab Beckman Laser Institute and Medical Clinic. University of California. Irvine, USA)

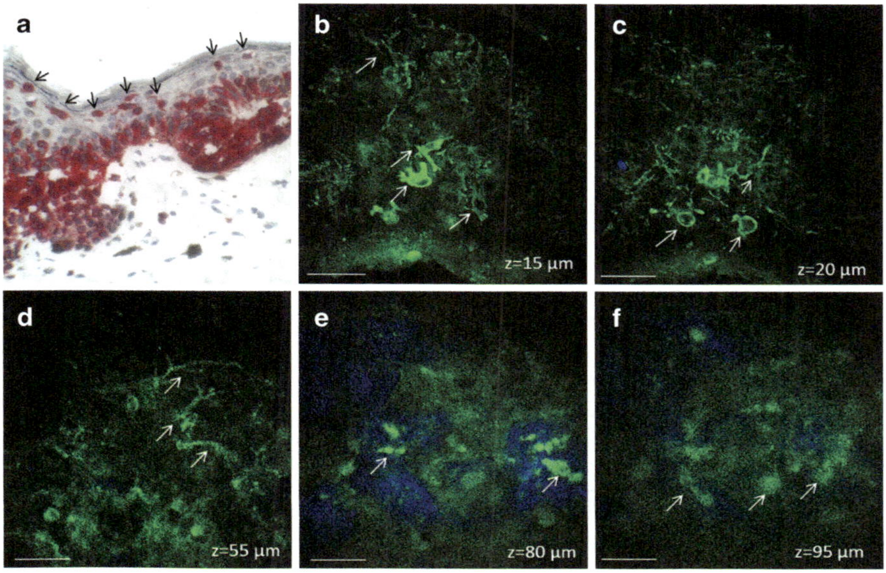

Fig. 9.20 Images of an invasive melanoma on MPM. (**a**) Histopathology image showing advanced melanocytes (arrows) in upper epidermal layers. (**b–f**) Horizontal MPM images (TPEF-green; SHG-blue) at different depths (z) showing: (**b**, **c**) migrating melanocytes (arrows) in upper epidermal layers; (**d**) proliferation of melanocytes (arrows) in the basal layer; (**e**, **f**) invasion of melanoma cells and probably melanophages in the dermis. The scale bar is 40 µm. (*Courtesy:* Mihaela Balu, PhD, Associate Researcher. Nonlinear Optical Microscopy Lab Beckman Laser Institute and Medical Clinic. University of California. Irvine, USA)

defined in the literature [53–56]. One study demonstrated a sensitivity of 75% and specificity of 80% for diagnosing melanoma based on these features [56]. However, large-scale clinical studies are necessary to validate this technique in clinics. Assessment of pigmentary skin disorders [57, 58], alopecia [59], cell metabolism, and monitoring effects of cosmetic treatment [60, 61] are additional indications of MPM.

Limitations include a small field of view and slow imaging speed. Also, similar to RCM imaging, shallow depth of imaging can only image superficial skin lesions.

Status of approval: MPTflex has obtained a CE-certified class 1 M/IIa medical product.

9.1.5 Combined Reflectance Confocal and Optical Coherence Tomography (RCM-OCT) Device

As discussed, all noninvasive devices have their advantages and limitations. None of the existing devices is perfect for imaging all types of skin lesions. Thus, the current focus is to provide a 'dream machine" to clinicians by combining various technologies. Combination devices include RCM-OCT, RCM-MPM, and RCM-Raman

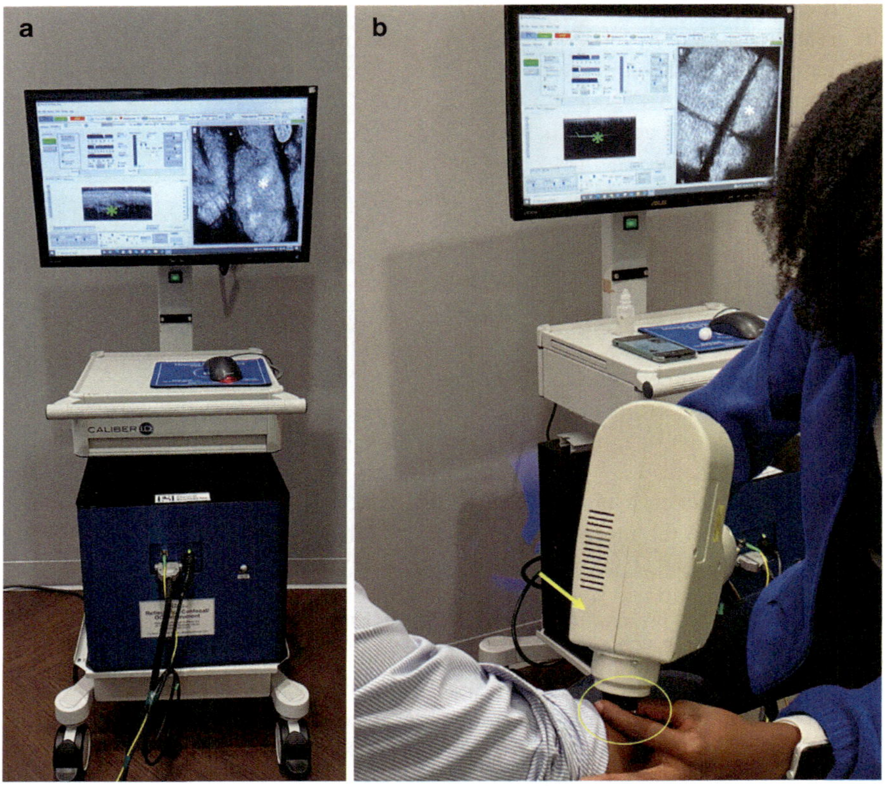

Fig. 9.21 Images of an RCM-OCT device. (**a**) RCM-OCT device on a wheelable trolley. The attached monitor shows an *en face* RCM image (white asterisk) and a vertical OCT image (green asterisk) being acquired simultaneously from the normal skin of a healthy volunteer. (**b**) Combined RCM-OCT handheld probe (yellow arrow) placed on the skin (yellow circle) for image acquisition

spectroscopy, among others. Here, we will only discuss the RCM-OCT device, as this prototype is available for imaging in clinics.

Principles: The OCT subsystem retrieves both the reflectance and birefringence information from the tissue, while the RCM subsystem uses a standard reflectance confocal scheme. A dichroic mirror combines RCM and OCT subsystems into the common optical imaging path to produce co-registered RCM and OCT images [62].

Currently available commercial devices and their imaging capabilities: Currently, only one prototype of this device is available from Physical Sciences, Inc., Andover, MA. This device simultaneously generates *en face* RCM images and cross-sectional OCT images. The FOV for the RCM image is 750 μm (similar to the handheld probe of RCM), while the FOV for OCT is 2 mm (similar to conventional OCT). RCM-OCT device can acquire several RCM stacks and OCT raster scans of 2 mm × 2 mm (multiple OCT cross-sectional scans with 5 μm separation) within a few minutes per lesion. Imaging depth on OCT is ~1 mm and on RCM is ~200 microns (Fig. 9.21) [63].

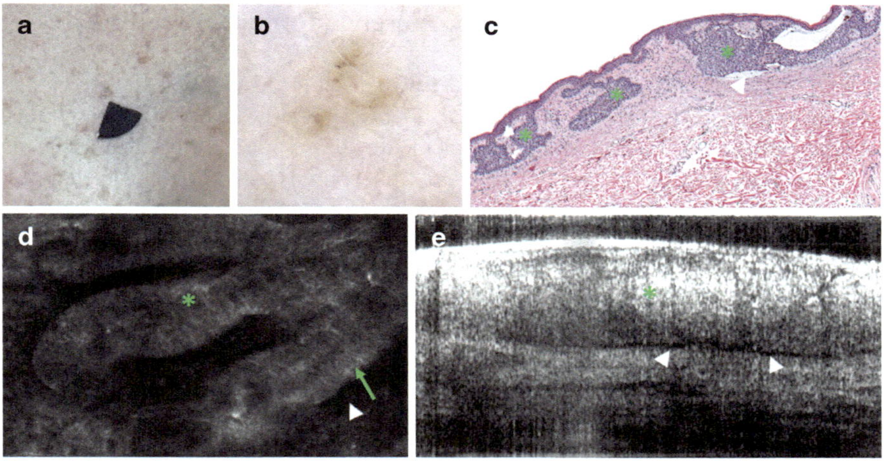

Fig. 9.22 Images of a BCC on an RCM-OCT device obtained from a pink papule on the chest of a 45-year-old female. (**a**) Clinical image. (**b**) Dermoscopy image shows an ovoid nest and pigmentation. (**c**) H&E image (20× mag.) of a superficial/early nodular BCC (green asterisk) and clefting (white arrowhead). (**d**) RCM image at the DEJ shows cords of BCC (green asterisk) with palisading (green arrow) and clefting (white arrowhead). (**e**) OCT image shows an oval grayish nodule in continuation with the epidermis and dark line of clefting at the lower edge (white arrowhead)

Clinical applications: This prototype is not yet commercialized. Initial clinical studies showed its utility for the management of BCC (Fig. 9.22) [64]. Recently, a clinical pilot study showed increased specificity to 100% (compared to RCM-alone) for detecting BCC in small, difficult-to-diagnose papules on dermoscopy [63]. Additional applications include delineating BCC margins during Mohs surgery and managing BCC lesions on the complex area of the head and neck [65, 66]. Future, large-scale clinical studies are warranted to establish its clinical potential.

Status of approval: Investigational device. Not yet FDA approved.

9.2 Ex Vivo Microscopy in Dermatology (EVM)

Ex vivo microscopy (EVM) is still a developing field in dermatology. Many existing IVM imaging devices can also image freshly excised tissues. Here, we will discuss two emerging commercially available EVM devices that show promising results in surgical settings: an OCT-based device and a confocal microscopy-based device. These devices can rapidly image thick, fresh tissue without requiring time-consuming and costly tissue processing, making it an alternative to frozen section analysis. Due to their compact design, the devices can be used in the operating room and dermatology suits. Moreover, since tissues are not cut, they can be saved for later molecular analysis.

9.2.1 Ex Vivo Full-Field Optical Coherence Tomography (FF-OCT)

Principles: A recent time-domain-based full-field (FF-OCT device) can evaluate excised tissues. This device has a crystal fiber light source that provides cellular-level images. Mirau interferometer makes the device compact for clinical use. This device uses Ce:YAG single-crystal fiber as a light source (445–560 nm wavelength). No fluorescent dye/contrast agent is used. The signals collected are backscattered light from the tissue [67].

Currently available commercial devices and their imaging capabilities: ApolloVue® B100 (Apollo Medical Optics, Taipei, Taiwan) is commercially available for imaging excised tissues. It has a high lateral and axial resolution of 1.1 μm and 1.5 μm to create cellular-resolution images. Large FOV mosaics are acquired (measuring ~1 mm × 1 mm) to provide architectural details. One mosaic takes around 6.5 min of acquisition time. The mosaic can be zoomed in digitally, in real-time, to evaluate lesions. The device comes with a cassette (similar to the tissue cassettes used for histopathology) to place tissues for imaging (Fig. 9.23) [67].

Clinical applications: So far, only one study has demonstrated its capability to image formalin-fixed, thick tissue sections [67]. In this study, novices and experts revealed 71–83% diagnostic accuracy for BCC detection [67]. Clinical studies are ongoing to assess diagnostic accuracy in fresh tissues obtained from Mohs surgery (Fig. 9.23).

Limitations include a learning curve due to the gray-scale nature of the images and the inability to use any dye to enhance the contrast.

Status of approval: FDA Class I listing.

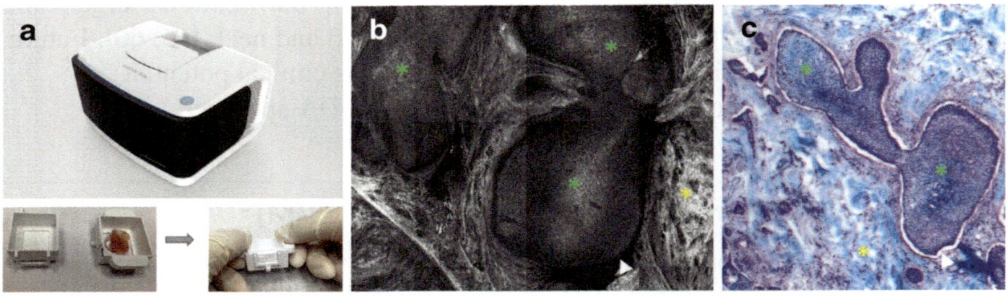

Fig. 9.23 Images of a nodular BCC on ex vivo full-field optical coherence tomography (FF-OCT). (**a**) The top panel shows a compact FFOCT device; the bottom panels show a regular pathology cassette for placing fresh tissue for imaging. (**b**) FFOCT image of BCC tumor nodules (green asterisks) with clefting (white arrowhead) seen in the bright collagenous dermis (yellow asterisk). (**c**) Corresponding toluidine blue histopathology image of the nodular BCC

9.2.2 Ex Vivo Confocal Microscopy (Reflectance and Fluorescence)

Principles: This device utilizes similar principles of in vivo confocal microscopy. Optically thin sections are created (without mechanical tissue cutting) within the fresh, thick piece of tissue by scanning a point source of light (laser) and rejecting out-of-focus light through a pinhole. For nuclear contrast, tissue is briefly (~30 s) dipped in acridine orange, a fluorescent dye. Other fluorescent dyes used for imaging are fluorescein and indocyanine. The device images tissues in both reflectance (830 nm wavelength) and fluorescent (488 nm or 658 nm wavelength) modes. The reflectance signal (originating from the keratin in the cytoplasm and collagen) is converted into a pink color, mimicking eosin staining. The fluorescent signal (from the nucleus) is converted to purple, mimicking hematoxylin staining. Thus, a digitally colored purple and pink image is created that simulates Haematoxylin and Eosin (H&E) staining on histopathology [68].

Currently available commercial devices and their imaging capabilities: Vivascope 2500 (Caliber I.D. Inc. Rochester, NY, USA; MAVIG GmbH, Munich, Germany) is the only commercial CM for imaging freshly excised tissues. This device images tissue in either *en face* (similar to RCM) or a cross-section view (similar to histology). An entire tissue measuring up to 20 mm × 20 mm can be imaged as a single mosaic and then digitally zoomed to get high-resolution cellular-level images. Furthermore, stacks (similar to in vivo RCM) are acquired in the areas of interest. The lateral and axial spatial resolutions are 1 μm and 3 μm, respectively. However, unlike in vivo RCM devices, ex vivo CM device is made for surface imaging and cannot image deeper than ~30 μm within the tissue. For imaging, the tissue is placed on a glass slide and then compressed using a mechanical pressing device or a foam to flatten the tissue, enabling good images even at the tissue edges (Fig. 9.24 and Video 9.3) [68]. Recently, an automated 3D mosaicking approach was created, and tissue flattening was achieved to improve the visualization of epidermal margins [69].

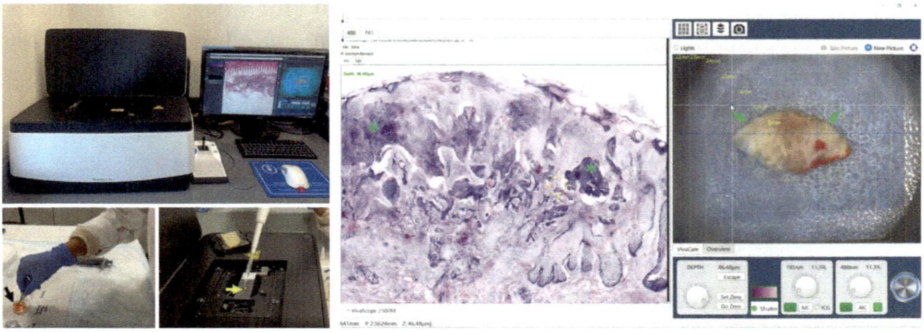

Fig. 9.24 Images of an ex vivo confocal microscope device (EVCM). (**Left image**) Top-panel shows an EVCM device with an attached monitor. The bottom left panel shows fresh tissue dipped in acridine orange dye (black arrow); the bottom right panel shows stained tissue (yellow arrow) mounted on a regular glass slide for imaging. (**Right image**) Digitally colored purple-pink EVCM image of a nodular BCC (green asterisks) from a freshly excised Mohs surgical tissue (green arrows)

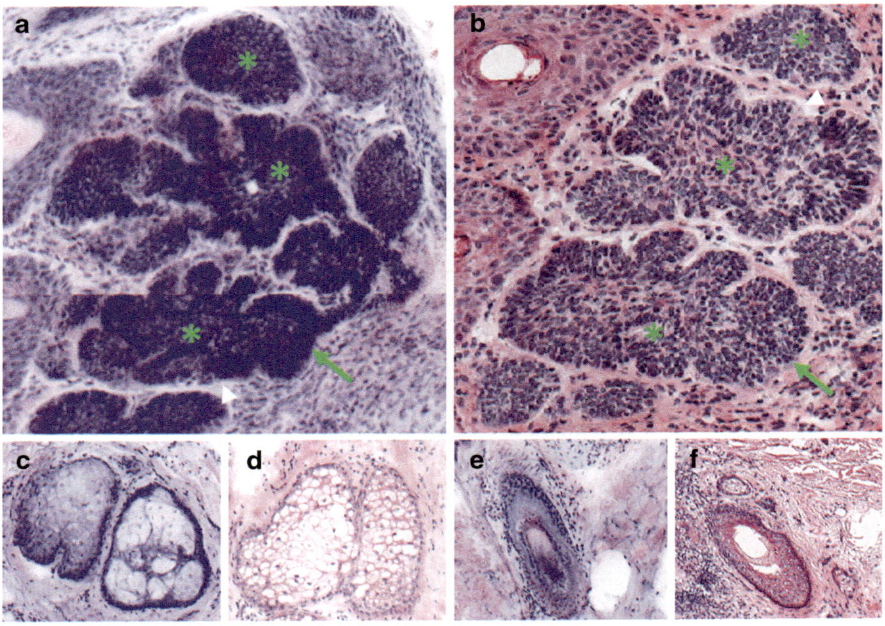

Fig. 9.25 Digitally colored purple-pink images from Mohs surgical margins on ex vivo confocal microscope device (EVCM). (**a**, **c**, **e**) EVCM images of (**a**) BCC nodules (green asterisks) with palisading (green arrow) and clefting (white arrowhead), (**c**) Sebaceous gland lobules, (**e**) A hair follicle in vertical section; and (**b**, **d**, **f**) their corresponding H&E-stained images. H&E = 10× magnification

Clinical applications: EVCM device is employed intra-operatively for tumor margin assessment of BCC during Mohs surgery. It has shown a high sensitivity of 88% and specificity of 99% for detecting residual BCCs (Fig. 9.25) [70–72]. Additionally, this device imaged surgical margins of SCCs [73, 74] and LM [75]. However, its role is not well-established for these malignancies. Furthermore, this device can rapidly evaluate melanocytic lesions [76], lesions of nails and hair, infectious diseases (such as viral and fungal infections), and inflammatory diseases [77]. It shows promise in the field of aesthetic medicine [77].

Status of approval: FDA Class 1 Medical Device.

9.3 Current Challenges for Clinical Integration of Noninvasive Imaging and Future Directions

Despite promising results, thus far, these devices have been used only in select large hospitals and academic centers. This limited use is mainly related to the lack of expert readers to analyze these images, the high cost of the devices, and the need for a dedicated and trained technician to acquire good-quality images. Steps such as teaching-training courses and building portable and cheaper devices [78–80] may aid in the expanding adoption of this technology (Fig. 9.26). Furthermore, AI algorithms were developed to assist the technicians in image acquisition and flagging suspicious lesions for untrained dermatologists [81–85]. Lastly, as all these devices acquire images in a digital format, they can be shared with an expert reader remotely for consultation (Fig. 9.27) [86, 87].

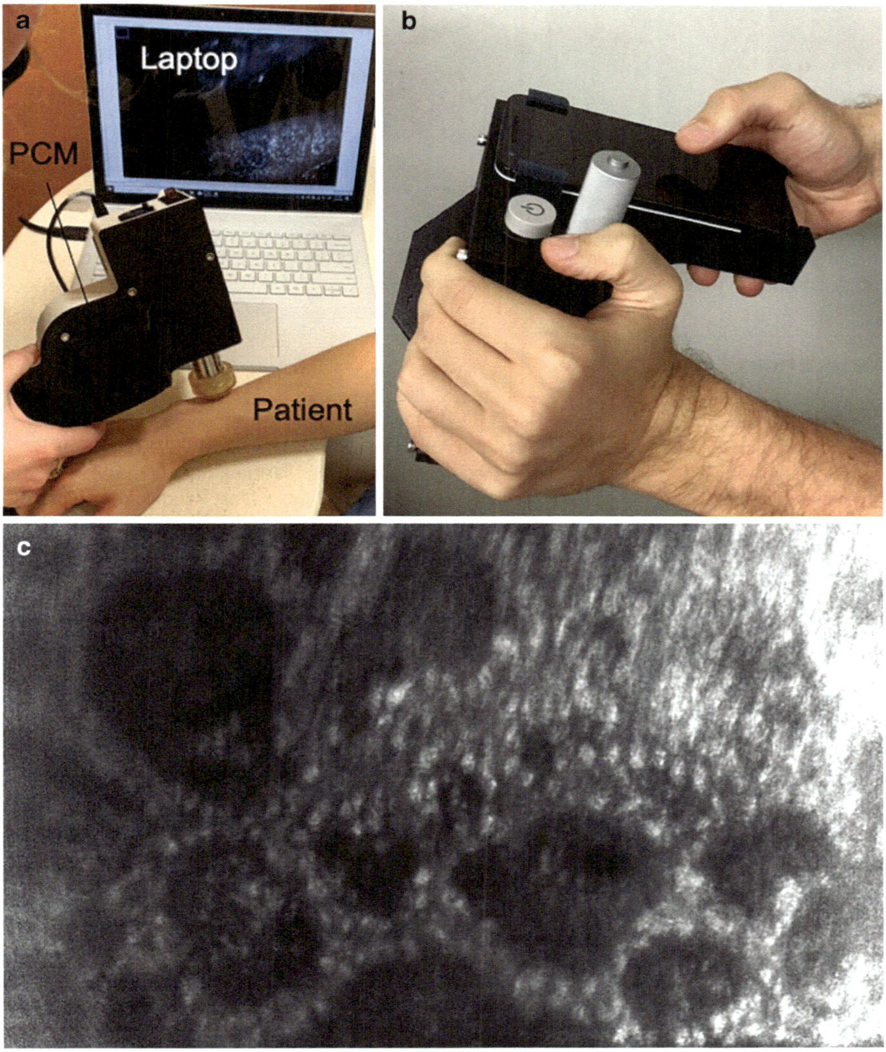

Fig. 9.26 Portable RCM devices. (**a**) Photo of a portable confocal microscope using near-infrared light. (**b**) Photo of a smartphone-based portable confocal microscope. (**c**) The RCM image showing a "ringed pattern" at the DEJ. The image quality is comparable with the commercial RCM devices. (*Courtesy:* Dongkyun Kang, PhD. Department of Biomedical Engineering. University of Arizona. Tucson, USA)

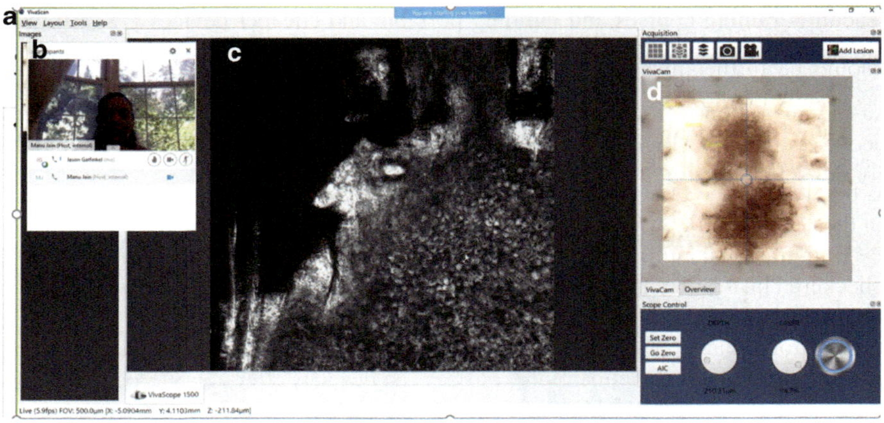

Fig. 9.27 Tele-reflectance confocal microscopy imaging session. (**a**) Screenshot of a live RCM imaging session shared with a remote expert reader (**b**). (**c**) RCM of the lesion, and (**d**) Dermoscopy (Vivacam) image of the same lesion

References

1. Choi JH, Kim YJ, Kim H, Nam SH, Choi YW. Distribution of basal cell carcinoma and squamous cell carcinoma by facial esthetic unit. Arch Plast Surg. 2013;40(4):387–91.
2. Al-Shakhli H, Harcourt D, Kenealy J. Psychological distress surrounding diagnosis of malignant and nonmalignant skin lesions at a pigmented lesion clinic. J Plast Reconstr Aesthet Surg. 2006;59(5):479–86.
3. Coldiron B, Ratnarathorn M. Scope of physician procedures independently billed by mid-level providers in the office setting. JAMA Dermatol. 2014;150(11):1153–9.
4. Nault A, Zhang C, Kim K, Saha S, Bennett DD, Xu YG. Biopsy use in skin cancer diagnosis: comparing dermatology physicians and advanced practice professionals. JAMA Dermatol. 2015;151(8):899–902.
5. Joyce K, Dorairaj J, Byrne M, Regan PJ, Kelly J, Jones D, et al. Are plastic surgeons excising too many benign lesions? Skin lesions excised in a tertiary referral centre. Int J Surg. 2012;10:S53–S109.
6. Buch J, Criton S. Dermoscopy Saga—a tale of 5 centuries. Indian J Dermatol. 2021;66(2):174–8.
7. Wozniak-Rito A, Zalaudek I, Rudnicka L. Dermoscopy of basal cell carcinoma. Clin Exp Dermatol. 2018;43:241–7.
8. Reiter O, Mimouni I, Gdalevich M, Marghoob AA, Levi A, Hodak E, et al. The diagnostic accuracy of dermoscopy for basal cell carcinoma: a systematic review and meta-analysis. J Am Acad Dermatol. 2019;80:1380–8.
9. Altamura D, Menzies SW, Argenziano G, Zalaudek I, Soyer HP, Sera F, et al. Dermatoscopy of basal cell carcinoma: morphologic variability of global and local features and accuracy of diagnosis. J Am Acad Dermatol. 2010;62:67–75.
10. Navarrete-Dechent C, Fischer C, Tkaczyk E, Jain M. Chapter 5. Principles of non-invasive diagnostic techniques in dermatology. vol 1. Section 2. Moschella and Hurley's dermatology. 4th ed. Jaypee Brothers Medical Publisher.
11. Levy J, Barrett DL, Harris N, Jeong JJ, Yang X, Chen SC. High-frequency ultrasound in clinical dermatology: a review. Ultrasound J. 2021;13(1):24.
12. Wortsman X. Common applications of dermatologic sonography. J Ultrasound Med. 2012;31:97–111. Sonography of cutaneous and ungual lumps and bumps. Wortsman, Ximena. Elsevier Inc. Ultrasound clinics, 2012–10, Vol. 7(4), p. 505–523.

13. Harland CC, Kale SG, Jackson P, Mortimer PS, Bamber JC. Differentiation of common benign pigmented skin lesions from melanoma by high-resolution ultrasound. Br J Dermatol. 2000;143(2):281–9.
14. Catalano O, Roldan FA, Varelli C, Bard R, Corvino A, Wortsman X. Skin cancer: findings and role of high-resolution ultrasound. J Ultrasound. 2019;22:423–31.
15. Welzel J, Lankenau E, Birngruber R, Engelhardt R. Optical coherence tomography of the human skin. J Am Acad Dermatol. 1997;37(6):958–63.
16. Sattler E, Kästle R, Welzel J. Optical coherence tomography in dermatology. J Biomed Opt. 2013;18(6):061224.
17. Wang YJ, Huang YK, Wang JY, Wu YH. In vivo characterization of large cell acanthoma by cellular resolution optical coherent tomography. Photodiagn Photodyn Ther. 2019;26:199–202.
18. Dubois A. High-resolution optical coherence tomography application in dermatology. In: Proceedings of imaging and applied optics 2019 (COSI, IS, MATH, pcAOP). OSA technical digest (Optical Society of America, 2019). Paper ITh2B.1.
19. Wan B, Ganier C, Du-Harpur X, et al. Applications and future directions for optical coherence tomography in dermatology. Br J Dermatol. 2021;184(6):1014–22.
20. Ferrante di Ruffano L, Dinnes J, Deeks JJ, et al. Optical coherence tomography for diagnosing skin cancer in adults. Cochrane Database Syst Rev. 2018;12(12):CD013189.
21. Ulrich M, von Braunmuehl T, Kurzen H, Dirschka T, Kellner C, Sattler E, et al. The sensitivity and specificity of optical coherence tomography for the assisted diagnosis of nonpigmented basal cell carcinoma: an observational study. Br J Dermatol. 2015;173(3):428–35.
22. Olsen J, Themstrup L, De Carvalho N, Mogensen M, Pellacani G, Jemec GB. Diagnostic accuracy of optical coherence tomography in actinic keratosis and basal cell carcinoma. Photodiagn Photodyn Ther. 2016;16:44–9.
23. Wang YJ, Wang JY, Wu YH. Application of cellular resolution full-field optical coherence tomography in vivo for the diagnosis of skin tumours and inflammatory skin diseases: a pilot study. Dermatology. 2022;238(1):121–31.
24. Ruini C, Schuh S, Gust C, Kendziora B, Frommherz L, French LE, et al. Line-field optical coherence tomography: in vivo diagnosis of basal cell carcinoma subtypes compared with histopathology. Clin Exp Dermatol. 2021;46(8):1471–81.
25. De Carvalho N, Ciardo S, Cesinaro AM, Gbe J, Ulrich M, Welzel J, et al. In vivo micro-angiography by means of speckle-variance optical coherence tomography (SV-OCT) is able to detect microscopic vascular changes in naevus to melanoma transition. J Eur Acad Dermatol Venereol. 2016;30(10):e67–8.
26. Morsy H, Kamp S, Thrane L, Behrendt N, Saunder B, Zayan H, et al. Optical coherence tomography imaging of psoriasis vulgaris: correlation with histology and disease severity. Arch Dermatol Res. 2010;302(2):105–11.
27. Abuzahra F, Spöler F, Först M, Brans R, Erdmann MHF, et al. Pilot study: optical coherence tomography as a noninvasive diagnostic perspective for real time visualisation of onychomycosis. Mycoses. 2010;53(4):334–9.
28. Rajadhyaksha M, Grossman M, Esterowitz D, Webb RH, Anderson RR, et al. In vivo confocal scanning laser microscopy of human skin: melanin provides strong contrast. J Invest Dermatol. 1995;104(6):946–52.
29. González S. Confocal reflectance microscopy in dermatology: promise and reality of non-invasive diagnosis and monitoring. Actas Dermosifiliogr. 2009;100(Suppl 2):59–69.
30. Levine A, Markowitz O. Introduction to reflectance confocal microscopy and its use in clinical practice. JAAD Case Rep. 2018;4(10):1014–23.
31. Jain M, Pulijal SV, Rajadhyaksha M, Halpern AC, Gonzalez S. Evaluation of bedside diagnostic accuracy, learning curve, and challenges for a novice reflectance confocal microscopy reader for skin cancer detection in vivo. JAMA Dermatol. 2018;154(8):962–5.
32. Sahu A, Cordero J, Wu X, Kossatz S, Harris U, Franca PDD, et al. Combined PARP1-targeted nuclear contrast and reflectance contrast enhances confocal microscopic detection of basal cell carcinoma. J Nucl Med. 2022;63(6):912–8.

33. Dinnes J, Deeks JJ, Chuchu N, Saleh D, Bayliss SE, Takwoingi Y, et al.; Cochrane Skin Cancer Diagnostic Test Accuracy Group. Reflectance confocal microscopy for diagnosing keratinocyte skin cancers in adults. Cochrane Database Syst Rev. 2018;12(12):CD013191.
34. Navarrete-Dechent C, Liopyris K, Monnier J, Aleissa S, Boyce LM, Longo C, et al. Reflectance confocal microscopy terminology glossary for melanocytic skin lesions: a systematic review. J Am Acad Dermatol. 2021;84(1):102–19.
35. Navarrete-Dechent C, DeRosa AP, Longo C, Liopyris K, Oliviero M, Rabinovitz H, et al. Reflectance confocal microscopy terminology glossary for nonmelanocytic skin lesions: a systematic review. J Am Acad Dermatol. 2019;80(5):1414–1427.e3.
36. Dinnes J, Deeks JJ, Saleh D, Chuchu N, Bayliss SE, Patel L, et al. Reflectance confocal microscopy for diagnosing cutaneous melanoma in adults. Cochrane Database Syst Rev. 2018;12(12):CD013190.
37. Nguyen KP, Peppelman M, Hoogedoorn L, Van Erp PE, Gerritsen MP. The current role of in vivo reflectance confocal microscopy within the continuum of actinic keratosis and squamous cell carcinoma: a systematic review. Eur J Dermatol. 2016;26(6):549–65.
38. Guitera P, Pellacani G, Crotty KA, Scolyer RA, Li LX, Bassoli S, et al. The impact of in vivo reflectance confocal microscopy on the diagnostic accuracy of lentigo maligna and equivocal pigmented and nonpigmented macules of the face. J Invest Dermatol. 2010;130:2080–91.
39. Yélamos O, Hibler BP, Cordova M, Hollmann TJ, Kose K, Marchetti MA, et al. Handheld reflectance confocal microscopy for the detection of recurrent extramammary Paget disease. JAMA Dermatol. 2017;153(7):689–93.
40. Grajdeanu IA, Statescu L, Vata D, Popescu IA, Porumb-Andrese E, Patrascu AI, et al. Imaging techniques in the diagnosis and monitoring of psoriasis. Exp Ther Med. 2019;18(6):4974–80.
41. Ardigo M, Longo C, Gonzalez S, International Confocal Working Group Inflammatory Skin Diseases Project. Multicentre study on inflammatory skin diseases from the international confocal working group: specific confocal microscopy features and an algorithmic method of diagnosis. Br J Dermatol. 2016;175(2):364–74.
42. Reingold RE, Monnier J, Ardigò M, Stoll JR, Pena MC, Nanda JK, et al. Real-time reflectance confocal microscopy of cutaneous graft-versus-host disease correlates with histopathology. Transplant Cell Ther. 2022;28(1):51.e1–51.e14.
43. Manfredini M, Mazzaglia G, Ciardo S, Simonazzi S, Farnetani F, Longo C, et al. Does skin hydration influence keratinocyte biology? In vivo evaluation of microscopic skin changes induced by moisturizers by means of reflectance confocal microscopy. Skin Res Technol. 2013;19(3):299–307.
44. Guida S, Pellacani G, Bencini PL. Picosecond laser treatment of atrophic and hypertrophic surgical scars: in vivo monitoring of results by means of 3D imaging and reflectance confocal microscopy. Skin Res Technol. 2019;25(6):896–902.
45. Ardigo M, Malizewsky I, Dell'anna ML, Berardesca E, Picardo M. Preliminary evaluation of vitiligo using in vivo reflectance confocal microscopy. J Eur Acad Dermatol Venereol. 2007;21(10):1344–50.
46. Ardigo M, Cameli N, Berardesca E, Gonzalez S. Characterization and evaluation of pigment distribution and response to therapy in melasma using in vivo reflectance confocal microscopy: a preliminary study. J Eur Acad Dermatol Venereol. 2010;24(11):1296–303.
47. Franceschini C, Persechino F, Ardigò M. In vivo reflectance confocal microscopy in general dermatology: how to choose the right indication. Dermatol Pract Concept. 2020;10(2):e2020032.
48. Masters BR, So PTC, Gratton E. Optical biopsy of in vivo human skin: multiphoton excitation microscopy. Laser Med Sci. 1998;13:196–203.
49. Konig K, Riemann I. High-resolution multiphoton tomography of human skin with subcellular spatial resolution and picosecond time resolution. J Biomed Opt. 2003;8(3):432–9.
50. Balu M, Mazhar A, Hayakawa CK, Mittal R, Krasieva TB, König K, et al. In vivo multiphoton NADH fluorescence reveals depth-dependent keratinocyte metabolism in human skin. Biophys J. 2013;104(1):258–67.
51. Pouli D, Balu M, Alonzo CA, Liu Z, Quinn KP, Rius-Diaz F, et al. Imaging mitochondrial dynamics in human skin reveals depth-dependent hypoxia and malignant potential for diagnosis. Sci Transl Med. 2016;8(367):367ra169.

52. Fast A, Lal A, Durkin AF, Lentsch G, Harris RM, Zachary CB, et al. Fast, large area multiphoton exoscope (FLAME) for macroscopic imaging with microscopic resolution of human skin. Sci Rep. 2020;10(1):18093.
53. Balu M, Kelly KM, Zachary CB, Harris RM, Krasieva TB, König K, et al. Distinguishing between benign and malignant melanocytic nevi by in vivo multiphoton microscopy. Cancer Res. 2014;74(10):2688–97.
54. Balu M, Zachary CB, Harris RM, Krasieva TB, König K, Tromberg BJ, et al. In vivo multiphoton microscopy of basal cell carcinoma. JAMA Dermatol. 2015;151(10):1068–74.
55. Lentsch G, Valdebran M, Saknite I, Smith J, Linden KG, König K, et al. Noninvasive optical biopsy by multiphoton microscopy identifies the live morphology of common melanocytic nevi. Pigment Cell Melanoma Res. 2020;33:869–77.
56. Dimitrow E, Ziemer M, Koehler MJ, Norgauer J, König K, Elsner P, et al. Sensitivity and specificity of multiphoton laser tomography for in vivo and ex vivo diagnosis of malignant melanoma. J Invest Dermatol. 2009;129:1752–8.
57. Saager RB, Balu M, Crosignani V, Sharif A, Durkin AJ, Kelly KM, et al. In vivo measurements of cutaneous melanin across spatial scales: using multiphoton microscopy and spatial frequency domain spectroscopy. J Biomed Opt. 2015;20:066005.
58. Lentsch G, Balu M, Williams J, Lee S, Harris RM, König K, et al. In vivo multiphoton microscopy of melasma. Pigment Cell Melanoma Res. 2019;32:403–11.
59. Lin J, Saknite I, Valdebran M, Balu M, Lentsch G, Williams JN, et al. Feature characterization of scarring and non-scarring types of alopecia by multiphoton microscopy. Lasers Surg Med. 2019;51:95–103.
60. Puschmann S, Rahn CD, Wenck H, Gallinat S, Fischer F. Approach to quantify human dermal skin aging using multiphoton laser scanning microscopy. J Biomed Opt. 2012;17:036005.
61. Quinn KP, Golberg A, Broelsch GF, Khan S, Villiger M, Bouma B, et al. An automated image processing method to quantify collagen fibre organization within cutaneous scar tissue. Exp Dermatol. 2015;24:78–80.
62. Iftimia N, Peterson G, Chang EW, Maguluri G, Fox W, Rajadhyaksha M. Combined reflectance confocal microscopy-optical coherence tomography for delineation of basal cell carcinoma margins: an ex vivo study. J Biomed Opt. 2016;21(1):16006.
63. Monnier J, De Carvalho N, Harris U, Garfinkel J, Saud A, Navarrete-Dechent C, et al. Combined reflectance confocal microscopy and optical coherence tomography to improve the diagnosis of equivocal lesions for basal cell carcinoma. J Am Acad Dermatol. 2022;86(4):934–6.
64. Sahu A, Yélamos O, Iftimia N, Cordova M, Alessi-Fox C, Gill M, et al. Evaluation of a combined reflectance confocal microscopy-optical coherence tomography device for detection and depth assessment of basal cell carcinoma. JAMA Dermatol. 2018;154(10):1175–83.
65. Aleissa S, Navarrete-Dechent C, Cordova M, Sahu A, Dusza SW, Phillips W, et al. Presurgical evaluation of basal cell carcinoma using combined reflectance confocal microscopy-optical coherence tomography: a prospective study. J Am Acad Dermatol. 2020;82:962–8.
66. Navarrete-Dechent C, Aleissa S, Cordova M, Liopyris K, Sahu A, Rossi AM, et al. Management of complex head-and-neck basal cell carcinomas using a combined reflectance confocal microscopy/optical coherence tomography: a descriptive study. Arch Dermatol Res. 2021;313(3):193–200.
67. Wang YJ, Chang WC, Wang JY, Wu YH. Ex vivo full-field cellular-resolution optical coherence tomography of basal cell carcinomas: a pilot study of quality and feasibility of images and diagnostic accuracy in subtypes. Skin Res Technol. 2020;26(2):308–16.
68. Jain M, Rajadhyaksha M, Nehal K. Implementation of fluorescence confocal mosaicking microscopy by "early adopter" Mohs surgeons and dermatologists: recent progress. J Biomed Opt. 2017;22:24002.
69. Sendín-Martín M, Kose K, Harris U, Rossi A, Lee E, Nehal K, et al. Complete visualization of epidermal margin during ex vivo confocal microscopy of excised tissue with 3-dimensional mosaicking and intensity projection. J Am Acad Dermatol. 2022;86(1):e13–4.
70. Bennàssar A, Carrera C, Puig S, Vilalta A, Malvehy J. Fast evaluation of 69 basal cell carcinomas with ex vivo fluorescence confocal microscopy: criteria description, histopathological correlation, and interobserver agreement. JAMA Dermatol. 2013;149(7):839–47.

71. Longo C, Pampena R, Bombonato C, Gardini S, Piana S, Mirra M, et al. Diagnostic accuracy of ex vivo fluorescence confocal microscopy in Mohs surgery of basal cell carcinomas: a prospective study on 753 margins. Br J Dermatol. 2019;180(6):1473–80.
72. Kose K, Fox CA, Rossi A, Jain M, Cordova M, Dusza SW, et al. An international 3-center training and reading study to assess basal cell carcinoma surgical margins with ex vivo fluorescence confocal microscopy. J Cutan Pathol. 2021;48(8):1010–9.
73. Longo C, Ragazzi M, Gardini S, Piana S, Moscarella E, Lallas A, et al. Ex vivo fluorescence confocal microscopy in conjunction with Mohs micrographic surgery for cutaneous squamous cell carcinoma. J Am Acad Dermatol. 2015;73:321–2.
74. Gareau D, Bar A, Snaveley N, Lee K, Chen N, Swanson N, et al. Tri-modal confocal mosaics detect residual invasive squamous cell carcinoma in Mohs surgical excisions. J Biomed Opt. 2012;17:066018.
75. Cinotti E, Belgrano V, Labeille B, Grivet D, Douchet C, Chauleur C, et al. In vivo and ex vivo confocal microscopy for the evaluation of surgical margins of melanoma. J Biophotonics. 2020;13(11):e202000179.
76. Debarbieux S, Hospod V, Depaepe L, Balme B, Poulalhon N, Thomas L. Perioperative confocal microscopy of the nail matrix in the management of in situ or minimally invasive subungual melanomas. Br J Dermatol. 2012;167:828–36.
77. Longo C, Ragazzi M, Rajadhyaksha M, Nehal K, Bennassar A, Pellacani G, et al. In vivo and ex vivo confocal microscopy for dermatologic and Mohs surgeons. Dermatol Clin. 2016;34(4):497–504.
78. Zhao J, Jain M, Harris UG, Kose K, Curiel-Lewandrowski C, Kang D. Deep learning-based denoising in high-speed portable reflectance confocal microscopy. Lasers Surg Med. 2021;53(6):880–91.
79. Curiel-Lewandrowski C, Stratton DB, Gong C, Kang D. Preliminary imaging of skin lesions with near-infrared, portable, confocal microscopy. J Am Acad Dermatol. 2021;85(6):1624–5.
80. Freeman EE, Semeere A, Laker-Oketta M, Namaganda P, Osman H, Lukande R, et al. Feasibility and implementation of portable confocal microscopy for point-of-care diagnosis of cutaneous lesions in a low-resource setting. J Am Acad Dermatol. 2021;84(2):499–502.
81. Campanella G, Navarrete-Dechent C, Liopyris K, Monnier J, Aleissa S, Minhas B, et al. Deep learning for basal cell carcinoma detection for reflectance confocal microscopy. J Invest Dermatol. 2022;142(1):97–103.
82. Combalia M, Garcia S, Malvehy J, Puig S, Mülberger AG, Browning J, et al. Deep learning automated pathology in ex vivo microscopy. Biomed Opt Express. 2021;12(6):3103–16.
83. Koller S, Wiltgen M, Ahlgrimm-Siess V, Weger W, Hofmann-Wellenhof R, Richtig E, et al. In vivo reflectance confocal microscopy: automated diagnostic image analysis of melanocytic skin tumours. J Eur Acad Dermatol Venereol. 2011;25:554–8.
84. Marvdashti T, Duan L, Aasi SZ, Tang JY, Ellerbee Bowden AK. Classification of basal cell carcinoma in human skin using machine learning and quantitative features captured by polarization sensitive optical coherence tomography. Biomed Opt Express. 2016;7:3721–35.
85. Sendín-Martín M, Lara-Caro M, Harris U, Moronta M, Rossi A, Lee E, et al. Classification of basal cell carcinoma in ex vivo confocal microscopy images from freshly excised tissues using a deep learning algorithm. J Invest Dermatol. 2022;142(5):1291–1299.e2.
86. Rubinstein G, Garfinkel J, Jain M. Live, remote control of an in vivo reflectance confocal microscope for diagnosis of basal cell carcinoma at the bedside of a patient 2500 miles away: a novel tele-reflectance confocal microscope approach. J Am Acad Dermatol. 2019;81(2):e41–2.
87. Witkowski A, Łudzik J, Soyer HP. Telediagnosis with confocal microscopy: a reality or a dream? Dermatol Clin. 2016;34(4):505–12.

Noise, Signal, and Confirmation Bias in Dermatological Diagnosis

10

Somesh Gupta

Dermatology is heavily dependent on visual pattern recognition for making a clinical diagnosis. While intuition-based judgment works well for dermatologists for common, straightforward cases, the same may not hold true for difficult-to-diagnose cases, or in conditions which are not common. Such cases need slow thinking. As described by Nobel Laureate Daniel Kahneman in his celebrated book, *Thinking, Fast and Slow*, human thinking can be divided into two broad categories: fast thinking is based on intuitive immediate judgment, and slow thinking is based on contemplating in the higher centers of the brain, cerebral cortex, and which is more likely to be based on sound logic [1].

Rare cases in dermatology pose rare challenges and need slow thinking. We need to exclude noise from the signals, and avoid confirmation bias, in which the clinician tends to find additional features to confirm initial intuitive diagnosis (heuristics) when they are not there. Confirmation bias is defined by Nickerson as *the tendency to search for, interpret, favor, and recall information in a way that confirms or supports one's prior beliefs or values*. In Dermatological diagnosis of rare, difficult-to-diagnose diseases, confirmation bias poses a significant challenge [2].

Keep and refine the useful information, and leave all the noise out.

In the weekly case conference, a patient with head and neck pigmentation also had whitish plaques in the oral cavity was referred. Intuitive thinking with confirmation bias made everyone conclude that everything fits well in a single diagnosis of lichen planus: lichen planus pigmentosus for facial pigmentation and mucosal lichen planus for oral plaques. However, as it turned out, the oral changes were better explained as tobacco-induced, and the facial pigmentation fitted well with pigmented contact dermatitis (fragrances-related). In this case, the oral cavity changes were noise, which parasitized the information processing system, the brain, leading

S. Gupta (✉)
Department of Dermatology and Venereology, AIIMS, New Delhi, India
e-mail: someshgupta@aiims.edu

S. Gupta et al. (eds.), *Critical Thinking in Contemporary Dermatology: Cognitive Essays*, https://doi.org/10.1007/978-981-97-0411-8_10

to a diagnostic error. None of the doctors took history of tobacco consumption as they thought the oral lesions were part of the lichenoid pathological process which was also there on the face. This is a case of confirmation bias, as well as a case of noise parasitizing on our mind, distracting us.

Another example of confirmation bias was seen in a patient who was also called to the weekly case conference. He had a linear lesion on the plantar aspect of his foot (Fig. 10.1). This was probably a case of linear psoriasis or verrucous inflammatory epidermal nevus. This patient also had hyperpigmented linearly arranged lesions on his forearms (Fig. 10.2). Everyone in a group of about 25 trained and trainee dermatologists thought that he had a systematized verrucous epidermal nevus, and the forearm lesions were milder extension of the same pathology which the child had on the sole, until a fellow faculty (Prof. Sujay Khandpur) cleaned the area using an alcohol swab to discover that it was completely removable. The forearm lesions were due to dermatitis neglecta. This is an astonishing example of how

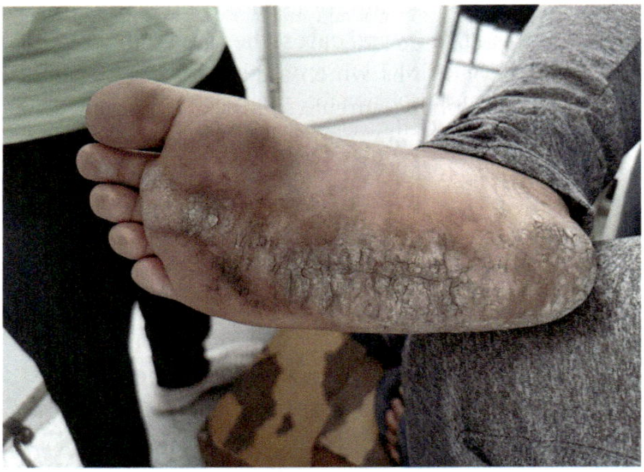

Fig. 10.1 Sole lesion of linear psoriasis (Signal)

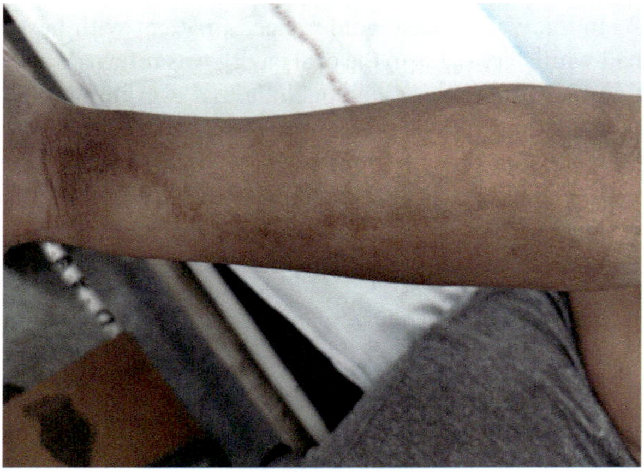

Fig. 10.2 The linear pigmentation due to dermatitis neglecta (Noise)

a large number of professionals can fall into the trap of confirmation bias and may fail to separate noise from the signal. We often look for information that supports our intuition-based diagnosis while ignoring those that don't. This hampers our slow thinking and impairs our ability to reach a correct diagnosis.

Unlearning the minute details of not-so-important information is important. An information handling system can be exploited—parasitized—by noise. We can allow our slow-thinking to sort through the noise and get to the real diagnosis if we remove the pressure of instant-diagnosis, and not fall into a trap of a "safe" diagnosis. It is acceptable or even desirable, to put a descriptive diagnosis when one is unsure, or to say that as of now you are unsure of the diagnosis but in the meantime you can help the patient feel better.

References

1. Kahneman D. Thinking, fast and slow. New York: Farrar, Straus and Giroux; 2011.
2. Dennett DC. Bacteria to Bach and Back: the evolution of minds. New York: W.W. Norton & Company; 2017.

Information Theory in the Diagnosis of Dermatological Disorders

11

Mansak Shishak and Somesh Gupta

11.1 Introduction to Information Theory and the Uncertainty Principle

In 1948, Claude Shannon presented a mathematical concept on how to efficiently transmit information to optimize information content. It has been a fundamental tool in science with a wide range of applications such as communication lines, data processing, machine learning and systems biology [1, 2]. Its application in medicine, however, has been less explored. Information theory explains that in a physical communication line, the goal is to decode the signals generated at the start or source of the line and reduce the "noise" that hampers network signals so that the message conveyed at the start is the same as that conveyed at the end.

Consider a noisy telephone line. By repeatedly saying a word over a noisy network in an attempt for the receiver to decode the correct word, the channel line does not become more efficient. Instead, energy gets "wasted" and entropy increases. The lesser the input, the higher the probability of each input yielding the right message and the higher the efficiency [3]. The key to understanding information theory is uncertainty. Uncertainty is the reason we need to decode the messages. If information was known with certainty, the diagnosis would be certain, and the challenge of making the correct diagnosis would be irrelevant. It is this very uncertainty principle that governs what information we try to decode to reach an endpoint, namely diagnosis [4, 5].

M. Shishak
ISIC Multispecialty Hospital, New Delhi, India

S. Gupta (✉)
ISIC Multispecialty Hospital, New Delhi, India

Department of Dermatology and Venereology, AIIMS, New Delhi, India
e-mail: someshgupta@aiims.edu

S. Gupta et al. (eds.), *Critical Thinking in Contemporary Dermatology: Cognitive Essays*, https://doi.org/10.1007/978-981-97-0411-8_11

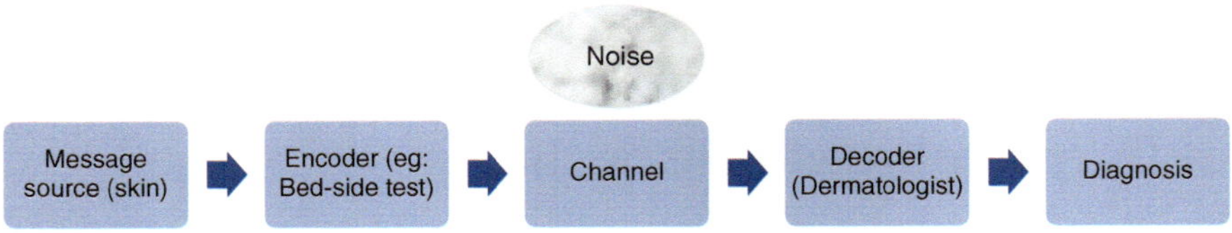

Fig. 11.1 Communication system in clinical dermatology setting—the basic model

Assume a hypothetical situation where only a single differential (variable) is known, say for a nodule on the scalp. What are the chances of error in diagnosis? None, as the probability of it being correct is 100. Assume now that two differentials exist for a nodule on the scalp. What are the chances of a correct diagnosis? It is less than 100 for each, as the probability is now lowered with the introduction of another variable. Compound the scenario to multiple variables, and the probability of correctly interpreting the information conveyed, and getting it correct, decreases. The more the number of differential diagnoses (variables), the smaller the probability of any one diagnosis being correct.

Consider also the following scenario—A violaceous papule at a peripheral site would mean a straightforward diagnosis. If more characteristics are added to it, such as multiple blisters, the decision to arrive at a concrete diagnosis gets trickier. We are now concerned about whether it is lichen planus coexisting with a blistering disease, the possibility of lichen planus pemphigoides, or the bullous variant of lichen planus. Or is it a blistering dermatosis that happens to be healing with lichenoid pigmentation? Note how the information processing to arrive at a decision gets impacted by the morphology of lesions, time of illness presentation and stage of disease evolution, particularly in waxing or waning nature. In this situation, if the lesions tend to be polymorphous, the chances of efficiently getting the correct diagnosis are further lowered.

We shall now reconstruct a basic dermatology communication system model, modified using the Shannon communication model (Fig. 11.1).

The starting point is the source of the message or information, namely, skin, while the end point is (attaining) the diagnosis. Each stage conveys information to the next step. The aim is to optimize the quality of information so that valuable and correct input is transmitted, conveyed, picked up, and not distorted via too much information, or "channel disturbance," increasing the likelihood of more errors being transmitted.

Encoder refers to a medium that conveys information from the source to the channel. For example, diascopy or dermoscopy.

The channel is an important route through which information is conveyed. Some examples are patient history (verbal information), internet (teledermatology or remote setting), and informed consent form (information conveyed and documented via written mode).

The decoder, which is the dermatologist, then decodes the information received and deduces a diagnosis from input using cognitive reasoning.

11.2 Interference in Inference

It is vital to note that at any stage of information transmission, there are inherent tendencies for errors and misinterpretation of signals. These interfering signals are collectively known as "noise," which can corrupt the channel. The higher the degree of the corrupt channel, the greater the impact on subsequent stages with increased chances of error [6].

At the site source of information, the skin itself may show great variation in presentation, which will be discussed later. The encoder carries the risk of error. For example, a bedside test shows variation in sensitivity due to observer interpretation. Grattage test to elicit auspitz's sign in psoriasis may be wrongly misinterpreted as "negative" in a resolving phase or "positive" by the observer in a case of highly inflammatory lesions of pityriasis rosea or a psoriasiform rash. The decoder may also be prone to cognitive bias, another source of noise. It is imperative to remember that the certainty of a variable itself is not 100% and is expressed by a probability. For example, the interpretation of a grattage test as "positive" is subjective and prone to inter-operator variability. In a patient with suspected genital herpes, identifying acantholytic cells and multinucleated giant cells in a Tzanck smear depends on the doctor's skills. The actual probability of Tzanck smear being positive in a true case of genital herpes is a combination of the intrinsic sensitivity of the test (measured with trained individuals) and the skill of the doctor performing the test in that case. The true effect size is not known in many scenarios. It might range from being insignificant to single-handedly tilting the favor in another differential. In a complex system, many such probabilities are compiled. The probability of making an incorrect diagnosis rises.

Besides, the expertise of the decoder (doctor or machine) in terms of knowledge, training, access to resources and the cognitive ability of the decoder to retrieve information plays a significant role in observer interpretation and high-quality transmission of input.

11.3 System Understanding and Decision-Making Process in Dermatology

Understanding systems is vital to knowing bits of information concerning the whole. The system here refers to the human body. Dealing with the human system is complex, as no two systems are identical in presenting symptoms, recovery and prognosis. A similar common template or situation may be present across all systems, but no two systems are completely identical, not even in identical twins. This means that each system will present with varying information. The more the information, the more the output is, based on system interactions, thereby more likely to be misinterpreted or wrongly understood.

This means that the nature of information within each system is not just highly variable, quantifiable or not, but also has an inherent nature of different order/complexities.

11.4 Applying the Cynefin Framework in Dermatology Conditions

In the preceding paragraph, it has been emphasized that the human biological system is complex. Corazza and Lenti explain the application of the cynefin framework (CF) in clinical reasoning and complexity in decision-making [7]. CF is a conceptual platform that explains how to make sense of complex information and explains situations into four main domains, namely, a) simple, b) complicated, c) complex, and d) chaotic. As we progress from simple to chaotic systems, the unknown variable increases [8, 9]. In the simple domain, the relationship between cause and effect is well established and requires no further reasoning or specialized lab tests. The complicated domain encompasses the majority of clinical cases where exact etiology (cause-effect) is difficult to pinpoint. However, clear diagnosis and treatment exist. Complex domain refers to those conditions where cause and effect are apparent only in retrospect. Conditions with protean manifestations, multi-system involvement and multiple chronic conditions come under the complex domain, while chaotic system refers to special situations where the cause-effect is not established. Pre-existing data and literature are scant. Urgent or innovative solutions are needed [10, 11].

Table 11.1 explains clinical scenarios in dermatology according to cynefin domains.

Having explained the communication model and CF, we shall now revisit the clinical situation previously described.

Situation A. A violaceous papule at a peripheral site would mean a straightforward diagnosis. (Read lichen planus, an example of a simple system) Assuming a classical presentation, and Wickham's striae on dermoscopy, let's say there are five differential diagnoses. The highest probability of correct diagnosis (lichen planus) would amount to around 96% and 1% each for the remaining differentials. The amount of uncertainty is less in a simple system.

Situation B. If more characteristics are added to it, such as multiple blisters, the decision to arrive at a concrete diagnosis gets trickier. We are now concerned about whether it is lichen planus coexisting with a blistering disease, the possibility of lichen planus pemphigoides, or bullous variant of lichen planus. Or is it a blistering dermatosis that happens to be healing with lichenoid pigmentation? In this case, let's assume again that there are five differential diagnoses. The probability of getting the correct diagnosis is now lowered as this is an example of a complicated domain with no clear cause-effect. There is increased clinical information at the source site, and the probability of each differential being correct is now spread more evenly, at around 20% for each. The degree of uncertainty is now higher than in Situation A.

Situation C. If this patient presents three years later with florid bullous involvement, oral ulcers, photoaggravated lesions with abdominal pain, and is on multiple drugs for recently diagnosed Type 2 Diabetes Mellitus and hypothyroidism, the situation now becomes an example of a complex system. Histopathology reveals inconsistent levels of intraepidermal and subepidermal bullae, plasma porphyrin

Table 11.1 Summary of the cynefin framework (CF) and application in dermatology domains

Domain	Characteristics (reasoning)	Clinical scenario
Simple	Cause-effect has a linear relationship. Basic examination and/or bedside test to confirm/refute diagnosis.	Sunburn or superficial thermal burn, acne vulgaris, herpes simplex. Management is straightforward.
Complicated	Has a clear diagnosis and effective management, but the exact cause-effect unknown.	A patient presenting with linear wheals along lines of pressure. Symptoms are aggravated with stress or physical exertion: Cholinergic dermographism. Other examples include pemphigus vulgaris, vitiligo. Protocols/guidelines are helpful.
Complex	The cause-effect becomes apparent only after retrospective analysis. Control of disease requires monitoring, follow-up, and change of therapeutics depending on response. It is a shifting situation with multi-disciplinary treatment.	A 46-year-old male presenting to the ER with high-grade fever, vasculitic lesions on distal limbs, septic arthritis and liver cirrhosis. Lab tests and multi-disciplinary interactions reveal disseminated gonococcal infection with decompensated liver disease. Protocols and guidelines less likely to help in the initial workup.
Chaotic	Cause effect not established. Urgent and novel therapeutics needed.	The recent COVID pandemic is an example of a chaotic system.

levels are mildly elevated and glycosylated Hb is at 12.6%. The information is now prone to more errors as we progress from site to diagnosis. The degree of uncertainty in predicting correct diagnosis is higher than in Situation B, and decision-making gets affected by more noise in the communication system.

This presents a massive plethora of unending options (information input as well as possible output options/diagnoses). Consider the information unit as i and human system h. Within a finite system, say 3 possible i units interacting with two h systems. The number of possibilities is 3^h. In the real-world clinical scenario, the number of possible interactions between i and h systems are limitless and infinite.

11.5 Dynamicity of the Skin as an Organ System and Variation with Different Human Systems

Clinical decision-making is not binary because the human system, in general, and dermatology disorders, in particular, involve a complex interplay with limitless capacity to display information. As dermatologists, we need to closely understand intra- and inter-system variation. Intra-system interaction refers to the interaction of the integumentary system with other organ systems within the same body (one human system), while inter-system variation is the biological differences between different bodies (two or more human systems).

11.6 Is Less Better?

The usual adage is that the more information we have at our disposal to decide, the better it is. As per the Dunning-Kruger effect, those with limited knowledge or competency tend to overestimate or be overconfident in their abilities. But does that overconfidence translate to fewer differentials and faster decision-making at a primary care level? A specialist is much more likely to keep the differentials of a hypertrophic dog and atrophic elephant in a case that is certainly a horse, as per a generalist. The one-off case or rare presentation that might have stumped a specialist sometimes might color his opinion in common cases and bias them to investigate that rare differential to get more information to exclude that differential. In a primary care setting, such an approach might not be required, and the cost of missing that one-off case can outweigh the benefit of not having to investigate all cases.

A specialist in a particular field might see all diseases through a particular tinged lens. An immunologist might keep vasculitis or connective tissue disease higher up in the differential list in a patient with respiratory symptoms. At the same time, a cardiologist might give priority to a heart issue. In these examples, categorizing the system as simple or complex and defining what constitutes noise might depend on the decoder's experience and specialization.

11.7 Conclusion

We have attempted to create an understanding of a communication system using information theory with respect to decisions in dermatology diagnosis. The information input is hardly perfect; the more the information input, the additive information carried from source to output increases the degree of disorder or uncertainty (entropy) within the system. Also, a system needing more information to understand is more difficult to understand. This has been illustrated via the cynefin framework model in dermatology. The probability/chances of the output (diagnosis) being correct is less error-prone in a simple system while in complicated and complex domains, the communication channel is ridden with more information as well as higher chances of noise or channel disturbance. The goal is to efficiently minimize input to yield higher chances of correct diagnosis (output), while understanding the unique complexities of the biological dermatology system.

References

1. Shannon CE. The mathematical theory of communication. 1963. MD Comput. 1997;14(4):306–17.
2. Krause P. Information theory and medical decision making. Stud Health Technol Inform. 2019;263:23–34.
3. Uda S. Application of information theory in systems biology. Biophys Rev. 2020;12(2):377–84.
4. Asch DA, Patton JP, Hershey JC. Prognostic information versus accuracy: once more with meaning. Med Decis Mak. 1991;11(1):45–7.
5. Benish WA. Relative entropy as a measure of diagnostic information. Med Decis Mak. 1999;19:202–6.
6. Eiseman NA, Bianchi MT, Westover MB. The information theoretic perspective on medical diagnostic inference. Hosp Pract (1995). 2014;42(2):125–38.
7. Corazza GR, Lenti MV. Diagnostic reasoning in internal medicine. Cynefin framework makes sense of clinical complexity. Front Med (Lausanne). 2021;8:641093.
8. Snowden DJ, Boone ME. A leader's framework for decision making. A leader's framework for decision making. Harv Bus Rev. 2007;85(11):68–76, 149.
9. Sturmberg JP, Martin CM. Knowing--in medicine. J Eval Clin Pract. 2008;14(5):767–70. Erratum in: J Eval Clin Pract. 2009;15(2):408.
10. Kempermann G. Cynefin as reference framework to facilitate insight and decision-making in complex contexts of biomedical research. Front Neurosci. 2017;11:634.
11. Gray B. The Cynefin framework: applying an understanding of complexity to medicine. J Prim Health Care. 2017;9(4):258–61.

12 Immune Dysregulation in Skin

Santosh Kurra, Shamima Akhtar, and Alpana Sharma

Abbreviations

4-F-Glc- NAc	4-fluorinated *N*-acetylglucosamine
ACD	Allergic contact dermatitis
APCs	Antigen-presenting cells
AMPs	Antimicrobial proteins
AHR	Aryl hydrocarbon receptor
b-FGF	Basic fibroblast growth factor
BB	Borderline borderline
BL	Borderline lepromatous
BT	Borderline tuberculoid
CCR	C-C Motif Chemokine Receptor
CCL	Chemokine ligand
CMKLR1	Chemokine like receptor 1
CAAR	Chimeric autoantibody receptor
CD	Cluster of differentiation
CLA	Cutaneous lymphocyte-associated antigen
CXCR	C-X-C chemokine receptor
CXCL	C-X-C motif chemokine ligand
CTLA-4	Cytotoxic T-lymphocyte-associated protein 4
dDCs	Dermal dendritic cells
DSG-3	Desmoglein 3

Santosh Kurra and Shamima Akhtar contributed equally with all other contributors.

S. Kurra · S. Akhtar · A. Sharma (✉)
Department of Biochemistry, AIIMS, New Delhi, India

S. Gupta et al. (eds.), *Critical Thinking in Contemporary Dermatology: Cognitive Essays*, https://doi.org/10.1007/978-981-97-0411-8_12

EGF	Epidermal growth factor
γδ-T cells	Gamma Delta T Cells
GM-CSF	Granulocyte-macrophage colony-stimulating factor
HBD-2	Human-β-defensin-2
HA	Hyaluronan
ILCs	Innate lymphoid cells
IGF-1	Insulin-like growth factor
IFN-γ	Interferon-γ
IL	Interleukin
KGF	Keratinocyte growth factor
LC	Langerhans cells
LL	Lepromatous
MCs	Mast cells
MMP	Matrix metalloproteinase
MCETs	MC extracellular traps
mo-MDSCs	Monocytic-MDSCs
MDT	Multidrug therapy
NK	Natural-killer
NGF	Neural growth factor
NRP	Neuropilin
NETs	Neutrophil extracellular traps
PBMC	Peripheral blood mononuclear cell
pDCs	Plasmacytoid dendritic cells
PD-1	Programmed cell death protein 1
PD-L1	Programmed death-ligand 1
ROR	RAR-related orphan receptor
Tregs	Regulatory T cells
S100A	S100 calcium-binding protein A
ST2	Suppressor of tumorigenicity 2
STAT	Signal transducer and activator of transcription
SCF	Stem cell factor
TIM	T cell immunoglobulin- and mucin-domain-containing molecules
T_{eff}	T effector cells
Tfh	T follicular helper
T_M	T memory cells
Th	T-helper
TSLP	Thymic stromal lymphopoietin
T_{RM}	Tissue resident memory CD8+ T cells
TLRs	Toll-like receptors
TGF	Transforming growth factor
TT	Tuberculoid
TNF-α	Tumor necrosis factor-α
TRP-1	Tyrosinase-related protein-1
UPR	Untranslated protein response

Skin acts as a fence between the immediate environment and our own body, forming the first line of defense. The integrity of this fence is preserved by a horde of immune and non-immune cells residing in or homing to the skin, which acts in sync with these cells. A breach in its integrity can allow pathogens, external hazards, or noxious substances to elicit an immune response. Immune dysregulation occurs when there's a failure to evoke an adequate immune response, which precipitates as different forms of skin diseases.

12.1 Cutaneous Immune Armature

The skin harbors a large repertoire of immune cells from innate and adaptive immune arms. The epidermis accommodates fewer immune cells, mainly skin-resident dendritic cells known as Langerhans cells (LC), resident T memory cells (T_M) of different phenotypes like regulatory T cells (Tregs), and resident $CD8^+$ T cells (T_{RM}). Langerhans cells originate from resident progenitor cells and remain in tight contact with epidermal keratinocytes through their radiating dendrites, permitting them to survey the epidermis while other cells remain dispersed in the epidermal layer. Skin-resident T_M cells are of αβ origin and stem from antigen-specific T effector cells (T_{eff}), which have infiltrated the skin in the past as a result of any injury. They are positioned essentially adjacent to LCs and are cutaneous lymphocyte-associated antigen (CLA) positive [1, 2].

The dermis houses distinct populations of immune cells like dermal dendritic cells (dDCs), natural-killer (NK) cells, macrophages, mast cells (MCs), $CD4^+$ T helper cells, $CD8^+$ T cells, gamma delta T Cells (γδ-T cells), innate lymphoid cells (ILCs) and eosinophils. The presence of B cells in the skin is still debatable. While the motility of immune cells is restricted in the epidermis, they are more motile in the dermis. The dDCs are derived from bone marrow progenitor cells and are replenished every 7–8 days. In humans, dDCs are mainly of 3 types: cDC1 ($CD141^+$), cDC2 ($CD1c^+$), and $CD14^+$ dDCs. Monocytes infiltrate the skin during any disease state and express CD163, the scavenger receptor and coagulation factor XIIIa; these are precursors of the skin-resident macrophages. The αβ-T cells are clustered and located primarily at post-capillary venules below the intersection of epidermis and dermis. Mast cells are abundantly present in the dermis, strongly expressing IgE receptors and complementing C5a (CD88). They are derived from Lin^-cKit^+ bone marrow progenitor cells, which mature in the presence of keratinocyte-derived stem cell factor (SCF). Dermal ILCs are also derived from bone marrow progenitor cells. ILC2 is the major skin-resident ILC expressing CD25 and suppressor of tumorigenicity 2 (ST2). NK cells in the skin are $CD56^+$ and $CD16^-$ and express CCR8, a homing receptor for the skin. Eosinophils are also detected in healthy skin [1, 2].

12.2 Skin Immune Homeostasis in Steady State

In the absence of an immune elicitor, skin-resident innate and adaptive immune cells secrete cytokines and growth factors aiding fellow immune and non-immune cells to survive and perform their steady-state functions. They also migrate to the skin-draining lymph node and express self-antigens, thus maintaining tolerance. Much of the functions of the immune cells in the skin have been deciphered using mice models.

Maintenance and survival of Langerhans cells depends on keratinocyte-derived IL-34. These cells remain anchored to keratinocytes by E-cadherin expression, which helps them appraise antigens under a steady state. Under a steady state, TGF-β secreted by LCs and other local cells is crucial for the expression of adhesion molecules (E-cadherin), LC survival, and phagocytic function. CXCR4 expressed on LCs facilitates their migration to skin-draining lymph nodes to promote tolerance via binding to its ligand, CXCL12, expressed on dermal fibroblast. These cells induce tolerance to keratinocyte antigens by boosting the expansion of anti-desmoglein 3 (DSG-3) specific Treg cells [3]. Similar to Langerhans cells, macrophages are also maintained by IL-34. They phagocytose the apoptotic cells and cellular debris in healthy skin and migrate to the draining lymph node, expressing self-antigens and consequently contributing to maintaining tolerance and homeostatic hair regeneration [3].

In normal skin, dDCs typically promote tolerance to external antigens, either topically applied antigens in the hair follicles or to the skin-resident commensal bacteria *Staphylococcus epidermidis.* Mast cells secrete cytokines, making the milieu favorable for themselves and other cells to survive. Under steady state, they release IL-2, IL-3, stem cell factor (SCF), epidermal growth factor (EGF) and neural growth factor (NGF). IL-2 promotes the growth, survival, and expansion of various subsets of skin-resident T cells ($CD4^+$, $CD8^+$ and Tregs). IL-3 and SCF exuded by keratinocytes and MCs themselves stimulate growth, differentiation, survival, and expansion of MCs; EGF and NGF do the same for fibroblasts, endothelial cells and neural cells, respectively [3, 4]. NK cells are also known to act as APCs. Hence, similar to LCs, NK cells also remove stressed cutaneous cells in non-inflamed skin by presenting antigens in skin-draining lymph nodes [5]. Healthy skin ILC2 entails keratinocyte-derived IL-7 and thymic stromal lymphopoietin (TSLP) for its survival [6]. ILC2 constitutively produces IL-13 and is positioned in close proximity to MCs in the dermis. IL-13 suppressed the function of MCs, such as degranulation [7]. Both types of T cells, αβ-T and γδ-T, require keratinocyte-produced IL-7, while the former also require IL-15 for their survival. These αβ-Tcells secrete keratinocyte growth factor (KGF), insulin-like growth factor (IGF-1), and IL-2. KGF and IGF-1 help keratinocytes proliferate and survive, while IL-2 does the same for γδ-T cells and themselves [2, 8]. Unlike αβ-T cells, γδ-T cells identify antigens derived from stressed or impaired cells, e.g., stressed keratinocytes, migrate to draining lymph nodes, thus maintaining tolerance in the skin. Similar to αβ-T cells, these cells also secrete IGF-1 which contributes to keratinocyte survival by upregulating Bcl-2 family members, thus preventing apoptosis [2, 8].

The function of eosinophils in normal skin remains to be explored (Fig. 12.1).

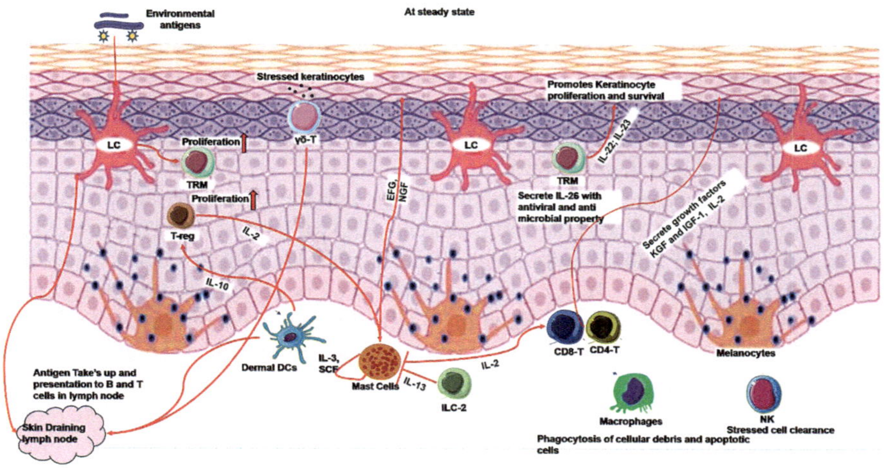

Fig. 12.1 Steady-state functions of skin-resident immune cells

12.3 Immune Dysregulation in Skin

Immune dysregulation underlies a plenitude of skin diseases. However, owing to the scope of this compendium, we are focusing on major skin disorders. These include autoimmune skin diseases (psoriasis, vitiligo, and pemphigus), allergic contact dermatitis and infectious diseases such as leprosy.

12.3.1 Autoimmune Skin Diseases

In autoimmune skin diseases, immune dysregulation occurs, leading to autoantibodies forming against skin self-antigens, resulting in skin damage. The trigger for autoimmune cutaneous disease can be genetic, biochemical, or environmental factors. Primarily, there is a defect in the central and peripheral tolerance.

12.3.1.1 Psoriasis

Psoriasis affects approximately 2–3% of the population globally. It is characterized by keratinocyte proliferation, resulting in erythematous plaques with large scaling, pruritus and pain. Histologically, a psoriatic lesion is typified by epidermal acanthosis, vascular proliferation and infiltration of immune cell populations dominated by neutrophils, MCs, T- cells and DCs. The etiology of the disease is still enigmatic [9, 10].

Psoriatic skin keratinocytes produce innate antimicrobial proteins (AMPs), i.e., psoriasin (S100A7), human-β-defensin-2 (HBD-2), S100 calcium-binding protein A1 (S100A), and Koebnerisin (S100A15) which attracts immune cells. AMPs bind to toll-like receptors (TLRs) expressed on skin-resident antigen-presenting cells

(APCs) such as LCs, which release chemokine CXCL16. CXCL16 aids the transmigration of neutrophils and MCs to the lesion site where they secrete extracellular traps like neutrophil and MC extracellular traps (NETs and MCETs). During the process these cells release IL-17A/F. In a positive feedback loop, extracellular traps upregulate AMP expression in keratinocytes. IL-1β and IL-23 can also induce MCET formation and degranulation of MCs [10, 11].

Macrophages are present in psoriatic lesions, and their numbers are further elevated in the absence of T cells. Skin resident (CD 163^+) macrophages are classically activated and release inflammatory molecules like tumor necrosis factor-α (TNF-α), IL-23p19, and IL-12/23p40, which is reduced by adoptive transfer of $FoxP3^+$ Tregs [12–14]. The number of classically activated intermediate monocytes ($CD16^+CD14^{++}$) expressing high levels of co-stimulatory molecule, CD86, is also increased in lesions and is positively related to disease severity [15]. Similarly, the frequency of $CD11c^+$ DCs is increased in psoriatic skin. Chemokine-like receptor 1-(CMKLR1) positive DCs are recruited from blood to the skin along the gradient of chemerin expressed by lesional skin and secrete IL-17 and interferon (IFN)-γ [16]. LC-specific expression of CXCL10 and CXCL9 aids in homing of inflammatory T cells to the psoriatic skin. While macrophages and DCs contribute to skin inflammation, NK cells in psoriatic lesions exhibit reduced degranulation and secreted minimally IFN-γ and TNF-α [10, 17]. Monocytic-MDSCs (mo-MDSCs) are increased in psoriasis with altered functionality. They release proinflammatory IL-8, matrix metalloproteinase MMP-8, MMP-1, CXCL1, and chemokine ligand CCL2; suppress $CD8^+$ T cells less efficiently; and abnormally convert Tregs from naïve T cells [18]. In response to IL-23 released by LCs, peripheral CLA+ and C-C motif chemokine receptor $CCR6^+$ Vγ9Vδ2 T-cells drift towards inflamed skin and contribute to ongoing inflammation by producing IL-17 and IL-22 as well as activating keratinocytes [19]. Another distinct type of immune cell, ILCs, is noted with higher frequency in psoriatic skin. These cells release proinflammatory cytokines IL-17A and IL-22 and are associated with disease severity. Skin-resident cell-derived IL-23 and IL-1β activate ILCs while therapeutic application of anti-TNF-α reduces them, implicating the pathogenic role of these cells in psoriasis [10, 20].

A main component of the adaptive immune response, T cells, are markedly increased in psoriasis. The intradermal proliferation of T cells is heightened in patients with active disease compared to patients in remission. However, patients in remission have a greater number of lesional T cells than healthy individuals, indicating a presence of immunologic memory [21].

Various inflammatory subsets of $CD4^+$ T helper cells are implicated in the pathogenesis of psoriasis. T-helper (Th)1, Th9, T follicular helper (Tfh)17, and Th17 subsets are increased in circulation as well as in lesions. This is supported by the presence of high levels of Th1 cytokines, IFN-γ, IL-2; Th9 cytokines IL-9, IL-13; and Th17 cytokines, IL-17, IL-22, in the circulation of patients [22]. Transcripts of T-bet, a transcription factor responsible for Th1 response, are upregulated in psoriatic patients' peripheral blood mononuclear cells (PBMCs) [23]. IL-27, which antagonizes IL-17 production, is remarkably reduced in circulation and lesions [24]. IL-36 and IL-21, liable for Th17 proliferation and differentiation, respectively, are augmented in the periphery and in lesions [25, 26]. Th17 cytokines, IL-17A and IL-22, increase AMP expression in keratinocytes, cause keratinocyte proliferation and decrease differentiation. IL-17A enhances the expression of chemokines, which recruit neutrophils (CXCL 1,3,5,6,8), DCs, and memory T cells (CCL20) [27]. IL-9 increases IL-17, IFN-γ and IL-13 production in a positive feedback loop [28]. CXCR3-CCR6^{+} Tfh17 cells are elevated and correlate well with disease severity and IL-21R expression on B cells [10, 29].

Contrarily, T cell subsets pertaining to anti-inflammation (Th2) and immune regulation (Tregs) are decreased in psoriasis. GATA-3, a transcription factor responsible for inducing Th2 response, is decreased in PBMCs of psoriatic patients. IL-10 and IL-4 levels are also lowered in patients [23]. Treg function is modulated in the inflammatory milieu of psoriasis. These cells acquire the Th17 profile via signal transducer and activator of transcription 3 (STAT3) phosphorylation and release inflammatory cytokines such as IFN-γ, TNF-α, and IL-17. Thus, Tregs become inefficient in downregulating T effector cell activation. Inhibiting STAT3 phosphorylation or adoptively transferring Tregs can reduce psoriasis by reducing macrophage infiltration [30]. Inhibitory immune checkpoints such as programmed cell death protein 1 (PD-1), programmed death-ligand 1 (PD-L1), cytotoxic T-lymphocyte-associated protein 4 (CTLA-4), CD69, and neuropilin (NRP)-1 are lowly expressed in severe psoriasis, thus failing to downregulate the ongoing inflammation. The expression of these cells is lowered in immune regulatory cells such as Mo-MDSCs

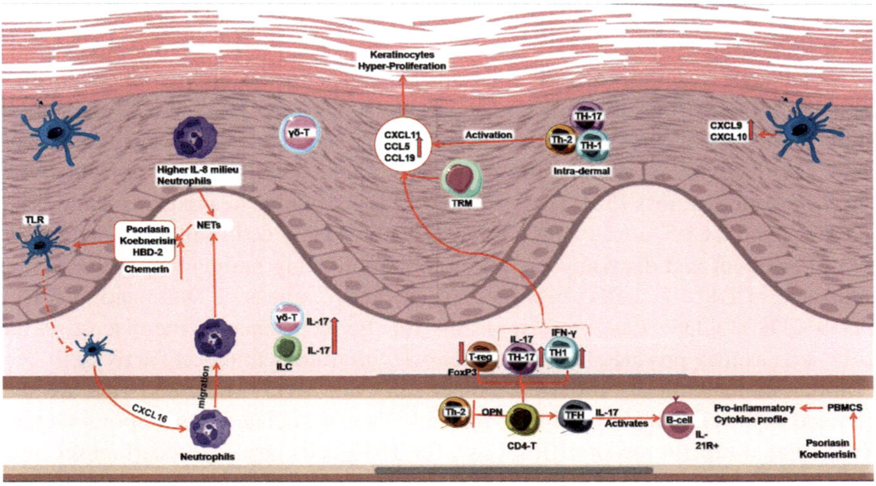

Fig. 12.2 Immune cell-mediated mechanism of psoriasis

and Tregs. Downregulation of these immune checkpoints is associated with increased expression of inflammatory cytokines such as IFN-γ [10, 31] (Fig. 12.2).

12.3.1.2 Vitiligo

Vitiligo is typified by melanocyte loss, leading to skin depigmentation primarily due to attacks by immune cells. Similar to psoriasis, this degeneration of melanocytes can be triggered by either biochemical, neural, and autoimmune mechanisms or combined. The biochemical trigger sets up the untranslated protein response (UPR) in melanocytes. Sequentially, UPR augments the secretion of proinflammatory cytokines IL-6 and IL-8 by the melanocytes [32]. Various subsets of DCs, i.e., LCs, dDCs, $LAMP^+$ DC, $CD1c^+$ DCs, plasmacytoid dendritic cells (pDCs) and $CD11c^+$ myeloid DCs, are implicated in pathogenesis of vitiligo [10]. In response to keratinocyte-specific chemokines CXCL9 and CXCL10, peripheral DCs and other immune cells home to the lesion site [33]. Granulocyte-macrophage colony-stimulating factor (GM-CSF), also secreted by keratinocytes, leads to the proliferation and maturation of myeloid DCs. Consequently, the frequency of DCs is increased in vitiligo lesions. pDCs-secreted IFN-γ correlates with the disease severity and in turn recruits $CXCR3^+$ immune cells to the lesion site [34]. Skin-resident LCs are also elevated in lesions with alterations in morphology, such as increased dendrites [35]. Activation of inflammasomes and elevation of IL-1β transcripts in LCs implicates the potential of LCs to drive Th17 activation [36].

The NK cell receptor has two potent ligands—NKR, its natural ligand, and NKG2D, elicited under inflammatory conditions. Attachment of tyrosinase-related protein-1 (TRP-1), a melanocyte antigen, with NKG2D, induces effective cytolytic activity in $CD8^+$ T cells against TRP-1 receptors, while binding with CD48 lowers the generation of reactive $CD8^+$ T cells, thus halting the progression of vitiligo. This is confirmed by the observation of elevated numbers of $NKG2D^+$ NK cells in vitiligo lesions [37].

Melanocyte-specific $CD8^+$ T cells are expanded in the circulation of vitiligo patients, followed by migration to lesion sites along the cytokine and chemokine gradient created by stressed keratinocytes and melanocytes. CXCL16 produced by these keratinocytes aids in migrating CXCR6 + CD8+ T cells to the lesion site, leading to melanocyte loss [38]. Early vitiligo lesion melanocytes express chemokine CXCL12 and CCL5, concurring with APCs and $CD8^+$ T cell infiltration, leading to loss of pigment and disease progression [39]. Following antigen exposure, few of infiltrated $CD8^+$ T cells becomes T_{RM}s and express CD69 and CD103. $CD69^+CD103^+CD8^+$ T_{RM}s are responsible for the recurrence of the disease in the same area as they produce IFN-γ and TNF-α with mild cytotoxicity activity.

Inflammatory subsets of $CD4^+$ T helper cells, i.e., Th17, Th22, and Th1, are also elevated in the circulation of vitiligo patients. Their associated transcription factors, RAR-related orphan receptor (ROR)-γt, for Th17 cells, aryl hydrocarbon receptor (AHR) for Th22 cells, and T-bet for Th1, are also upregulated. Concurrently, cytokines IL-17A, IL-22, IL-21 and IL-2 are augmented in the serum of the vitiligo patients. The lesion area positively correlates with the number of $IL\text{-}17A^+CD4^+$ T cells in the lesions. Moreover, the presence of IL-17A⁺Th17 cells at the leading edge of the lesions indicates their pathogenic role in spreading the disease [40].

The role of anti-inflammatory $CD4^+$ Th subset, Th2 and regulatory $CD4^+$ Th cells (Tregs), in the pathogenesis of vitiligo is ambiguous. In one study, Th2 cells and associated cytokines were comparable between the patients and healthy individuals; in another study, they were decreased. Similarly, peripheral $CD4^+CD25^+FoxP3^+$ Treg cells, expressing transforming growth factor (TGF)-β1 and CCL2, were reduced in patients' circulation but increased in the perilesional skin of the patients. These cells, however, were inefficient in suppressing the proliferation and cytolytic function of autologous $CD8^+$ T cells. Reduced Tregs frequency negatively correlated with VIDA score and body surface area [41]. Yet in another study no significant difference between Treg number, FOXP3 expression, and TGF-β1 levels was observed between patients and healthy controls [36]. Nonetheless, it specifies that elevation of the inflammatory $CD4^+$Th cells with concomitant functional impairment of Tregs cells drives the disease.

Contribution of immune checkpoints, T cell immunoglobulin- and mucin-domain containing molecules (TIM) and programmed cell death 1 (PD-1) is implicated in the pathogenesis of vitiligo. Augmented percentage of circulating $CD3^+CD4^+TIM3^+$ Th1 cells in vitiligo occurs, which is positively associated with the percentage body surface area involvement in patients. Simultaneously, ligands for TIM-3 and Galectin-9 are elevated in lesional skin [42]. The presence of $TIM\text{-}3^+$ cells in lesional and perilesional skin implies their involvement in melanocyte destruction. Although Tregs are decreased in vitiligo, $PD\text{-}1^+$ Tregs are increased in generalized vitiligo, indicating the PD-1/PD-L1 pathway might cause Treg exhaustion [41] (Fig. 12.3).

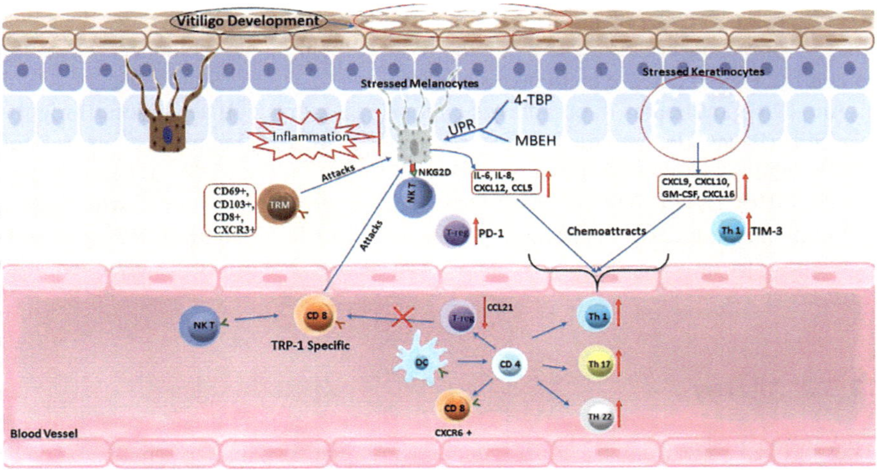

Fig. 12.3 Immune cell-derived mechanism of vitiligo

12.3.1.3 Pemphigus

Pemphigus, a blistering mucocutaneous disease, is mediated by autoantibodies (IgG subtype) primarily against autoantigens, Desmoglein-1 (DSG1) and Desmoglein-3 (DSG3). The hallmark clinical feature of pemphigus is "acantholysis." Similar to other skin autoimmune diseases, the trigger for autoantibody formation is still unclear. Nonetheless, the disease initiates with exposure to desmogleins, which are recognized by LCs as antigens. LCs present DSG antigens to T-cells, thus initiating a deregulated cell-mediated immune response [10].

NK cells function as prime APCs in pemphigus. This is evidenced by co-culturing experiments wherein $CD56^{+}CD3^{-}$ NK cells from patients steered the proliferation of $CD4^{+}$T helper (Th) cells in the presence of DSG-3 peptides. NK cells further induce $CD4^{+}$T cells to release proinflammatory cytokines IL-6, IL-8, and IFN-γ [42]. Recently, γδ-T cells are also detected in pemphigus. These cells exhibited high Th1 type and low Th2 type profile, indicating their plasticity which is required for sustaining high autoantibody titers [43].

In parallel with other autoimmune skin diseases, various inflammatory subsets of $CD4^{+}$ Th cells, i.e., Th1, Th17, and Tfh, are augmented in pemphigus with concomitant decrease in Th2 and Tregs. Accordingly, IFN-γ, IL-17, IL-23, IL-8, IL-6 and IL-21 cytokines are elevated in the patient, and IL-10, IL-2, IP-10, and CCL11 are diminished, implicating dysregulation of the immune response [44–46]. T cell co-stimulatory molecule, CD28 is essential for Treg activation and suppressive function. Heightened expression of CD28 on Th cells and a minimal expression on Tregs indicate a faulty activation and proliferation of Tregs in the patients. In-vivo expanded Tregs significantly diminished the DSG3-specific T-cell responses as well as IgG production [47]. Skin-homing receptor-ligand pair for Treg, CCR4-CCL22 is diminished, impairing their homing to the lesional sites, thus making them incapable of regulating the immune response [45]. While the role of $CD4^{+}$ T cells in pemphigus is well-defined, the function of $CD8^{+}$ T cells is still unclear. In a sole study on mice, eliminating $CD8^{+}$ T cells reduced pemphigus incidence, indicating its contribution to disease pathogenesis [48].

Anti-DSG antibodies in pemphigus patients indicate B-cell activation. B regulatory cells (Bregs) dampen the immune responses in mice and humans by expressing FOXP3 and releasing anti-inflammatory cytokines IL-10 and TGF-β. Elevated levels of $CD19^{+}CD24^{hi}CD38^{hi}$ Bregs are observed in pemphigus patients, which, upon stimulation, produces IL-10. However, they are unable to suppress IFN-γ expression and Th1 immune response, indicating reduced suppressive function [49] (Fig. 12.4).

12.3.2 Allergy

Allergy is an unwarranted and exaggerated immune response to small molecules known as "haptens," which are experienced repeatedly by the person in their environment. After combining with larger protein molecules, haptens form neoantigens which instigate an immune response. The incidence of allergic contact dermatitis

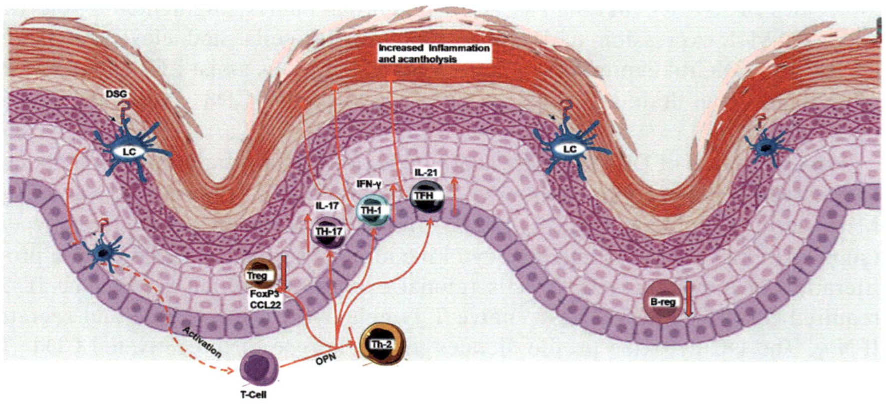

Fig. 12.4 Immunologic network in pemphigus

(ACD) is progressively increasing, with an occurrence rate of 1 in every 7 individuals every year [50].

12.3.2.1 Allergic Contact Dermatitis (ACD)

ACD is the most common form of the occupation-related disease which manifests as erythema, pruritus, redness, edema, and lesions in the affected skin, and is primarily diagnosed by the patch test. A plenitude of compounds is known to elicit ACD, such as nickel, dust mite (*Dermatophagoides*), pollen, chemicals from leaves and trichomes, parthenin and sesquiterpene lactones from the cosmopolitan weed *Parthenium hysterophorus*, etc. ACD is a typical example of a cell-mediated hypersensitivity reaction exemplified by sensitization or "afferent phase" and elicitation phase or "efferent phase."

The *sensitization/afferent phase* initiates with the haptenization of host cutaneous proteins, which is the covalent binding of low molecular weight molecules with host proteins. Following haptenization, the host proteins become immunogenic. LCs and dDCs, the professional APCs of skin, sense these immunogenic hapten-protein complexes. Lipophilic haptens can infiltrate the APCs and attach to cytoplasmic proteins, get processed by proteasomes and are expressed by MHC class I molecules. Alternatively, hydrophilic haptens bind to extracellular proteins which are taken up by APCs, processed and presented on MHC class II molecules. Thus, lipophilic molecules will activate $CD8^+$ T lymphocytes while hydrophilic molecules will activate $CD4^+$ T lymphocytes [51, 52]. The antigenic encounter induces a series of morphological and functional changes in LCs and dDCs, including expression of co-stimulatory molecules (CD86, ICAM-1) and secretion of proinflammatory molecules, IL-1β and TNF-α. These cytokines stimulate keratinocytes to release IL-1α, GM-CSF, IL-18, IL-8, IL-23, and TNF-α. Together, these cytokines induce changes in the microenvironment such as reduced expression of E-cadherin on keratinocytes, increased expression of MMPs which degrade basement membrane, increased interaction between DC-specific adhesion molecules LFA-1, ICAM1, and VLA-6 with dermal matrix, augmented E-selectin and VCAM-1 expression of lymphatic endothelial cells, and elevated CCR7, CCR4, and CXCR4 expression on DCs. These alterations assist LCs and dDCs in migrating to skin-draining lymph nodes to activate naive $CD8^+$ and $CD4^+$ T lymphocytes [50, 53].

Post-migration of DCs to the paracortical region of skin-draining lymph nodes, they establish connections with naïve $CD8^+$ and $CD4^+$ T lymphocytes via TCR-MHC-antigen complex (signal 1) and co-stimulatory molecules on both cell types (signal 2). This interaction and the cytokine milieu created by DCs lead to a proliferation of hapten-specific T-cells (clonal expansion), which secrete the IL-2 required for their growth. $CD8^+$ naïve T lymphocytes get activated and secrete IFN-γ. The DC cytokine profile dictates the phenotype of the activated $CD4^+$ T cells. DC-specific IL-12/TNF-α leads to Th1 type cells, IL-17 triggers Th17 cell formation, IL22/IL-23 results in Th22 cells, and IL-4 and IL-10 produce Th2 cells while IL-10 causes Treg generation [54]. In support of this theory, *Parthenium* dermatitis patients in the Indian cohort were noted to have elevated serum levels of Th1 and Th17 cytokines and decreased levels of Treg and Th2 cytokines, indicating an ongoing inflammation [55, 56]. Activated T cells also expressed CCR4 and CLA, which aid in homing to the site of action. At the site, $CD8^+$ T cells mediate cytotoxicity of hapten-loaded keratinocytes while Th1/Th17 cells mount an immune response and get converted to hapten-specific memory T cells and reside there [50, 54]. In the sensitization phase, appearance of clinically relevant symptoms is rare.

The *elicitation/efferent phase* initiates with re-exposure of the individuals already sensitized to the same hapten. This time the hapten can be taken up by other "non-professional" APCs like macrophages, MCs and keratinocytes which activate hapten-specific skin-resident memory $CD8^+$ and $CD4^+$ T cells as well as central memory T cells. While skin-resident memory cells are responsible for immediate contact hypersensitivity, central memory T cells result in delayed hypersensitivity reactions. These cells also release proinflammatory cytokines like IFN-γ, TNF-α, IL-4, IL-13, IL-17, and IL-22, activating keratinocytes and innate immune cells. Keratinocytes also secretes chemokines i.e. CXCL9/10, CCL17, CCL20, CCL27which attract T lymphocytes. Thus, an immune response is mounted. Increased inflammation induces Fas expression on keratinocytes, making them more prone to become apoptotic via the Fas-FasL pathway. Apoptosis of keratinocytes makes the tissue spongiotic, and vesicles are formed. Loss of keratinocytes and desquamation removes the antigen, resulting in the resolution of inflammation [54, 57] (Fig. 12.5).

12.3.3 Infection

Infectious skin diseases embody a vast array of conditions that range in severity from mild to life-threatening. The clinical presentation in infectious skin diseases

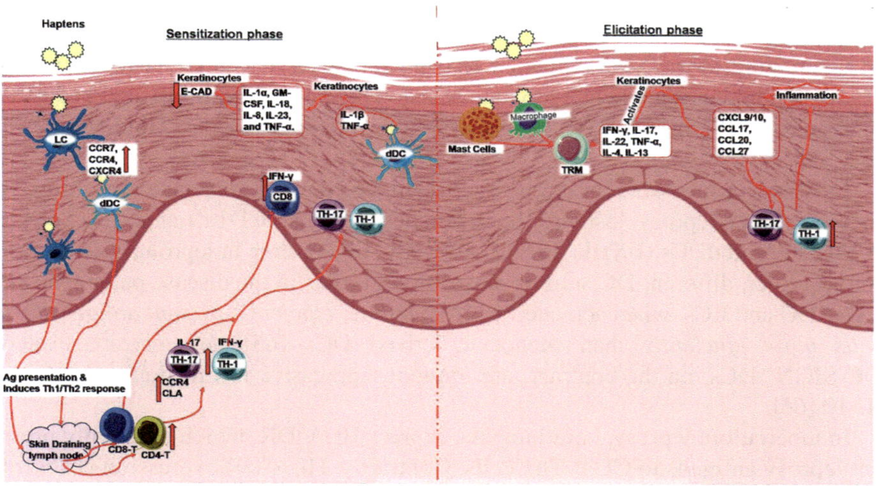

Fig. 12.5 Immune cell-derived mechanism in allergic contact dermatitis

depends on the pathogen involved, i.e., viral, bacterial, fungal or parasitic. Among them, bacterial skin infections are the most common infectious skin diseases [58].

12.3.3.1 Leprosy

Leprosy, or Hansen's disease, is a chronic infectious disease caused by *Mycobacterium leprae*, a microorganism that preferentially infects skin and nerves. Mankind has been known to be afflicted with this disease for ages. Despite the continuous efforts of the World Health Organisation (WHO) for widespread usage of multidrug treatment for leprosy, it is still endemic in many areas, including Southeast Asia and the Americas. More than 200,000 new cases of leprosy are recorded each year globally [59]. Based on the immunological response, leprosy is classified into five types: tuberculoid (TT), borderline tuberculoid (BT), borderline borderline (BB), borderline lepromatous (BL), and lepromatous (LL) [60]. WHO has categorized leprosy based on the extent of skin and nerve involvement in the disease into two types: multibacillary and paucibacillary [61]. Once the infection is established, sporadic episodes of acute inflammation occur where cytokines and chemokines are released by immune and non-immune cells, which decides the disease course. A Th1-type response to *M. leprae* leads to cellular immune response and is seen in unstable borderline patients (BT, BB, and BL). In contrast, a Th2 response directs humoral immune response and is frequently seen in BL and LL patients [59]. Lack of an ideal animal model for the disease is the main hurdle in delineating the pathophysiology of the disease. Nonetheless, identifying different immune cells with varied phenotypes in the patient lesions has increased our understanding of the disease.

Macrophages are abundantly found in the lesions of tuberculosis patients. Depending on the type of lesions, they are polarized to either M1 or M2 phenotype. In tuberculoid lesions, inflammatory M1 macrophages ($CD68^{+}CD163^{-}$) secreting IL-15 predominates while in lepromatous lesion lipid-loaded anti-inflammatory M2 macrophages ($CD68^{+}CD163^{+}$) known as foamy cells, releasing IL-10 predominate [62, 63].

DCs are indispensable for setting a cell-mediated immune response. Accordingly, in tuberculoid leprosy lesions, the frequency of LCs ($CD1a^{+}Langerin^{+}$), pDCs ($CD123^{+}$), and dDCs ($FXIIIa^{+}$) are significantly higher than in lepromatous lesions [64]. Further, different DC subsets play different roles in the disease pathogenesis. $CD1^{+}$ DC and LCs, when activated with *M. leprae, efficiently present antigens to T cells more efficiently* than monocyte-derived DCs [65]. *M. leprae*-activated DC-$SIGN^{+}$ DCs, on the contrary, are immunosuppressive in function and release IL-10 [66].

In tuberculoid leprosy, keratinocytes express HLA-DR, which efficiently present leprosy antigens to $CD4^{+}$ Th1 cells. Contrarily, HLA-DR expression is absent in keratinocytes from lepromatous lesions [67]. Consistent with it, intercellular adhesion molecules between keratinocytes (ICAM-1) and T-lymphocytes (LFA-1) are co-localized and overexpressed in tuberculoid lesions [68]. This further supports the notion that a cell-mediated immune reaction occurs in tuberculoid leprosy. Infected keratinocytes release AMP, cathelicidin and an inflammatory cytokine, TNF-α [69].

Th1/Th2 lymphocytes are the major players in deciding the disease outcome in leprosy. Th1 cells secreting IL-2 and IFN-γ polarize macrophages to the microbicidal M1 phenotype, restricting the bacilli and disease progression in tuberculoid lesions. Th2-type cells release IL-4, IL-5 and IL-10, which induce M2 macrophage polarization which curtails microbicidal activity, thus promoting bacilli dissemination and disease progression in lepromatous lesions. Accordingly, PBMCs of patients also showed a Th1/Th2 polarization depending on the disease phenotype [59, 70]. Nevertheless, Th1/Th2 reactions are irreversible in patients. Like Th1/Th2 cells, Treg, and Th17 cells also exhibit polarization in leprosy lesions. Tregs expressing IL-10, [71] TGF-β, [72] and IL-35 [73] are elevated in tuberculoid lesions while Th17-related cytokines are prominent in lepromatous lesions [74]. Similar divergence was observed in PBMC of patients when stimulated with *M. leprae* antigens [75]. Unlike Th1/Th2 paradigm, lepromatous patient derived-Tregs can be reversed to Th17 in vitro by supplementing exogenous rIL-23 [76], implicating a novel regime for reducing immunosuppression in lepromatous patients.

Yet another subset of T lymphocyte, Th9 cells, secreting IL-9, with cytotoxicity activity, was augmented in tuberculoid lesions [77, 78], while Th22 cells, releasing IL-22 and basic fibroblast growth factor (b-FGF), were found in high frequency in lepromatous lesions [79]. $CD8^{+}$ T cells are also identified in leprosy lesions. In lepromatous lesions, they are $CD28^{-}$ suggesting an immunosuppressive phenotype, while in tuberculoid lesions, though low in number, they are $CD28^{+,}$ implicating a cytotoxic nature [80]. $CD8^{+}$ T cells in lepromatous lesions secrete immunosuppressive cytokines IL-4, IL-5, and IL-10 [81]. In addition to $\alpha\beta$-T cells, $\gamma\delta$ T cells are

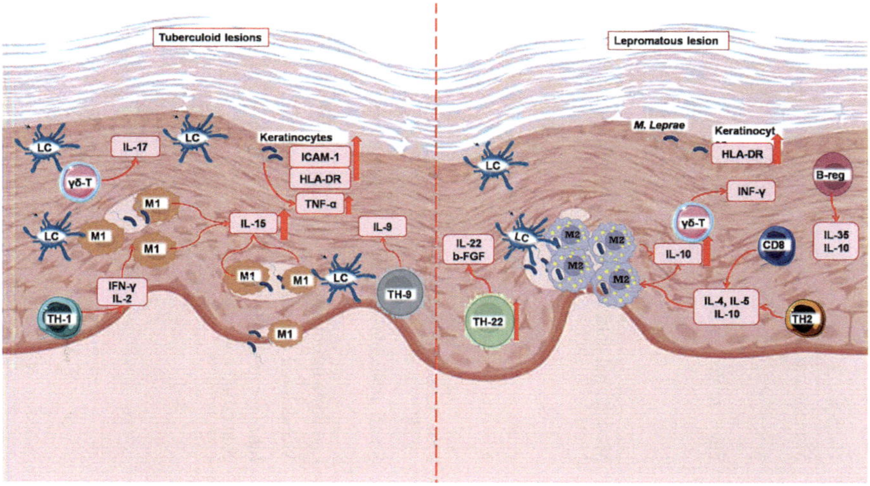

Fig. 12.6 Immune cell-mediated mechanism in leprosy

also detected in large numbers in leprosy lesions. While γδ-T cells secreting IL-17 and IFN-γ were present in both tuberculoid and lepromatous skin, CD4$^+$FOXP3$^+$γδ T was identified in only lepromatous lesions [82–84].

B lymphocytes are the major players of the humoral immune system and are implicated in lepromatous lesions. In recent years, Breg sub-types, i.e., IL-35 [73] and IL-10 [85] secretions, have been identified in lepromatous lesions and in patient PBMCs. Additionally, memory Bregs with immunosuppressive function are also present in lepromatous lesions [86]. IL-10 secreting Bregs interact with effector T cells and convert them to Tregs with enhanced function [85]. All of them contribute to the immunosuppressive milieu in lepromatous lesions (Fig. 12.6).

12.4 Immune Cells as Therapeutic Targets in Cutaneous Disease

Our progressive understanding of the pathophysiology of the various cutaneous diseases has shown that immune cells and/or immune cell-derived cytokines/chemokine-receptor pairs and associated signaling molecules are critical players in the disease progression. These molecules are increasingly targeted for therapeutic intervention for managing skin diseases with improved efficacy (Table 12.1).

12.4.1 Autoimmune Skin Diseases

Initially, general immunosuppressants such as corticosteroids, azathioprine, methotrexate, mycophenolate mofetil, etc., were administered to patients with

Table 12.1 Immune cell-based therapeutic strategies in autoimmune skin disorders

Disease	Strategy	Target	Therapeutic agent	Status
Psoriasis	*Cytokine blockade (inflammatory arm)*	TNF-α, IL-17A, IL-17RA, IL-12/IL-23p40, IL-23p19, IL-1α, IL-1β, IL-1R	Monoclonal antibody	FDA- approved
	Signaling blockade (inflammatory arm)	JAK1, JAK1/2, JAK1/3, TYK2	Small molecule inhibitors	Clinical trial
	Co-inhibitory stimulation (regulatory arm)	PD-1 agonist		Clinical trial
Pemphigus	*Cellular depletion (inflammatory arm)*	CD20	Monoclonal antibody	FDA- approved
	Cellular therapy (regulatory arm)	Polyclonal Treg, CAAR T cells		Clinical trial
	Tolerogenic vaccine (regulatory arm)	PI-0824	Small DSG-3 peptide	Clinical trial
Vitiligo	*Cytokine blockade (inflammatory arm)*	IL-15	Monoclonal antibody	Clinical trial
	Signaling blockade (inflammatory arm)	JAK1, JAK1/3, JAK2, TYK2	Small molecule inhibitors	Clinical trial
ACD	*Cytokine blockade (inflammatory arm)*	IL-8, IL-12/23p40, IL-23 (p19), TNF-α,	Cytokine inhibitors	Clinical trial
		IL-17	Monoclonal antibody	
		IL-1β	Inhibitor of IL-1β converting enzyme	
	Induction of immune tolerance (regulatory arm)	$CD4^+$ $CD25^+$ Treg cell		Clinical trial
		CD45 RO/RB binding molecule on DCs		Clinical trial
		Antisense oligonucleotide to CFLAR		Clinical trial

	Inhibitors of immune cell migration and infiltration (inflammatory arm)	4-fluorinated N-Acetylglucosamine (4-F-Glc-NAc)	Inhibitor of selectins	Clinical trial
Leprosy	*Muti-drug treatment (inflammatory arm)*	MDT (clofazimine, dapsone & rifampicin)	Antibiotics	WHO approved
	Immune checkpoint inhibitors (regulatory arm)	PD-1, CTLA-4, LAG-3, TIGIT	Monoclonal antibodies	Animal studies

autoimmune skin disorders, which impaired the entire immune system to down-regulate the inflammation. Nonetheless, these drugs have potentially severe side-effects [87].

Studies have shown that drugs targeting the innate and adaptive arms of the immune system can efficiently impede the progression of autoimmune disease, but their effects are only short-lived. Researchers have targeted the immune system's regulatory arm to achieve long-term remission, which increases tolerance and reinstates homeostasis. In psoriasis, proinflammatory cytokines such as IL-17, IL-23, and TNF-α are overly expressed and participate in disease progression. Similarly, the IL-15 pathway is aimed at remedial involvement in vitiligo; hence, monoclonal antibodies targeting this cytokines-receptor axis have been developed, and many have been FDA-approved for clinical usage [87, 88]. The binding of the cytokine to its receptor mainly induces JAK-STAT signaling, which induces a distinct gene expression profile. Hence, this signaling pathway is also therapeutically targeted by small molecule inhibitors in psoriasis and vitiligo. Another avenue is to inhibit T-cell activation by blocking T-cell-specific CD28 and APC-specific CD80/CD86 interaction with inhibitory immune checkpoint molecules, e.g., CTLA-4, which has the same affinity as co-stimulatory molecules CD80/CD86 [87].

A cellular depletion strategy has been adopted for treating pemphigus. Depleting $CD20^+$ mature B cells with rituximab or ofatumumab [89] has shown efficacy in managing the disease; however, it has its own side effects. This strategy limits only $CD20^+$ mature B cells; however, B cell precursors and plasma cells which actively participate in disease progression and are $CD20^-$ remain unaffected. Hence, disease recurrence is a common problem. Further, adoptive cell transfer of polyclonally expanded Tregs in patients has been seen to suppress IFN-γ and is yet another recent development in the treatment of pemphigus. Another potential approach is using autoantigen-specific chimeric autoantibody receptor T cells (CAART). This method utilizes engineered effector T cells to spot the anti-DSG3 B cells, thus eliminating them without diminishing other B cell subsets. PI-0824, a synthetic peptide of DSG-3, was developed to generate tolerance against autoantigens. Nonetheless, this strategy was not successful, as no difference in autoantibodies was observed between treated and untreated groups. The major limitation of this strategy was that the autoantigens and initiators of pemphigus must be known [87].

12.4.2 Allergic

Initially, acute symptoms of ACD were treated by administration of systemic and topical steroids, but avoidance of allergens was recognized as the ideal way to treat this disease. Owing to the side effects of steroids, other approaches to managing the disease have evolved. The foremost alternative approach used antisense RNA against functional human CFLAR (CASP8 and FADD-like apoptosis regulator) in lymphocytes to induce tolerance. CFLAR is an anti-apoptotic protein upregulated in T cells following T-cell activation and plays a crucial role in cell survival. Like autoimmune diseases, inflammatory cytokine blockade has been a recent approach to managing ACD. Targeting immune cell adhesion and migration is yet another strategy to curb inflammation. 4-fluorinated *N*-acetylglucosamine (4-F-Glc- NAc) downregulates E- and P-selectin expression on activated T cells, which concurred with anti-inflammatory efficacy. Similarly, hyaluronic acid (HA) is implicated in the homing of immune cells via binding to CD44. Small peptide inhibitors of HA effectively reduce immune cell infiltration and thus the disease severity. Another treatment strategy with long-term effects is the induction of immunologic tolerance, which is mediated mainly by IL-10$^+$ Tregs. Treating lesional skin with haptens or modified haptens induces expansion of IL-10-producing Tregs, which inhibits CD8$^+$ T cell function. Moreover, the binding of small molecules to CD45RO/RB on DCs inhibits their activation, leading to the formation of tolerogenic DCs implicated in the attenuation of inflammation [90].

12.4.3 Infectious Skin Disorder

Current treatment regimens for leprosy include the administration of multidrug therapy (MDT) which includes antibiotics clofazimine, dapsone and rifampicin. This approach focuses on limiting the infectious *Mycobacterium leprae*. Nonetheless, recent emphasis is on inhibiting immune checkpoints such as CTLA- 4, LAG-3, PD-1, and TIGIT to accentuate T effector function, thus curtailing the tolerogenic features observed in lepromatous leprosy patients. The success of this approach is presently limited to animal models as patient studies are yet to be started [91].

12.5 Conclusion

Our understanding of the immune system and immune dysregulation has evolved in the past two decades. The unveiling of novel immune cell types in both innate and adaptive arms, such as Th17, Th9, and Th22, and ILCs, have unfolded the complexity of the pathogenesis of various skin diseases. Likewise, the availability of animal models for different skin-related diseases has improved our understanding of their pathophysiology and mechanism. Different subtypes of JAK and STAT signaling molecules seem to play a crucial role in immune cell activation, thus expressing a unique set of proteins in different skin diseases. The discovery of immune checkpoints has added another layer of complexity. Hence, the therapeutic strategies in skin diseases have also progressed from local or systemic immunosuppressants to a more targeted approach, i.e., human monoclonal antibodies against different cytokines, small molecules against JAK and STAT subtypes and immune checkpoints or administration of ex-vivo expanded Tregs and CAAR T cells as cellular therapy. Advancement in the knowledge of immune dysregulation in different skin diseases has shifted the treatment strategy towards novel therapeutic approaches for better management with fewer side effects.

References

1. Pasparakis M, Haase I, Nestle FO. Mechanisms regulating skin immunity and inflammation. Nat Rev Immunol. 2014;14(5):289–301.
2. Nestle FO, Di Meglio P, Qin JZ, Nickoloff BJ. Skin immune sentinels in health and disease. Nat Rev Immunol. 2009;9(10):679–91.
3. Nguyen AV, Soulika AM. The dynamics of the Skin's immune system. Int J Mol Sci. 2019;20(8):1811.
4. Mukai K, Tsai M, Saito H, Galli SJ. Mast cells as sources of cytokines, chemokines, and growth factors. Immunol Rev. 2018;282(1):121–50.
5. Ebert LM, Meuter S, Moser B. Homing and function of human skin gammadelta T cells and NK cells: relevance for tumor surveillance. J Immunol. 2006;176(7):4331–6.
6. Kobayashi T, Voisin B, Kim DY, Kennedy EA, Jo JH, Shih HY, et al. Homeostatic control of sebaceous glands by innate lymphoid cells regulates commensal bacteria equilibrium. Cell. 2019;176(5):982–97 e16.
7. Roediger B, Kyle R, Yip KH, Sumaria N, Guy TV, Kim BS, et al. Cutaneous immunosurveillance and regulation of inflammation by group 2 innate lymphoid cells. Nat Immunol. 2013;14(6):564–73.
8. Cruz MS, Diamond A, Russell A, Jameson JM. Human alphabeta and gammadelta T cells in skin immunity and disease. Front Immunol. 2018;9:1304.
9. Richmond JM, Harris JE. Immunology and skin in health and disease. Cold Spring Harb Perspect Med. 2014;4(12):a015339.
10. Das D, Akhtar S, Kurra S, Gupta S, Sharma A. Emerging role of immune cell network in autoimmune skin disorders: an update on pemphigus, vitiligo and psoriasis. Cytokine Growth Factor Rev. 2019;45:35–44.
11. Kakeda M, Schlapbach C, Danelon G, Tang MM, Cecchinato V, Yawalkar N, et al. Innate immune cells express IL-17A/F in acute generalized exanthematous pustulosis and generalized pustular psoriasis. Arch Dermatol Res. 2014;306(10):933–8.
12. Leite Dantas R, Masemann D, Schied T, Bergmeier V, Vogl T, Loser K, et al. Macrophage-mediated psoriasis can be suppressed by regulatory T lymphocytes. J Pathol. 2016;240(3):366–77.

13. Fuentes-Duculan J, Suarez-Farinas M, Zaba LC, Nograles KE, Pierson KC, Mitsui H, et al. A subpopulation of CD163-positive macrophages is classically activated in psoriasis. J Invest Dermatol. 2010;130(10):2412–22.
14. Yawalkar N, Tscharner GG, Hunger RE, Hassan AS. Increased expression of IL-12p70 and IL-23 by multiple dendritic cell and macrophage subsets in plaque psoriasis. J Dermatol Sci. 2009;54(2):99–105.
15. Nguyen CTH, Kambe N, Yamazaki F, Ueda-Hayakawa I, Kishimoto I, Okamoto H. Upregulated expression of CD86 on circulating intermediate monocytes correlated with disease severity in psoriasis. J Dermatol Sci. 2018;90(2):135–43.
16. Zaba LC, Fuentes-Duculan J, Eungdamrong NJ, Abello MV, Novitskaya I, Pierson KC, et al. Psoriasis is characterized by accumulation of immunostimulatory and Th1/Th17 cell-polarizing myeloid dendritic cells. J Invest Dermatol. 2009;129(1):79–88.
17. Fujita H, Shemer A, Suarez-Farinas M, Johnson-Huang LM, Tintle S, Cardinale I, et al. Lesional dendritic cells in patients with chronic atopic dermatitis and psoriasis exhibit parallel ability to activate T-cell subsets. J Allergy Clin Immunol. 2011;128(3):574–82; e1–12.
18. Soler DC, Young AB, Fiessinger L, Galimberti F, Debanne S, Groft S, et al. Increased, but functionally impaired, CD14(+) HLA-DR(−/low) myeloid-derived suppressor cells in psoriasis: a mechanism of dysregulated T cells. J Invest Dermatol. 2016;136(4):798–808.
19. Yoshiki R, Kabashima K, Honda T, Nakamizo S, Sawada Y, Sugita K, et al. IL-23 from Langerhans cells is required for the development of imiquimod-induced psoriasis-like dermatitis by induction of IL-17A-producing gammadelta T cells. J Invest Dermatol. 2014;134(7):1912–21.
20. Ward NL, Umetsu DT. A new player on the psoriasis block: IL-17A- and IL-22-producing innate lymphoid cells. J Invest Dermatol. 2014;134(9):2305–7.
21. Khairutdinov VR, Mikhailichenko AF, Belousova IE, Kuligina ES, Samtsov AV, Imyanitov EN. The role of intradermal proliferation of T-cells in the pathogenesis of psoriasis. An Bras Dermatol. 2017;92(1):41–4.
22. Priyadarssini M, Divya Priya D, Indhumathi S, Rajappa M, Chandrashekar L, Thappa DM. Immunophenotyping of T cells in the peripheral circulation in psoriasis. Br J Biomed Sci. 2016;73(4):174–9.
23. Zhu K, Ye J, Wu M, Cheng H. Expression of Th1 and Th2 cytokine-associated transcription factors, T-bet and GATA-3, in peripheral blood mononuclear cells and skin lesions of patients with psoriasis vulgaris. Arch Dermatol Res. 2010;302(7):517–23.
24. Chen W, Gong Y, Zhang X, Tong Y, Wang X, Fei C, et al. Decreased expression of IL-27 in moderate-to-severe psoriasis and its anti-inflammation role in imiquimod-induced psoriasis-like mouse model. J Dermatol Sci. 2017;85(2):115–23.
25. Arakawa A, Vollmer S, Besgen P, Galinski A, Summer B, Kawakami Y, et al. Unopposed IL-36 activity promotes clonal CD4(+) T-cell responses with IL-17A production in generalized pustular psoriasis. J Invest Dermatol. 2018;138(6):1338–47.
26. Wang Y, Wang LL, Yang HY, Wang FF, Zhang XX, Bai YP. Interleukin-21 is associated with the severity of psoriasis vulgaris through promoting CD4+ T cells to differentiate into Th17 cells. Am J Transl Res. 2016;8(7):3188–96.
27. Nograles KE, Zaba LC, Guttman-Yassky E, Fuentes-Duculan J, Suarez-Farinas M, Cardinale I, et al. Th17 cytokines interleukin (IL)-17 and IL-22 modulate distinct inflammatory and keratinocyte-response pathways. Br J Dermatol. 2008;159(5):1092–102.
28. Schlapbach C, Gehad A, Yang C, Watanabe R, Guenova E, Teague JE, et al. Human TH9 cells are skin-tropic and have autocrine and paracrine proinflammatory capacity. Sci Transl Med. 2014;6(219):219ra8.
29. Wang Y, Wang L, Yang H, Yuan W, Ren J, Bai Y. Activated circulating T follicular helper cells are associated with disease severity in patients with psoriasis. J Immunol Res. 2016;2016:7346030.
30. Yang L, Li B, Dang E, Jin L, Fan X, Wang G. Impaired function of regulatory T cells in patients with psoriasis is mediated by phosphorylation of STAT3. J Dermatol Sci. 2016;81(2):85–92.
31. Bartosinska J, Purkot J, Kowal M, Michalak-Stoma A, Krasowska D, Chodorowska G, et al. The expression of selected molecular markers of immune tolerance in psoriatic patients. Adv Clin Exp Med. 2018;27(6):721–5.

32. Toosi S, Orlow SJ, Manga P. Vitiligo-inducing phenols activate the unfolded protein response in melanocytes resulting in upregulation of IL6 and IL8. J Invest Dermatol. 2012;132(11):2601–9.
33. Richmond JM, Bangari DS, Essien KI, Currimbhoy SD, Groom JR, Pandya AG, et al. Keratinocyte-derived chemokines orchestrate T-cell positioning in the epidermis during vitiligo and may serve as biomarkers of disease. J Invest Dermatol. 2017;137(2):350–8.
34. Bertolotti A, Boniface K, Vergier B, Mossalayi D, Taieb A, Ezzedine K, et al. Type I interferon signature in the initiation of the immune response in vitiligo. Pigment Cell Melanoma Res. 2014;27(3):398–407.
35. Itoi S, Tanemura A, Kotobuki Y, Wataya-Kaneda M, Tsuruta D, Ishii M, et al. Coexistence of Langerhans cells activation and immune cells infiltration in progressive nonsegmental vitiligo. J Dermatol Sci. 2014;73(1):83–5.
36. Wang CQ, Cruz-Inigo AE, Fuentes-Duculan J, Moussai D, Gulati N, Sullivan-Whalen M, et al. Th17 cells and activated dendritic cells are increased in vitiligo lesions. PLoS One. 2011;6(4):e18907.
37. Zloza A, Lyons GE, Chlewicki LK, Kohlhapp FJ, O'Sullivan JA, Lacek AT, et al. Engagement of NK receptor NKG2D, but not 2B4, results in self-reactive CD8+ T cells and autoimmune vitiligo. Autoimmunity. 2011;44(8):599–606.
38. Li S, Zhu G, Yang Y, Jian Z, Guo S, Dai W, et al. Oxidative stress drives CD8(+) T-cell skin trafficking in patients with vitiligo through CXCL16 upregulation by activating the unfolded protein response in keratinocytes. J Allergy Clin Immunol. 2017;140(1):177–89 e9.
39. Rezk AF, Kemp DM, El-Domyati M, El-Din WH, Lee JB, Uitto J, et al. Misbalanced CXCL12 and CCL5 chemotactic signals in vitiligo onset and progression. J Invest Dermatol. 2017;137(5):1126–34.
40. Zhen Y, Yao L, Zhong S, Song Y, Cui Y, Li S. Enhanced Th1 and Th17 responses in peripheral blood in active non-segmental vitiligo. Arch Dermatol Res. 2016;308(10):703–10.
41. Tembhre MK, Parihar AS, Sharma VK, Sharma A, Chattopadhyay P, Gupta S. Alteration in regulatory T cells and programmed cell death 1-expressing regulatory T cells in active generalized vitiligo and their clinical correlation. Br J Dermatol. 2015;172(4):940–50.
42. Tembhre MK, Parihar AS, Sharma A, Gupta S, Chattopadhyay P, Sharma VK. Participation of T cell immunoglobulin and mucin domain-3 (TIM-3) and its ligand (galectin-9) in the pathogenesis of active generalized vitiligo. Immunol Res. 2015;62(1):23–34.
43. Das D, Anand V, Khandpur S, Sharma VK, Sharma A. T helper type 1 polarizing gammadelta T cells and scavenger receptors contribute to the pathogenesis of pemphigus vulgaris. Immunology. 2018;153(1):97–104.
44. Satyam A, Khandpur S, Sharma VK, Sharma A. Involvement of T(H)1/T(H)2 cytokines in the pathogenesis of autoimmune skin disease-pemphigus vulgaris. Immunol Investig. 2009;38(6):498–509.
45. Asothai R, Anand V, Das D, Antil PS, Khandpur S, Sharma VK, et al. Distinctive Treg associated CCR4-CCL22 expression profile with altered frequency of Th17/Treg cell in the immunopathogenesis of pemphigus vulgaris. Immunobiology. 2015;220(10):1129–35.
46. Hennerici T, Pollmann R, Schmidt T, Seipelt M, Tackenberg B, Mobs C, et al. Increased frequency of T follicular helper cells and elevated Interleukin-27 plasma levels in patients with pemphigus. PLoS One. 2016;11(2):e0148919.
47. Schmidt T, Willenborg S, Hunig T, Deeg CA, Sonderstrup G, Hertl M, et al. Induction of T regulatory cells by the superagonistic anti-CD28 antibody D665 leads to decreased pathogenic IgG autoantibodies against desmoglein 3 in a HLA-transgenic mouse model of pemphigus vulgaris. Exp Dermatol. 2016;25(4):293–8.
48. Giurdanella F, Fania L, Gnarra M, Toto P, Di Rollo D, Sauder DN, et al. A possible role for CD8+ T lymphocytes in the cell-mediated pathogenesis of pemphigus vulgaris. Mediat Inflamm. 2013;2013:764290.
49. Zhu HQ, Xu RC, Chen YY, Yuan HJ, Cao H, Zhao XQ, et al. Impaired function of CD19(+) CD24(hi) CD38(hi) regulatory B cells in patients with pemphigus. Br J Dermatol. 2015;172(1):101–10.
50. Brys AK, Rodriguez-Homs LG, Suwanpradid J, Atwater AR, MacLeod AS. Shifting paradigms in allergic contact dermatitis: the role of innate immunity. J Invest Dermatol. 2020;140(1):21–8.

51. Cavani A, Hackett CJ, Wilson KJ, Rothbard JB, Katz SI. Characterization of epitopes recognized by hapten-specific CD4+ T cells. J Immunol. 1995;154(3):1232–8.
52. Kohler J, Martin S, Pflugfelder U, Ruh H, Vollmer J, Weltzien HU. Cross-reactive trinitrophenylated peptides as antigens for class II major histocompatibility complex-restricted T cells and inducers of contact sensitivity in mice. Limited T cell receptor repertoire. Eur J Immunol. 1995;25(1):92–101.
53. Kimber I, Cumberbatch M, Dearman RJ. Langerhans cell migration: not necessarily always at the center of the skin sensitization universe. J Invest Dermatol. 2009;129(8):1852–3.
54. Brites GS, Ferreira I, Sebastiao AI, Silva A, Carrascal M, Neves BM, et al. Allergic contact dermatitis: from pathophysiology to development of new preventive strategies. Pharmacol Res. 2020;162:105282.
55. Akhtar N, Satyam A, Anand V, Verma KK, Khatri R, Sharma A. Dysregulation of T(H) type cytokines in the patients of Parthenium induced contact dermatitis. Clin Chim Acta. 2010;411(23–24):2024–8.
56. Akhtar N, Verma KK, Sharma A. Study of pro- and anti-inflammatory cytokine profile in the patients with parthenium dermatitis. Contact Derm. 2010;63(4):203–8.
57. Martins LE, Reis VM. Immunopathology of allergic contact dermatitis. An Bras Dermatol. 2011;86(3):419–33.
58. Dawson AL, Dellavalle RP, Elston DM. Infectious skin diseases: a review and needs assessment. Dermatol Clin. 2012;30(1):141–51; ix-x.
59. Mi Z, Liu H, Zhang F. Advances in the immunology and genetics of leprosy. Front Immunol. 2020;11:567.
60. Ridley DS, Jopling WH. Classification of leprosy according to immunity. A five-group system. Int J Lepr Other Mycobact Dis. 1966;34(3):255–73.
61. Pannikar V. Enhanced global strategy for further reducing the disease burden due to leprosy: 2011-2015. Lepr Rev. 2009;80(4):353–4.
62. Fachin LR, Soares CT, Belone AF, Trombone AP, Rosa PS, Guidella CC, et al. Immunohistochemical assessment of cell populations in leprosy-spectrum lesions and reactional forms. Histol Histopathol. 2017;32(4):385–96.
63. Montoya D, Cruz D, Teles RM, Lee DJ, Ochoa MT, Krutzik SR, et al. Divergence of macrophage phagocytic and antimicrobial programs in leprosy. Cell Host Microbe. 2009;6(4):343–53.
64. Hirai KE, Aarao TL, Silva LM, de Sousa JR, de Souza J, Dias LB Jr, et al. Langerhans cells (CD1a and CD207), dermal dendrocytes (FXIIIa) and plasmacytoid dendritic cells (CD123) in skin lesions of leprosy patients. Microb Pathog. 2016;91:18–25.
65. Hunger RE, Sieling PA, Ochoa MT, Sugaya M, Burdick AE, Rea TH, et al. Langerhans cells utilize CD1a and langerin to efficiently present nonpeptide antigens to T cells. J Clin Invest. 2004;113(5):701–8.
66. Kumar S, Naqvi RA, Bhat AA, Rani R, Ali R, Agnihotri A, et al. IL-10 production from dendritic cells is associated with DC SIGN in human leprosy. Immunobiology. 2013;218(12):1488–96.
67. Mutis T, De Bueger M, Bakker A, Ottenhoff TH. HLA class II+ human keratinocytes present mycobacterium leprae antigens to CD4+ Th1-like cells. Scand J Immunol. 1993;37(1):43–51.
68. Sullivan L, Sano S, Pirmez C, Salgame P, Mueller C, Hofman F, et al. Expression of adhesion molecules in leprosy lesions. Infect Immun. 1991;59(11):4154–60.
69. Lyrio EC, Campos-Souza IC, Correa LC, Lechuga GC, Vericimo M, Castro HC, et al. Interaction of mycobacterium leprae with the HaCaT human keratinocyte cell line: new frontiers in the cellular immunology of leprosy. Exp Dermatol. 2015;24(7):536–42.
70. Misra N, Murtaza A, Walker B, Narayan NP, Misra RS, Ramesh V, et al. Cytokine profile of circulating T cells of leprosy patients reflects both indiscriminate and polarized T-helper subsets: T-helper phenotype is stable and uninfluenced by related antigens of mycobacterium leprae. Immunology. 1995;86(1):97–103.
71. Kumar S, Naqvi RA, Ali R, Rani R, Khanna N, Rao DN. CD4+CD25+ T regs with acetylated FoxP3 are associated with immune suppression in human leprosy. Mol Immunol. 2013;56(4):513–20.

72. Saini C, Ramesh V, Nath I. Increase in TGF-beta secreting CD4(+)CD25(+) FOXP3(+) T regulatory cells in anergic lepromatous leprosy patients. PLoS Negl Trop Dis. 2014;8(1):e2639.
73. Tarique M, Saini C, Naqvi RA, Khanna N, Rao DN. Increased IL-35 producing Tregs and CD19(+)IL-35(+) cells are associated with disease progression in leprosy patients. Cytokine. 2017;91:82–8.
74. Saini C, Ramesh V, Nath I. CD4+ Th17 cells discriminate clinical types and constitute a third subset of non Th1, non Th2 T cells in human leprosy. PLoS Negl Trop Dis. 2013;7(7):e2338.
75. Sadhu S, Khaitan BK, Joshi B, Sengupta U, Nautiyal AK, Mitra DK. Reciprocity between regulatory T cells and Th17 cells: relevance to polarized immunity in leprosy. PLoS Negl Trop Dis. 2016;10(1):e0004338.
76. Tarique M, Saini C, Naqvi RA, Khanna N, Sharma A, Rao DN. IL-12 and IL-23 modulate plasticity of FoxP3(+) regulatory T cells in human leprosy. Mol Immunol. 2017;83:72–81.
77. de Sousa JR, Pagliari C, de Almeida DSM, Barros LFL, Carneiro FRO, Dias LB Jr, et al. Th9 cytokines response and its possible implications in the immunopathogenesis of leprosy. J Clin Pathol. 2017;70(6):521–7.
78. Finiasz MR, Franco MC, de la Barrera S, Rutitzky L, Pizzariello G, del Carmen SM, et al. IL-9 promotes anti-mycobacterium leprae cytotoxicity: involvement of IFNgamma. Clin Exp Immunol. 2007;147(1):139–47.
79. de Lima SE, de Sousa JR, de Sousa Aarao TL, Fuzii HT, Dias Junior LB, Carneiro FR, et al. New immunologic pathways in the pathogenesis of leprosy: role for Th22 cytokines in the polar forms of the disease. J Am Acad Dermatol. 2015;72(4):729–30.
80. Modlin RL, Mehra V, Wong L, Fujimiya Y, Chang WC, Horwitz DA, et al. Suppressor T lymphocytes from lepromatous leprosy skin lesions. J Immunol. 1986;137(9):2831–4.
81. Yamamura M, Uyemura K, Deans RJ, Weinberg K, Rea TH, Bloom BR, et al. Defining protective responses to pathogens: cytokine profiles in leprosy lesions. Science. 1991;254(5029):277–9.
82. Saini C, Tarique M, Ramesh V, Khanna N, Sharma A. Gammadelta T cells are associated with inflammation and immunopathogenesis of leprosy reactions. Immunol Lett. 2018;200:55–65.
83. Sridevi K, Neena K, Chitralekha KT, Arif AK, Tomar D, Rao DN. Expression of co-stimulatory molecules (CD80, CD86, CD28, CD152), accessory molecules (TCR alphabeta, TCR gammadelta) and T cell lineage molecules (CD4+, CD8+) in PBMC of leprosy patients using mycobacterium leprae antigen (MLCWA) with murabutide and T cell peptide of Trat protein. Int Immunopharmacol. 2004;4(1):1–14.
84. Tarique M, Naqvi RA, Ali R, Khanna N, Rao DN. CD4(+) TCRgammadelta(+) FoxP3(+) cells: an unidentified population of immunosuppressive cells towards disease progression leprosy patients. Exp Dermatol. 2017;26(10):946–8.
85. Tarique M, Naz H, Kurra SV, Saini C, Naqvi RA, Rai R, et al. Interleukin-10 producing regulatory B cells transformed CD4(+)CD25(−) into Tregs and enhanced regulatory T cells function in human leprosy. Front Immunol. 2018;9:1636.
86. Negera E, Walker SL, Bekele Y, Dockrell HM, Lockwood DN. Increased activated memory B-cells in the peripheral blood of patients with erythema nodosum leprosum reactions. PLoS Negl Trop Dis. 2017;11(12):e0006121.
87. Vesely MD. Getting under the skin: targeting cutaneous autoimmune disease. Yale J Biol Med. 2020;93(1):197–206.
88. Hawkes JE, Yan BY, Chan TC, Krueger JG. Discovery of the IL-23/IL-17 signaling pathway and the treatment of psoriasis. J Immunol. 2018;201(6):1605–13.
89. Izumi K, Bieber K, Ludwig RJ. Current clinical trials in pemphigus and pemphigoid. Front Immunol. 2019;10:978.
90. Alase A, Wittmann M. Therapeutic strategies in allergic contact dermatitis. Recent Patents Inflamm Allergy Drug Discov. 2012;6(3):210–21.
91. Lima HR, Gasparoto TH, de Souza Malaspina TS, Marques VR, Vicente MJ, Marcos EC, et al. Immune checkpoints in leprosy: immunotherapy as a feasible approach to control disease progression. Front Immunol. 2017;8:1724.

Vitiligo: A Patch on Skin and the Mind

13

Jung Min Bae and Hyun Jeong Ju

13.1 Introduction

Vitiligo is a pigmentary disorder characterized by well-demarcated chalky-white patches of variable size on any part of the body, affecting 0.5–2.0% of general populations worldwide [1]. The disease was first described prior to 1500 B.C. in the earliest Vedic and Egyptian literatures [2]. Ancient texts referred to white patches on the skin as leprosy; the confusion triggered social stigma from the very beginning in many communities. By the end of the nineteenth century, vitiligo was finally defined as a distinct pigmentary disorder. Our current understanding of vitiligo, based on advanced translational studies, supports the autoimmune nature of vitiligo, but much remains to be elucidated [3].

Various treatments for vitiligo are mentioned in historical texts, of which phototherapy was the mainstay of treatment from ancient times to the present day. Egyptian and Indian writings depict the application of the psoralen-containing plants *Ammi majus* and *Psoralen corylifolia* to white skin, followed by exposure to sunlight which became the basis of modern psoralen photochemotherapy (PUVA) [4]. The introduction of narrowband UVB (NBUVB) phototherapy replaced PUVA therapy because of the superior cosmetic result, fewer side effects, and ease of administration [5].

In the current era of biologics, many treatment options are available for patients with atopic dermatitis or psoriasis, but vitiligo has long been neglected in the development of medicine, probably because it was regarded as merely a cosmetic problem, especially in Western countries. However, the burden of vitiligo is comparable to those of other skin diseases; patients with vitiligo often present with depression,

J. M. Bae (✉) · H. J. Ju
Department of Dermatology, St. Vincent's Hospital, College of Medicine, The Catholic University of Korea, Seoul, South Korea

S. Gupta et al. (eds.), *Critical Thinking in Contemporary Dermatology: Cognitive Essays*, https://doi.org/10.1007/978-981-97-0411-8_13

anxiety, and other psychiatric comorbidities [6]. Thus, a better understanding of the disease and the development of more effective treatments are essential.

Vitiligo is a disfiguring disease associated with various autoimmune conditions. Although subjective symptoms like pruritus and pain are absent, vitiligo profoundly impacts the quality of life (QoL) [7]. Vitiligo patients suffer from various psychosocial issues, including low self-esteem, stigmatization, a poor body image, difficulties with social interactions, and employment inequality. QoL impairment is particularly serious when vitiligo involves visible body parts [8]. Patients are concerned that the condition will spread because the progression of vitiligo is unpredictable. In a recent study, vitiligo patients reported a significantly higher willingness to pay for treatment than did those with other chronic skin disorders, revealing the enormous psychosocial burden of vitiligo patients [9].

Also, children and adolescents with vitiligo often suffer from low self-esteem, difficulties with friendships and schoolwork, and teasing and bullying [10]. Thus, psychological evaluation is particularly important when managing children with vitiligo.

According to the distribution patterns and extent of lesions, vitiligo can be roughly classified into focal, nonsegmental, segmental, and mixed types (Fig. 13.1). Focal vitiligo is defined as a few small, acquired isolated depigmented lesions without segmental distribution with a maximum diameter of 5 cm [11]. Many patients with initially limited disease may eventually have more extensive involvement. In a prospective study, 23% of patients with focal vitiligo developed nonsegmental vitiligo within 2–5 years after initial onset [12].

Nonsegmental vitiligo is the most common type, comprising 85–90% of cases. It is characterized by bilateral white patches symmetrically distributed on any part of the body. White patches appear around the facial orifices and acral sites in acrofacial vitiligo. Vitiligo vulgaris, the most common subtype, further involves the trunk and extremities, often beginning in areas exposed to repeated pressure or irritation. The entire skin is affected in the universal subtype.

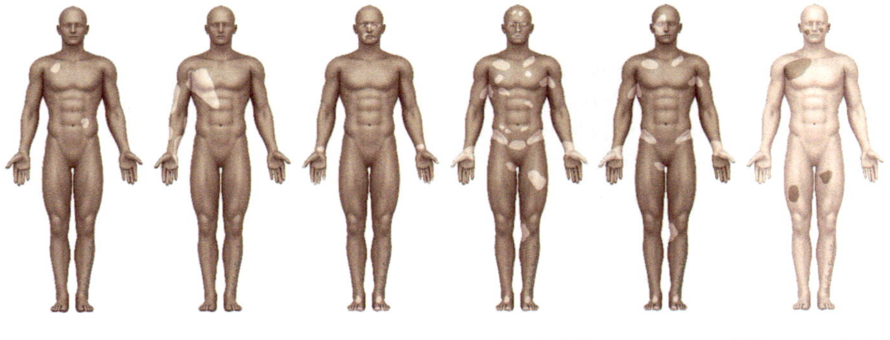

Fig. 13.1 Classification of vitiligo. From left to right, focal vitiligo, segmental vitiligo, acrofacial vitiligo, vitiligo vulgaris, mixed type, vitiligo universalis. Acrofacial, vulgaris, and universal subtypes are also collectively referred to as nonsegmental vitiligo

Segmental vitiligo is a distinct type of vitiligo characterized by a unilateral distribution of white patches along various distinct patterns, including the Blaschko's lines, rarely crossing the midline. It rapidly spreads within the affected area, stabilizes, and persists throughout life. It accounts for 5–16% of all vitiligo; the majority of cases develop before 30 years of age. The face is the most frequently involved site, reported in 71.3% of 956 patients with segmental vitiligo. Meanwhile, recurrence after stabilization for at least 6 months was noted in 11.9% of patients [13]. Mixed-type vitiligo refers to an overlap of segmental and nonsegmental vitiligo in an individual.

Facial vitiligo requires special attention apart from body involvement because vitiligo in the exposed area compromises the QoL significantly more than vitiligo elsewhere. Distinguishing specific subtypes with distinct clinical features would allow us to manage the condition properly by predicting the clinical course. Facial vitiligo could be classified into three distinct subtypes: centrofacial, panfacial, and hairline vitiligo (Fig. 13.2). Centrofacial vitiligo involving the periorificial areas is the most common, exemplifying the typical facial involvement of generalized vitiligo. Panfacial vitiligo with extensive involvement of the face is a distinct subtype with onset in older age and little involvement of other body parts. This subtype tends to respond well to phototherapy but often recurs. Hairline vitiligo is another distinct subtype with an onset in old age and poor response to conventional phototherapy [14].

Some rarer variants of vitiligo are important to recognize.

Inflammatory vitiligo is a rare variant with an erythematous, scaly, raised rim at the periphery of a hypopigmented or depigmented patch. This localized inflammation can precede the onset of classical vitiligo or can appear even several months later. Histological examination of the active margin reveals a typical interface dermatitis with a lichenoid inflammation featuring T cells [15].

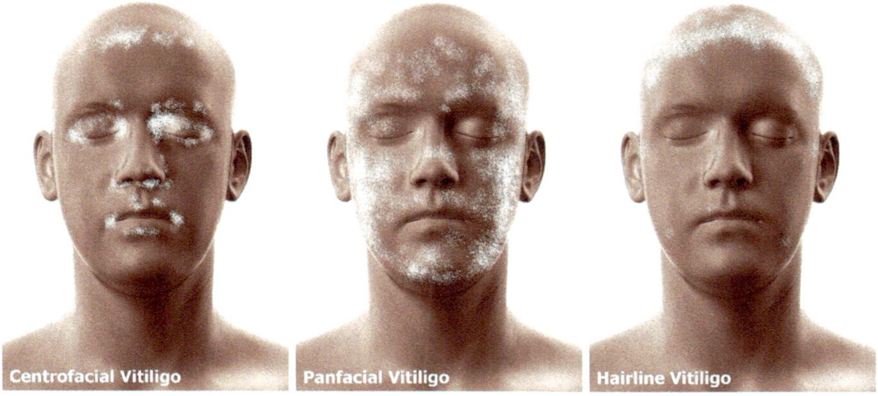

Fig. 13.2 Facial vitiligo. Facial vitiligo is classified into three distinct subtypes: centrofacial, panfacial, and hairline vitiligo. A relevant classification system could help us to anticipate the prognosis and manage the condition in patients with vitiligo

Chemical vitiligo, also termed occupational or contact vitiligo by reference to etiological factors, is induced by contact with phenols or other chemicals. Initial depigmentation usually commences within the exposed area and progresses to remote areas into a typical pattern of vitiligo. Of commercial products that induce vitiligo, cosmetics containing rhododendrol have been of special concern as they were shown to induce melanocyte-specific cytotoxicity and oxidative stress [16]. Because it is indistinguishable from vitiligo in terms of both clinical presentation and histological features, it is considered a chemically induced vitiligo [17].

13.2 Etiology of Vitiligo

Complex interactions between genetic, environmental, and immune systems account for the development of vitiligo. Early studies focused on melanocyte abnormalities and degeneration. Melanocytes from vitiligo patients proliferated more slowly than healthy controls and were more susceptible to oxidative stress [18]. Recently, advanced research has shed light on our understanding of the pathogenesis. Vitiligo patients showed increased melanocyte-specific autoreactive CD8+ cytotoxic T cells, especially on the borders of active disease. Experimental studies revealed that melanocyte reactive T cells produce IFN-γ, which induces local keratinocytes to produce CXCL9 and CXCL10 [19]. These inflammatory chemokines recruited CD8+ T cells to the skin via the CXCR3 receptor of pathogenic T cells [20]. During vitiligo progression, IFN-γ stimulated the JAK/STAT pathway, thus further upregulating IFN-γ-dependent chemokine expression, creating a positive feedback loop (Fig. 13.3).

In terms of the maintenance and relapse of vitiligo, several studies have shown that CD8+ T cells with a resident memory phenotype (TRM cells) were present in vitiligo lesions [21]. IL-15 signaling is required to promote the function and maintenance of TRM cells; IL-15 inhibition may offer a future strategy to prevent disease recurrence [22].

Nonsegmental vitiligo varies in terms of the disease course and the treatment responses by the anatomical region. A recent study found that the dermal fibroblasts of different anatomical regions exhibited different IFN-γ responses, which may contribute to the anatomical preference and therapeutic responses among body sites [23].

Meanwhile, segmental vitiligo is considered to have a distinct mechanism from that of nonsegmental vitiligo. In the past, a neuronal hypothesis was widely accepted; however, the characteristic pattern along the Blaschko line is suggestive of cutaneous mosaicism. The disease may be caused by somatic mutations of developing melanocytes. Recent research has suggested that autoimmunity also contributes to the pathogenesis of segmental vitiligo [24].

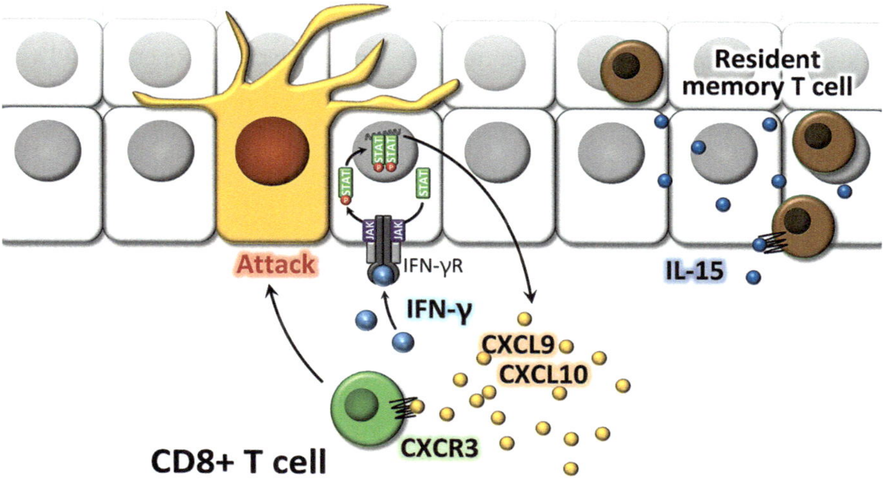

Fig. 13.3 Immunological responses in vitiligo. IFN-γ induces keratinocytes to produce chemokines such as CXCL9 and CXCL10, which recruit autoreactive CD8+ cytotoxic T cells to attack melanocytes. Resident memory T (TRM) cells contribute to the relapse of vitiligo, where IL-15 signaling is critical for TRM cell survival

13.3 Treatment

The treatment strategy of vitiligo seeks to stop disease activity, retain pigmentation, and prevent recurrence. As early intervention can decide the disease prognosis, proactive steps by both patients and physicians are essential. The optimal method should be selected according to the location, extent, and severity of vitiligo.

Currently, NBUVB phototherapy is the gold standard treatment for generalized vitiligo since Westerhof and Krobotova first reported its efficacy in 1997 [25]. NBUVB features a narrow emission peak at a wavelength of 311 nm, which greatly reduced unwanted side effects such as erythema and burning associated with broadband UVB. The safety profile is excellent; NBUVB can be administered to children and pregnant women.

NBUVB successfully repigments vitiligo lesions by stimulating melanocyte differentiation, proliferation, and migration. NBUVB upregulates basic fibroblast growth factor, endothelin-1, and stem cell factor. In addition, melanocyte stem cells differentiate into melanoblasts in response to Wnt/β-catenin signaling, migrate along the outer root sheath, and repopulate towards the epidermis. Also, NBUVB stabilizes vitiligo by inducing the apoptosis of epidermal and dermal T cells and upregulating regulatory T cells.

In most patients who respond to NBUVB, repigmentation is evident in 1–2 months; if no response is noted by 3–6 months, disease status should be reassessed. One meta-analysis [26] reported 75% repigmentation was noted in 13% of patients by 3 months, 19.2% by 6 months, and 35.7% by 12 months. The treatment response depends on the anatomical site; the face responds best, and the hands and feet poorest (Fig. 13.4).

The 308 nm xenon chloride excimer laser (EL) is currently the treatment of choice for localized vitiligo. The EL emits at a monochromatic wavelength of 308 nm and induces photobiological effects similar to NBUVB. The irradiance (mW/cm^2), rather than fluence (mJ/cm^2), was revealed to play a major role in UVB-induced development of immature melanocytes. The EL may induce primitive melanoblasts better than NBUVB.

The EL may yield better cosmetic results than NBUVB, especially in patients with facial vitiligo, as the EL can prevent unnecessary hyperpigmentation of uninvolved skin. Furthermore, children would be good candidates for laser treatment because it does not require entering a phototherapy unit, which may distress them. EL is associated with faster repigmentation onset than NBUVB, showing an initial repigmentation after an average of six treatment sessions. A recommended protocol is shown in Table 13.1.

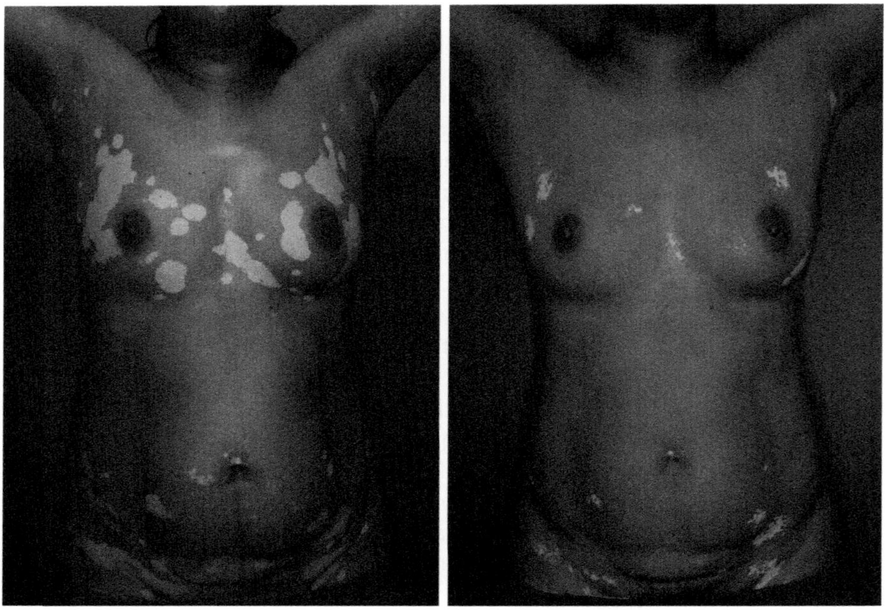

Fig. 13.4 Narrowband UVB phototherapy. Phototherapy has been the mainstay of treatment for vitiligo for decades. Longer treatment duration should be encouraged to enhance the treatment response, and a period of at least 6 months is required to assess the responsiveness to phototherapy

Table 13.1 The proposed 308 nm excimer laser treatment protocol for vitiligo

Body region	Initial dose	Dose increment when erythema is absent
Face and neck	100 mJ/cm²	20–50 mJ/cm²
Trunk and extremities	200 mJ/cm²	50 mJ/cm²
Hands and feet	300 mJ/cm²	50 mJ/cm²
Post-treatment response		*Dose modification*
No erythema		See above
Transient asymptomatic erythema in 48 h		Maintain dose
Persistent asymptomatic erythema over 48 h		Decrease dose by 50–100 mJ/cm²
Persistent symptomatic erythema with pain or blistering		Stop treatment until resolved, then reduce dose by 100 mJ/cm²
General treatment principles		
• A dose that induces asymptomatic erythema for 24–48 h after treatment is ideal • Treatment should be performed on 2 non-consecutive days per week • Sunscreens should be removed from the treatment area because they absorb UVB light • EL treatment can be performed with the eyes closed if the lesions are on the eyelids • The protocols can be adjusted by reference to individual age and condition		

A gain-switched titanium:sapphire laser (TSL) that emits UV light at a 311 nm wavelength was developed recently. The TSL showed comparable efficacy to the EL and exhibited good safety profiles in several clinical studies [27]. Unlike the EL, the TSL requires no periodic gas charging because a solid laser medium is employed.

Topical calcineurin inhibitors (TCIs), including tacrolimus and pimecrolimus, are first-line treatments for localized vitiligo [28]. TCIs possess a dual mechanism action for the treatment of vitiligo: immunosuppressive effects and melanocyte regeneration. A meta-analysis showed that at least mild repigmentation was achieved by 55.0% of patients on TCI monotherapy [29]. A combination therapy of TCI and phototherapy significantly increased the response compared to either therapy alone. Also, TCIs successfully reduced the recurrence rate of vitiligo [30]. Thus, TCIs are recommended for the management of vitiligo after successful repigmentation.

Corticosteroids are well known for anti-inflammatory and immunosuppressive effects. High-potency topical corticosteroids such as clobetasol and betamethasone have long been used to treat localized vitiligo. Several studies have found that topical corticosteroids were as effective as tacrolimus or pimecrolimus in repigmentation of vitiligo [31, 32]. Topical corticosteroid, in combination with NBUVB phototherapy, further enhanced the treatment response [33].

In patients with active vitiligo, systemic therapy is required. Systemic corticosteroids suppress immunity, leading to the disease's arrest and facilitating repigmentation. Low-dose oral prednisolone (0.3 mg/kg daily) for 2 months stabilized 87.7% of 81 active vitiligo patients [34]. Oral minipulse therapy of betamethasone (5–10 mg on two consecutive days weekly) halted disease in 91.8% of 408 patients at 13.2 weeks [35]. Recent studies showed that administration of systemic steroids combined with NBUVB was superior to either monotherapy alone, even in patients with stable vitiligo, reducing the number of total phototherapy sessions and relapses [36]. Furthermore, combination therapy of short-term systemic corticosteroids and phototherapy stabilized and repigmented segmental vitiligo, which often responds poorly to conventional phototherapy [37].

Several studies have suggested that oral calcineurin inhibitors may arrest disease progression and induce pigmentation. Cyclosporine (3 mg/kg/day) not only halted disease progression but also induced repigmentation by 12 weeks [38]. Another randomized controlled study showed that cyclosporine led to disease stabilization even faster than oral steroid minipulse therapy in patients with active progressive vitiligo [39]. In another study, cyclosporine combined with noncultured melanocyte transplantation significantly reduced perigraft halo formation; cyclosporine may effectively target perilesional CD8+ T cells [40].

Although the efficacy of methotrexate (MTX) has been little studied in vitiligo, a randomized controlled trial found that low-dose MTX (10 mg/week) was as effective as dexamethasone oral minipulse therapy in terms of disease arrest [41]. MTX decreased the number of T cells capable of TNF-α production and increased the numbers of T cells producing IL-10 [42]. MTX may be useful for patients with active vitiligo for whom corticosteroids are contraindicated.

JAK inhibitors have shown promising results consistent with the functional importance of IFN-γ/CXCL10/CXCR3 signaling pathway in vitiligo pathogenesis. IFN-γ signals through JAK1 and JAK2; inhibition of either JAK would be expected to reduce IFN-γ signaling. Topical ruxolitinib (a JAK1/2 inhibitor) 1.5% (w/w) cream twice daily was associated with a substantial repigmentation up to 52 weeks of treatment [43]. In a recent study, ritlecitinib (a JAK3/TEC inhibitor) showed a significant repigmentation, suggesting that cytokine signaling dependent on other JAK families might also contribute to vitiligo pathogenesis. Concurrent NBUVB phototherapy appeared to improve the efficacies of both topical and oral forms of JAK inhibitors [44, 45].

As nonsurgical treatment is not always successful, surgical interventions may be required for patients with refractory vitiligo. Surgical treatment is a method in which melanocytes of normal skin are transplanted into vitiligo lesions and provided as a source of repigmentation. It is primarily divided into tissue and cellular grafting, depending on the nature of the graft.

Selection of patients with stable vitiligo that has not spread for more than 12 months is the most critical factor that decides the surgical outcome. It is also important to choose an appropriate surgical modality for each patient; a combination of procedures often improves the overall outcome. Punch grafting is a traditional surgical option for vitiligo; 1–2 mm punch grafts are transferred from normal skin to a vitiligo area. This is the most convenient and least expensive method, but the major limitations include the long procedure time required and cobblestoning. Recently, 0.5–0.8 mm motorized micropunch grafting has been introduced and markedly reduced both the time required and complications (Fig. 13.5) [46]. Repigmentation spreading from each punch graft is evident by 2–3 weeks after

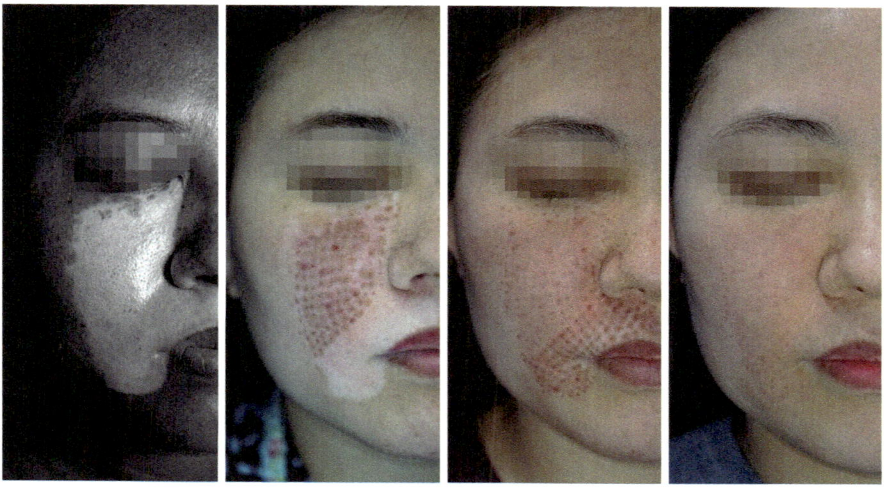

Fig. 13.5 Micropunch grafting. Micropunch grafting using 0.5–0.8 mm motorized micropunches can markedly reduce both operation time and complications such as cobblestone appearance. Preferred indications are face and neck vitiligo, children, and small scattered lesions

transplantation. The preferred indications are face and neck vitiligo, childhood vitiligo, and small scattered lesions.

In another method, suction blister grafting, blisters created on normal skin using suction cups or syringes are transplanted to the denuded vitiligo lesions. Suction blisters induced by negative pressure cause the split precisely at the dermal-epidermal junction; it is possible to harvest only the epidermal sheets where the melanocytes are located. Repigmentation is usually evident within weeks of the procedure. The limitations include perigraft haloes and the long time required to create blisters. Also, the donor:recipient ratio is 1:1, so it is difficult to perform on large areas requiring many blisters.

Cell transplantation allows smooth margins and better cosmetic results due to the small transplantation unit. It is a surgical method that separates melanocytes and keratinocytes from normal skin and transplants them into vitiligo lesions as a cell suspension. For extensive vitiligo, cellular grafting has the advantage of treating a large area at once. The area of non-cultured epidermal cell suspension transplantation (NCES) can be five to ten-fold that of the donor area. NCES features four steps: harvesting of normal epidermis, cell separation, preparation of a cell suspension, and transplantation. NCES requires 4–5 h of operation time and a skilled team for a satisfactory result.

Several modifications have been described to enhance the outcome of NCES. The addition of dermal cell suspensions enhanced the responses in patients whose vitiligo durations were less than 12 months [47]. Hair follicle outer root sheath cell suspension achieved repigmentation comparable to that of NCES [48, 49].

Cultured epidermal cell suspensions can be innovatively used to treat extensive areas of stable vitiligo; autologous melanocytes and keratinocytes are cultured and

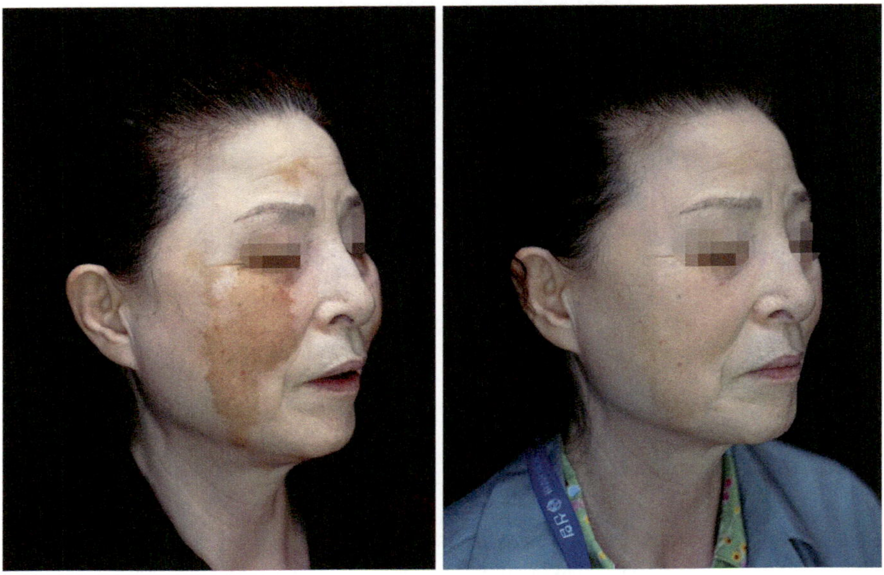

Fig. 13.6 Depigmentation therapy using monobenzyl ether of hydroquinone (MBEH). When vitiligo spreads extensively and is difficult to treat with standard treatments, depigmentation therapy can help patients improve their quality of life. The application of MBEH 20% ointment is effective, but caution is required as it may cause depigmentation in the area if it is applied to other family members

transplanted. This is an expensive and complicated procedure requiring a dedicated laboratory and instrumentation. However, it can cover the largest recipient area up to 10- to 60-fold that of the donor area [50]. Although it remains experimental, many patients and physicians look forward to the future development of the method.

Depigmentation can be considered for patients whose vitiligo involves over 60–80% of the total body surface area and who do not respond to conventional treatments. The monobenzyl ether of hydroquinone (MBEH) is the only FDA-approved depigmenting agent. Residual melanocytes are destroyed by the application of 20% (w/w) MBEH cream twice daily; complete depigmentation requires 2–8 months (Fig. 13.6). The possible side effects include erythema, burning, itching, and systemic absorption. Special care must be taken to ensure that family members do not contact the cream.

13.3.1 Dihydroxyacetone

Camouflage is a good option as a tide-over while other therapies take effect and cover visible remnant areas. Dihydroxyacetone (DHA), the principal component of self-tanning products, contains sugars that bind to amino acids in the stratum corneum to produce melanoidin, a brown high-molecular-weight polymer. The color fades as the stratum corneum exfoliates over 3–6 days. DHA creams are available at concentrations of 5–15% (w/w) for skins of different colors.

Micropigmentation, also termed semi-permanent make-up, features fine-needle insertion of pigment particles into the epidermis and upper dermis. This can be an alternative option for patients with acral vitiligo resistant to conventional treatments. Inserted pigments remain in the papillary dermis for 2–3 years [51]. The procedure has several limitations. It is difficult to treat extensive lesions and the texture and color change seasonally. Careful color selection and an appropriate implantation depth are important.

13.4 Conclusion

Vitiligo is a major skin disease that profoundly impacts patients' lives, especially those of people of color. Although the treatment of vitiligo is not easy, conventional treatments afford significant improvements in most patients. Thus, it is important to understand all possible therapeutic options and choose an optimal treatment modality considering the patient's age, condition, and disease subtype and activity. Surgical or camouflage options may be useful for patients resistant to nonsurgical interventions. Vitiligo is more than just a cosmetic disease; comprehensive management is required, with special attention to the psychological burden. As vitiligo treatment is usually prolonged, patient encouragement is required to enhance treatment adherence. The more we understand the patient's suffering, the better physicians can respectfully and knowledgeably assist our patients.

References

1. Krüger C, Schallreuter KU. A review of the worldwide prevalence of vitiligo in children/adolescents and adults. Int J Dermatol. 2012;51:1206–12.
2. Cunliffe WJ, Hall R, Newell DJ, et al. Vitiligo, thyroid disease and autoimmunity. Br J Dermatol. 1968;80:135–9.
3. Jin Y, Andersen G, Yorgov D, et al. Genome-wide association studies of autoimmune vitiligo identify 23 new risk loci and highlight key pathways and regulatory variants. Nat Genet. 2016;48:1418–24.
4. El-Mofty AM. Observations on the use of Ammi majus Linn. In vitiligo. Br J Dermatol. 1952;64:431–41.
5. Zubair R, Hamzavi IH. Phototherapy for Vitiligo. Dermatol Clin. 2020;38:55–62.
6. Elbuluk N, Ezzedine K. Quality of Life, Burden of Disease, Comorbidities, and Systemic Effects in Vitiligo Patients. Dermatol Clin. 2017;35:117–28.
7. Bae JM, Hong BY, Lee JH, et al. The efficacy of 308-nm excimer laser/light (EL) and topical agent combination therapy versus EL monotherapy for vitiligo: A systematic review and meta-analysis of randomized controlled trials (RCTs). J Am Acad Dermatol. 2016;74:907–15.
8. Bae JM, Lee SC, Kim TH, et al. Factors affecting quality of life in patients with vitiligo: a nationwide study. Br J Dermatol. 2018;178:238–44.
9. Bae JM, Kim JE, Lee RW, et al. Beyond quality of life: A call for patients' own willingness to pay in chronic skin disease to assess psychosocial burden-A multicenter, cross-sectional, prospective survey. J Am Acad Dermatol. 2021;85:1321–4.

10. Silverberg JI, Silverberg NB. Quality of life impairment in children and adolescents with vitiligo. Pediatr Dermatol. 2014;31:309–18.
11. Ezzedine K, Lim HW, Suzuki T, et al. Revised classification/nomenclature of vitiligo and related issues: the Vitiligo Global Issues Consensus Conference. Pigment Cell Melanoma Res. 2012;25:E1–13.
12. Lommerts JE, Schilder Y, de Rie MA, et al. Focal vitiligo: long-term follow-up of 52 cases. J Eur Acad Dermatol Venereol. 2016;30:1550–4.
13. Oh J, Lee RW, Lee HR, et al. Classification of facial and truncal segmental vitiligo and its clinical courses including recurrence rate and patterns: a retrospective review of 956 patients. Br J Dermatol. 2021;184:750–3.
14. Bae JM, Jung YS, Jung HM, et al. Classification of facial vitiligo: A cluster analysis of 473 patients. Pigment Cell Melanoma Res. 2018;31:585–91.
15. Attili VR, Attili SK. Lichenoid inflammation in vitiligo—a clinical and histopathologic review of 210 cases. Int J Dermatol. 2008;47:663–9.
16. Matsunaga K, Suzuki K, Ito A, et al. Rhododendrol-induced leukoderma update I: Clinical findings and treatment. J Dermatol. 2021;48:961–8.
17. Rodrigues M, Ezzedine K, Hamzavi I, et al. New discoveries in the pathogenesis and classification of vitiligo. J Am Acad Dermatol. 2017;77:1–13.
18. Frisoli ML, Essien K, Harris JE. Vitiligo: Mechanisms of Pathogenesis and Treatment. Annu Rev. Immunol. 2020;38:621–48.
19. Rashighi M, Agarwal P, Richmond JM, et al. CXCL10 is critical for the progression and maintenance of depigmentation in a mouse model of vitiligo. Sci Transl Med. 2014;6:223ra223.
20. Richmond JM, Masterjohn E, Chu R, et al. CXCR3 Depleting Antibodies Prevent and Reverse Vitiligo in Mice. J Invest Dermatol. 2017;137:982–5.
21. Boniface K, Jacquemin C, Darrigade AS, et al. Vitiligo Skin Is Imprinted with Resident Memory CD8 T Cells Expressing CXCR3. J Invest Dermatol. 2018;138:355–64.
22. Richmond JM, Strassner JP, Zapata L Jr, et al. Antibody blockade of IL-15 signaling has the potential to durably reverse vitiligo. Sci Transl Med. 2018;10(450):eaam7710.
23. Xu Z, Chen D, Hu Y, et al. Anatomically distinct fibroblast subsets determine skin autoimmune patterns. Nature. 2021;601:118–24.
24. Speeckaert R, Lambert J, Bulat V, et al. Autoimmunity in Segmental Vitiligo. Front Immunol. 2020;11:568447.
25. Westerhof W, Nieuweboer-Krobotova L. Treatment of vitiligo with UV-B radiation vs. topical psoralen plus UV-A. Arch Dermatol. 1997;133:1525–8.
26. Bae JM, Jung HM, Hong BY, et al. Phototherapy for Vitiligo: A Systematic Review and Meta-analysis. JAMA Dermatol. 2017;153:666–74.
27. Bae JM, Eun SH, Lee HN, et al. Comparison of 311-nm Titanium:Sapphire laser and 308-nm excimer laser treatment for vitiligo: A randomized controlled non-inferiority trial. Lasers Surg Med. 2019;51:239–44.
28. Stinco G, Piccirillo F, Forcione M, et al. An open randomized study to compare narrow band UVB, topical pimecrolimus and topical tacrolimus in the treatment of vitiligo. Eur J Dermatol. 2009;19:588–93.
29. Lee JH, Kwon HS, Jung HM, et al. Treatment Outcomes of Topical Calcineurin Inhibitor Therapy for Patients With Vitiligo: A Systematic Review and Meta-analysis. JAMA Dermatol. 2019;155:929–38.
30. Cavalié M, Ezzedine K, Fontas E, et al. Maintenance therapy of adult vitiligo with 0.1% tacrolimus ointment: a randomized, double blind, placebo-controlled study. J Invest Dermatol. 2015;135:970–4.
31. Bagherani N. Comparison of pimecrolimus with clobetasol propionate in the treatment of localized vitiligo. Dermatol Ther. 2016;29:288.
32. Mumtaz H, Anis S, Akhtar A, et al. Efficacy of Tacrolimus Versus Clobetasol in the Treatment of Vitiligo. Cureus. 2020;12:e11985.

33. Bapur Erduran F, Adışen E. Comparison of the efficacy of 308-nm excimer lamp monotherapy with topical tacrolimus or clobetasol 17-propionate combination therapies in localized vitiligo. Photodermatol Photoimmunol Photomed. 2016;32:247–53.
34. Kim SM, Lee HS, Hann SK. The efficacy of low-dose oral corticosteroids in the treatment of vitiligo patients. Int J Dermatol. 1999;38:546–50.
35. Kanwar AJ, Mahajan R, Parsad D. Low-dose oral mini-pulse dexamethasone therapy in progressive unstable vitiligo. J Cutan Med Surg. 2013;17:259–68.
36. El Mofty M, Essmat S, Youssef R, et al. The role of systemic steroids and phototherapy in the treatment of stable vitiligo: a randomized controlled trial. Dermatol Ther. 2016;29:406–12.
37. Bae JM, Yoo HJ, Kim H, et al. Combination therapy with 308-nm excimer laser, topical tacrolimus, and short-term systemic corticosteroids for segmental vitiligo: A retrospective study of 159 patients. J Am Acad Dermatol. 2015;73:76–82.
38. Taneja A, Kumari A, Vyas K, et al. Cyclosporine in treatment of progressive vitiligo: An open-label, single-arm interventional study. Indian J Dermatol Venereol Leprol. 2019;85:528–31.
39. Mehta H, Kumar S, Parsad D, et al. Oral cyclosporine is effective in stabilizing active vitiligo: Results of a randomized controlled trial. Dermatol Ther. 2021;34:e15033.
40. Mutalik S, Shah S, Sidwadkar V, et al. Efficacy of Cyclosporine After Autologous Noncultured Melanocyte Transplantation in Localized Stable Vitiligo-A Pilot, Open Label. Comparative Study. Dermatol Surg. 2017;43:1339–47.
41. Singh H, Kumaran MS, Bains A, et al. A Randomized Comparative Study of Oral Corticosteroid Minipulse and Low-Dose Oral Methotrexate in the Treatment of Unstable Vitiligo. Dermatology. 2015;231:286–90.
42. Rudwaleit M, Yin Z, Siegert S, et al. Response to methotrexate in early rheumatoid arthritis is associated with a decrease of T cell derived tumour necrosis factor alpha, increase of interleukin 10, and predicted by the initial concentration of interleukin 4. Ann Rheum Dis. 2000;59:311–4.
43. Rosmarin D, Pandya AG, Lebwohl M, et al. Ruxolitinib cream for treatment of vitiligo: a randomised, controlled, phase 2 trial. Lancet. 2020;396:110–20.
44. Liu LY, Strassner JP, Refat MA, et al. Repigmentation in vitiligo using the Janus kinase inhibitor tofacitinib may require concomitant light exposure. J Am Acad Dermatol. 2017;77:675–682.e671.
45. Phan K, Phan S, Shumack S, et al. Repigmentation in vitiligo using janus kinase (JAK) inhibitors with phototherapy: systematic review and Meta-analysis. J Dermatolog Treat. 2020;33(1):173–7.
46. Bae JM, Lee JH, Kwon HS, et al. Motorized 0.8-mm micropunch grafting for refractory vitiligo: A retrospective study of 230 cases. J Am Acad Dermatol. 2018;79:720–727.e721.
47. Thakur V, Kumar S, Kumaran MS, et al. Efficacy of Transplantation of Combination of Noncultured Dermal and Epidermal Cell Suspension vs. Epidermal Cell Suspension Alone in Vitiligo: A Randomized Clinical Trial. JAMA Dermatol. 2019;155:204–10.
48. Vinay K, Dogra S, Parsad D, et al. Clinical and treatment characteristics determining therapeutic outcome in patients undergoing autologous non-cultured outer root sheath hair follicle cell suspension for treatment of stable vitiligo. J Eur Acad Dermatol Venereol. 2015;29:31–7.
49. Kumar P, Bhari N, Tembhre MK, et al. Study of efficacy and safety of noncultured, extracted follicular outer root sheath cell suspension transplantation in the management of stable vitiligo. Int J Dermatol. 2018;57:245–9.
50. Hong WS, Hu DN, Qian GP, et al. Ratio of size of recipient and donor areas in treatment of vitiligo by autologous cultured melanocyte transplantation. Br J Dermatol. 2011;165:520–5.
51. Ju HJ, Eun SH, Lee HN, et al. Micropigmentation for vitiligo on light to moderately colored skin: Updated evidence from a clinical and animal study. J Dermatol. 2020;47:464–9.

Autoinflammatory Disorders: Under-Discussed Pathologies in Dermatology

14

Bhavya Swarnkar

Autoinflammatory diseases are rare disorders characterized by recurrent or persistent systemic inflammation in the form of recurrent fever, mucocutaneous lesions, serositis, osteoarticular, and various other symptoms, in the absence of infectious, neoplastic, or autoimmune triggers [1]. Though these disorders have been known for quite a long time, their detailed understanding has been of recent interest. These unprovoked episodes of systemic inflammation are caused by the defective innate immune response unlike autoimmune disorders where acquired immunity is the culprit. Majority of these disorders are monogenic, seen predominantly during childhood, and caused by amutation or polymorphism in genes controlling innate immune response. There is excessive production of acute phase reactants and inflammatory cytokines like IL-1 β, IL-6 in the autoinflammatory disorders [2].

The clinical presentations of these disorders include fever, skin rash, mucosal ulcers, arthritis, vasculopathy/vasculitis, ocular involvement, organomegaly, and lymphadenopathy. Few or all clinical features occur in periodicity, forming the crux of the diagnosis, especially after ruling out diseases like infections, malignancy, and autoimmunity. Cutaneous manifestations are quite common in many of these diseases and might indicate a higher likelihood of a particular autoinflammatory disorder over the others.

In 1999, Kastner et al. first described the term "autoinflammation" describing two diseases characterized by recurrent episodes of systemic inflammation without any identifiable trigger: TNF Receptor-Associated Periodic Syndrome (TRAPS) and Familial Mediterranean Fever (FMF) [3].

No specific triggers, such as an infection or malignancy has been identified yet. Self-directed inflammation due to a predominantly inherited or acquired monogenic/polygenic alteration in innate immunity leads to recurrent or periodic systemic inflammation. Underlying inflammation may be persistent without overt clinical signs and symptoms leading to complications like amyloidosis.

B. Swarnkar (✉)
Department of Dermatology, Apollo Hospitals, Bilaspur, Chhattisgarh, India

S. Gupta et al. (eds.), *Critical Thinking in Contemporary Dermatology: Cognitive Essays*, https://doi.org/10.1007/978-981-97-0411-8_14

Inflammasomes are critical to the pathogenesis (inflammasomopathies) but recently, nuclear factor (NF)-kB-mediated disorders (Relopathies) and type 1 interferonopathies have been studied [4].

The most common mechanism involving inflammasomes (pattern recognition receptors) is mentioned in Flowchart 14.1:

As has been mentioned before, the cluster of clinical features occurring periodically after excluding infections, malignancy and autoimmunity forms the basis of the diagnosis of autoinflammatory disorders. There is no one clinical feature; rather, the combination (fever, skin rash, arthritis, etc.) helps in making the diagnosis. Sometimes it is difficult to recognize the pattern of these features and diagnosis is delayed. A high index of suspicion is key to early diagnosis. Although the majority of these syndromes have recurrent fever, some of them have no fever or show persistent fever, further complicating the process of making a diagnosis. Some other clues include positive family history, childhood onset, and raised acute phase reactants like ESR and CRP, especially during the episodes [1, 5].

As skin rash is quite common in these disorders, we as dermatologists need to be aware of them to help in the diagnosis and treatment of such patients. Urticarial lesions (so-called atypical urticaria) are the commonest dermatological manifestation. Autoinflammatory urticaria differs from idiopathic urticaria in lesions being polymorphic (patches or purpura may be present), with no surrounding flare, no associated angioedema, predominant symmetrically involving trunk and extremities with relative sparing of face, longer-lasting (sometimes exceeding 24 h), being asymptomatic or burning or pruritic, and showing poor response to conventional antihistamines. Atypical urticaria lacks dermal edema and shows neutrophilic predominance rather than eosinophilic predominance in histopathology [6]. Other dermatological manifestations include erysipelas-like, cellulitis-like rash, erythematous papuloplaques, periorbital edema, mucosal ulcers, vasculitis/vasculopathic lesions, neutrophilic dermatosis-like rash, pustules, nodules, and granulomatous lesions.

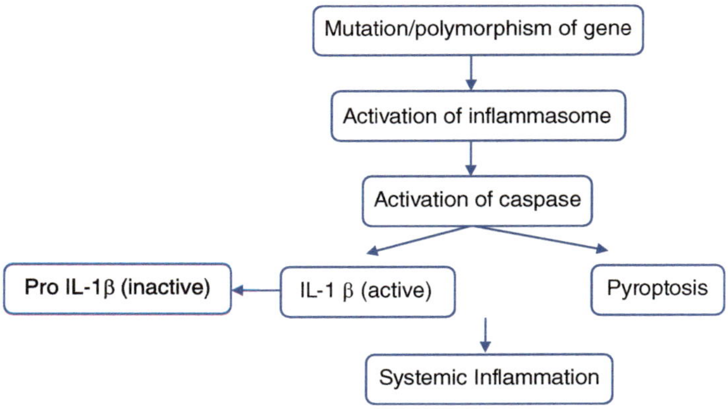

Flowchart 14.1 Inflammasome-mediated autoinflammation

The concept of systemic autoinflammatory diseases has expanded over time to include recognition of a continuum between autoinflammatory and autoimmune disorders. It also includes polygenic disorders like neutrophilic dermatosis, acne, vitiligo, psoriasis, alopecia areata, atopic and contact dermatitis, and systemic lupus erythematosus [7]. This is mentioned in Flowchart 14.2 [8].

Autoinflammatory disorders (AIDs) can be classified based on the involved pathogenic mechanism as mentioned in Table 14.1: [9, 10].

Various classifications have been proposed over time based on clinical and histopathological features of cutaneous manifestations of monogenic autoinflammatory disorders.

A new classification depicting nine dermatologic categories as suggested by Figueras-Nart et al. is mentioned in Table 14.2: [10].

The diagnosis of autoinflammatory syndromes is mainly clinical, while genetic analysis is only used to confirm the clinical suspicion. Autoinflammatory diseases during *adulthood* are usually of milder phenotypes, seem to be driven by mild genotypes, and develop because of low-penetrance mutations or polymorphisms of respective genes as compared to the onset in children [11]. It is difficult to reach the diagnosis not only because of its rarity but also because of overlap with diseases like infections, malignancy, and autoimmunity.

General signs of chronic inflammation in children include growth retardation and organomegaly. Anemia of chronic disease is seen in all age groups. During the attacks, there is elevation of total leukocyte count and acute phase reactants like ESR, CRP, ferritin, and serum amyloid A protein. In between the attacks, these components may be elevated or normal.

In older times, in untreated cases, the risk of systemic amyloidosis was as high as 60%, but with the availability of good treatment options the incidence of

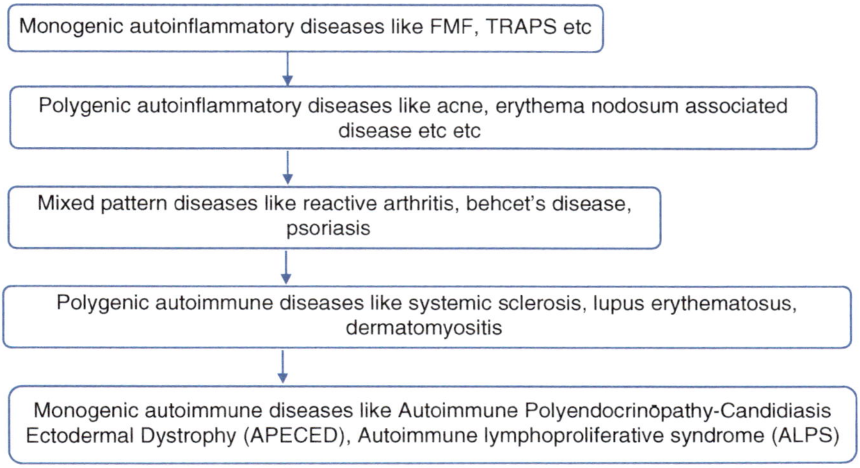

Flowchart 14.2 Spectrum of immunological diseases

Table 14.1 Autoinflammatory disorders based on pathogenic mechanism

Disease		Mutation
Inflammasomopathies/ Monogenic recurrent fevers	Familial Mediterranean fever (FMF)	MEFV, autosomal recessive
	Mevalonate kinase deficiency/ hyper IgD syndrome (MKD/HIDS)	MVK, autosomal recessive
	TNF receptor-associated periodic fever syndrome (TRAPS)	TNFRSF1A, autosomal dominant
	Cryopyrin-associated periodic syndrome (CAPS)	NLRP3, autosomal dominant
	Pyogenic arthritis, pyoderma gangrenosum, acne syndrome (PAPA)	PSTPIP1, autosomal dominant
New inflammasomopathies	NLRC4-inflammasomopathies including autoinflammation and infantile enterocolitis (AIFEC) fever and familial cold autoinflammatory syndrome 4 (FCAS4)	NLRC4, autosomal dominant
	NLRP1-associated autoinflammation with arthritis and dyskeratosis (NAIAD)	NLRP1, autosomal dominant and autosomal recessive
	NALP12 periodic fever syndrome	NALP12, autosomal dominant
	Pyrin-associated autoinflammation with neutrophilic dermatosis (PAAND)	S242R autosomal dominant mutation of MEFV gene
	Autoinflammation and PLCγ2-associated antibody deficiency and immune dysregulation (APLAID)/PLAID (FCAS3)	PLCG2
	Periodic fever immunodeficiency and thrombocytopenia (PFIT)	WDR1
	C/EBP + -associated autoinflammation and immune impairment of neutrophils (CAIN)	CEBPE, autosomal recessive
Relopathies/nuclear factor kappa-B (NFk-B)-related AIDs	NOD2/CARD 15-associated diseases: Blau syndrome/early onset sarcoidosis	NOD2, autosomal dominant
	NOD2/CARD 15-associated diseases: NOD2-associated autoinflammatory disease (NAID) or Yao syndrome	NOD2/CARD15
	NLRP12-associated autoinflammatory disease (NLRP12-AD) (FCAS2)	NLRP12, autosomal dominant
	Familial pityriasis rubra pilaris/CARD14-associated psoriasis	CARD14, autosomal dominant
	NFKB1-associated autoinflammatory diseases (NFKB1-AD)	NFKB1, autosomal dominant
	RELA haploinsufficiency	RELA, autosomal dominant

Table 14.1 (continued)

Disease		Mutation
	ADAM17 deficiency	ADAM17, autosomal recessive
Ubiquitinopathies	Autoinflammation/immunodeficiency associated with mutations in LUBAC proteins	HOIP, autosomal recessive HOIL, autosomal dominant
	A20 protein haploinsufficiency (HA20)	TNFAIP3, autosomal dominant
	Otulin deficiency (ORAS)	FAM105B, autosomal recessive
Interferonopathies	Aicardi Goutieres syndrome (AGS)	TREX1, NASEH2, SAMHD1, ADAR1, autosomal recessive, IFIH1, autosomal dominant
	STING-associated vasculopathy with onset in infancy (SAVI)	TMEM173, autosomal Dominant
	Proteasome-associated autoinflammatory syndromes (PRAAS)/ chronic atypical neutrophilic dermatitis with lipodystrophy and elevated temperature syndrome (CANDLE)	PSMB8, PSMB4 PSMA3, PSMB9, POMP, autosomal dominant
	Familial chilblain lupus	TREX1, SAMHD1, TMEM173, autosomal dominant
	Singleton-Merten syndrome (SMS)	IFIH1 DDX58, autosomal dominant
	POMP-related autoinflammation and immune dysregulation disease (PRAID)	POMP
	Spondyloenchondrodysplasia with immune dysregulation (SPENCDI)	ACP5, autosomal recessive
Other monogenic AIDs	Adenosine deaminase 2 (ADA2) deficiency	ADA2, autosomal recessive
	Sideroblastic anemia, immunodeficiency, fevers and developmental Delay (SIFD)	TRNT1, autosomal recessive
	Deficiency of IL-36 receptor antagonist (DITRA)	IL36RN, autosomal recessive
	H syndrome	SLC29A3, autosomal recessive
	Vibratory urticaria	ADGRE2, autosomal dominant
	AP1S3 and autoinflammatory psoriasis	AP1S3

(continued)

Table 14.1 (continued)

Disease		Mutation
	Monogenic forms of inflammatory bowel disease (IL-10 signaling defects)	IL10RA, IL10RB, and IL10, autosomal recessive
Autoinflammatory diseases without an identified monogenic etiology	Systemic-onset juvenile idiopathic arthritis (SoJIA)	Polygenic Monogenic early onset associated to mutation of LACC1/FAMIN
	Idiopathic pericarditis	Polygenic
Autoinflammatory bone disorders	Chronic recurrent multifocal osteomyelitis (CRMO)	Polygenic
	Majeed syndrome	LPIN2
	Deficiency of IL-1 receptor antagonist (DIRA)	IL1RN, autosomal recessive
	Cherubism	SH3BP2, autosomal dominant

systemic amyloidosis has drastically decreased. So, if there is a suspicion or as a part of regular screening, urine 24-h protein should be analysed. Rectalor abdominal fat pad biopsy, renal biopsy, and iodine-123-labeled serum amyloid P scan-which is highly sensitive-can be considered for ruling out systemic amyloidosis [12].

There is no **one** specific cutaneous histopathological finding. The findings vary depending upon specific disease and its cutaneous manifestation. For example, in FMF, erysipelas-like lesions show dermal edema with perivascular lymphohistiocytic and neutrophilic infiltrate. DIF (direct immunofluorescence) shows IgM, C3, and fibrinogen in the capillaries of papillary dermis. In cryopyrin-associated autoinflammatory syndrome (CAPS), there is evidence of neutrophilic urticaria where neutrophils predominate in eccrine ducts and the epidermis [13].

We shall be discussing some of the common autoinflammatory syndromes here.

Table 14.2 A classification depicting nine categories of dermatologic manifestations

S. No.	Main cutaneous manifestation	Disease
1.	Urticarial rashes	Cryopyrin-associated periodic syndromes (CAPS) NLRP12-associated autoinflammatory disease (NLRP12-AD) PLCγ2-associated antibody deficiency and immune Dysregulation (PLAID) NLRC4-associated autoinflammatory diseases (NRLC4-AD) Vibratory urticaria
2.	Maculopapular rashes or inflammatory plaques	Familial Mediterranean fever (FMF) TNF receptor-associated periodic syndrome (traps) Hyper-IgD syndrome/mevalonate kinase deficiency (HIDS/MKD) Otulipenia/OTULIN-related autoinflammatory Syndrome (ORAS) HOIL-1 deficiency
3.	Pustular, pyogenic, or neutrophilic dermatosis-like rashes	Pyogenic sterile arthritis, pyoderma gangrenosum, and acne (PAPA) Syndromic forms of pyoderma gangrenosum Deficiency of IL-1 receptor antagonist (DIRA) Deficiency of IL-36 receptor antagonist (DITRA) CARD-14-mediated psoriasis (CAMPS) Majeed syndrome Pyrin-associated autoinflammation with neutrophilic dermatosis (PAAND) Singleton-Merten syndrome (SMS) ADAM17 deficiency AP1S3 and autoinflammatory psoriasis NFKB1-associated sterile familial autoinflammatory necrotizing fasciitis (FANF)
4.	Vasculitis or vasculopathy	Deficiency of adenosine deaminase 2 (DADA2) STING-associated vasculopathy with onset in infancy (SAVI) Familial chilblain lupus Aicardi-Goutières syndrome (AGS) 1–7 Spodyloenchondrodysplasia with immune dysregulation (SPENCDI)
5.	Panniculitis or subcutaneous nodules	Blau syndrome / early-onset sarcoidosis Chronic atypical neutrophilic dermatitis with Lipodystrophy and elevated temperature (CANDLE)
6.	Hyperpigmented lesions	H syndrome
7.	Hyperkeratotic lesions	NLRP-1-associated disease (NAIAD)

(continued)

Table 14.2 (continued)

S. No.	Main cutaneous manifestation	Disease
8.	Aphthous lesions	Haploinsufficiency of A20 (HA20) Autoinflammatory periodic fever, immunodeficiency, and thrombocytopenia (PFIT) C/EBP + -associated autoinflammation and immune impairment of neutrophils (CAIN) NFKB1-associated Behcet-like disease RELA haploinsufficiency Monogenic forms of inflammatory bowel disease (IL-10 signaling defects)
9.	Bullous lesions	Autoinflammation and PLCγ2-associated antibody deficiency and immune dysregulation (APLAID)

14.1 Inflammasomopathies [9, 10]: A Few of Them Are Tabulated in Table 14.3

1. FMF is the most frequent monogenic autoinflammatory disease.
2. TRAPS is the most frequent autosomal dominant autoinflammatory disease.
3. CAPS includes familial cold autoinflammatory syndrome (FCAS) (mildest), chronic infantile neutrophilic cutaneous and articular or neonatal onset multisystem inflammatory disease (CINCA/NOMID) (most severe form), and Muckle-Wells syndrome (MWS), which has a severity in between.

14.1.1 Other Inflammasomopathies

NLRC4-inflammasomopathies: Related to mutations of NLR-family CARD domain-containing protein 4 (NLRC4) gene.

Autoinflammation and infantile enterocolitis (AIFEC) fever is characterized by recurrent episodes of multiorgan autoinflammatory syndrome and very early onset enterocolitis. There is elevated serum IL-18 during the attacks.

Familial cold autoinflammatory syndrome 4 (FCAS4) presents with neonatal-onset, cold-induced urticaria and arthralgia resembling FCAS [14].

NLRP1-associated autoinflammation with arthritis and dyskeratoisis (NAIAD): Early onset oligo/polyarthritis, recurrent fever, vitamin A deficiency, immunological dysfunction in the form of chronic or recurrent infections, and dyskeratotic skin lesions. Acitretin has been used for dyskeratosis with variable results.

NALP12 periodic fever syndrome- Very early onset, recurrent fever, arthralgia, headache, triggered by cold exposure.

Pyrin-associated autoinflammation with neutrophilic dermatosis (PAAND): Early onset of febrile episodes along with arthalgia, myalgia, and neutrophilic dermatosis. Pyoderma gangrenosum, neutrophilic abscesses, severe acne, and neutrophilic small vessel vasculitis are other dermatological manifestations. Anakinra and anti-TNF α agents are used for the treatment [15].

Table 14.3 Inflammasomopathies

Disease	Onset	Fever	Cutaneous manifestations	Other features	Treatment
FMF[1]	Childhood	Attack lasting 12–72 h	**Erysipelas like rash on lower limbs**, Diffuse palmoplantar erythema and purpuric papules involving the face, trunk, and extremities	Non-deforming oligoarthritis of lower limbs, myalgia, less commonly: destructive arthritis, serositis, aseptic meningitis, systemic vasculitis, etc.	Colchicine, anti-IL-1 agents
MVK/HIDS	Infancy	Attack lasting 3–7 days	70% patients, **Aphthous stomatitis**, Non-migratory maculopapular, urticarial rash, macules, papules, nodules, cellulitis like rash, erythema nodosum, petechiae, purpura, erythema elevatum diutinum, neutrophilic dermatosis	Cervical lymphadenopathy Myalgia, arthralgia, diarrhea, vomiting, neurological involvement Increased serum IgD, IgA, urine mevalonic acid level during attacks	Glucocorticoids, anti-IL-1 agents, etanercept, tocilizumab
TRAPS[2]	Childhood	Attacks lasting up to 3–4 weeks	80% patients, **migratory pseudo-cellulitis rash**, periorbital edema, urticaria-like plaques, generalized serpiginous plaques, and small-sized vessel vasculitis	Myalgia associated with pseudo-cellulitic rash, arthralgia, serositis	NSAIDs, glucocorticoids, Anti-IL-1 agents, etanercept, tocilizumab
FCAS[3]	Childhood	<24 h	Cold-induced urticaria	Conjunctivitis Arthralgia	Anti-IL-1 agents like anakinra, canakinumab
MWS[3]	Childhood	2–3 days	Urticarial rash	Sensorineural hearing loss, arthralgia, episcleritis, conjunctivitis	Anti-IL-1 agents
CINCA/ NOMID[3]	Childhood	Continuous	Urticarial rash	Hypertrophic arthropathy of long bones, Facial dysmorphism, chronic arthritis, aseptic chronic meningitis, uveitis, conjunctivitis	Anti-IL-1 agents
PAPA	Childhood		Severe cystic acne Pyoderma gangrenosum Hydradenitis Suppurativa	Sterile pyogenic arthritis, hepatosplenomegaly, growth failure, pancytopenia	Glucocorticoids, IL-1 blockers, and anti-TNF agents

Autoinflammation and PLCγ2-associated antibody deficiency and immune dysregulation (APLAID): Cellulitis, recurrent skin blistering (epidermolysis bullosa-like), erythematous plaques, vesicopustular lesions, interstitial pneumonia, enterocolitis, arthralgia, ocular erosions, recurrent sinopulmonary infections, low serum IgM and IgA. It shows good response to oral corticosteroids.

PLAID: Recurrent itchy cold-induced evaporative urticaria, **presence of autoantibodies like ANA**, immunoglobulin deficiencies. Other cutaneous findings include nasal tip ulceration in neonates, erosions and papules over fingers and toes, and granulomatous inflammatory lesions.

Periodic fever immunodeficiency and thrombocytopenia (PFIT): Early onset of recurrent fever (of up to 7 days duration), thrombocytopenia, mucosal ulceration, thrombocytopenia, and recurrent infections. Corticosteroid, colchicine, anakinra, and hematopoietic stem cell transplantation are the treatment options [16].

Pyoderma Gangrenosum-Associated Syndromes: [10]

PASH syndrome: Pyoderma gangrenosum, acne, and hidradenitis suppurativa. Dapsone, cyclosporine, infliximab, adalimumab, and IL-1 inhibitors are the treatment options.

PAPASH syndrome: Pyogenic/psoriasis arthritis, pyoderma gangrenosum, acne, and hidradenitis suppurativa. Glucocorticoids, cyclosporine, anakinra, adalimumab, infliximab, and secukinumab are the available treatment options.

PsAPASH syndrome: Psoriatic arthritis, pyoderma gangrenosum, acne, and hidradenitis suppurativa. Can be treated with glucocorticoids, cyclosporine, anakinra, adalimumab, and infliximab.

PASS syndrome: Pyoderma gangrenosum, acne, hidradenitis suppurativa, and seropositive spondyloarthropathy. Infliximab is a treatment option.

14.2 Relopathies/Nuclear Factor Kappa-B (NFk-B)-Related AIDs: Some of Them Are Depicted in Table 14.4

Table 14.4 Relopathies/nuclear factor Kappa-B (NFk-B)-related AIDs

Disease	Clinical features	Treatment
NOD2/CARD 15-associated diseases	Blau syndrome (autosomal dominant)/ early onset sarcoidosis (de novo) shows triad of **granulomatous erythematous skin rash**, granulomatous uveitis, symmetrical polyarthritis of early onset [17] Yao syndrome develops in adulthood (around 40 years) and is characterized by recurrent fever, **erythematous patches and plaques**, arthralgia/ non-erosive arthritis, diarrhea, abdominal pain, dry eyes	Corticosteroid, anti-IL-1, IL-6 agents
Familial pityriasis rubra pilaris/CARD14-associated psoriasis	**Pityriasis rubra pilaris-like follicular papules/ psoriasiform lesions** develop in early childhood	Ustekinumab, secukinumab
NFKB1-associated autoinflammatory diseases (NFKB1-AD) [18]	**Behcet's-like disease, necrotizing fasciitis**, recurrent respiratory tract infection, lymphadenopathy, autoimmunity, hypogammaglobulinemia	Anti-IL-1, TNFα agents
ADAM17 deficiency [19]	Neonatal onset **pustular psoriasis**, cutaneous infections, fragile/short hair, wiry eyebrows, eyelashes, cardiomyopathy, chronic bloody diarrhea, thickened nails with episodes of paronychia	Anti-IL-1, IL-6 agents

14.3 Ubiquitinopathies: Some Are Described in Table 14.5

14.4 Interferonopathies: Some of Them Are Mentioned in Table 14.6

Table 14.5 Ubiquitinopathies

Disease	Clinical features	Treatment
Autoinflammation/ immunodeficiency associated with mutations in LUBAC proteins [20, 21]	HOIP mutation causes **lymphangiectasia**, splenomegaly and B,T cell defects leading to increased risk of infections HOIL patients have lymphadenopathy, hepatosplenomegaly, defective B cell function	Anti-TNFα, IL-1 agents
A20 protein haploinsufficiency (HA20)	Childhood onset **oral and genital ulcers**, **polymorphic skin lesions** like erythematous papules, folliculitis, abscesses, fever, uveitis, arthritis, diarrhea, respiratory tract infection, autoimmune features	Colchicine, methotrexate, azathioprine, thalidomide, cyclophosphamide, anti-TNFα, IL-1, IL-6 agents
Otulin deficiency (ORAS) [22]	Onset within 3 months of age, **lipodystrophy, pustules, nodules, panniculitis, non-specific painful erythematous rash**, fever, diarrhea, arthritis	Anti-TNFα, IL-1 agents

Table 14.6 Interferonopathies

Disease	Clinical features	Treatment
Aicardi Goutieres syndrome (AGS)	Neonatal onset of recurrent fever, **chilblains, livedo reticularis**, basal ganglia calcification, subacute leukoencephalopathy	JAK inhibitors
Proteasome-associated autoinflammatory syndromes (PRAAS) [23]	JMP syndrome: Joint contractures, muscle atrophy, microcytic anemia and panniculitis-induced lipodystrophy Nakajo Nishimura syndrome: Pernio-like lesions, recurrent fever, nodular skin eruption, lipodystrophy Of extremities and joint contractures Japanese autoinflammatory syndrome with lipodystrophy (JASL): Nodular erythema, lipodystrophy, fever, bony deformities, basal ganglia calcification Chronic atypical neutrophilic dermatosis with lipodystrophy and elevated temperature (CANDLE): Recurrent fever, purpuric skin lesions, progressive lipodystrophy, atypical facies, failure to thrive	
STING-associated vasculopathy with onset in infancy (SAVI)	**Vasculopathy of extremities, livedo reticularis, Raynaud's phenomenon**, fever, interstitial lung disease, failure to thrive	
Singleton-Merten syndrome (SMS) [24]	**Psoriasis**, early onset osteoporosis, dental dysplasia, arthropathy, tendon rupture, glaucoma, neurological abnormalities	

14.5 Other Monogenic AIDs

Adenosine deaminase 2 (ADA2) deficiency: Early childhood vasculopathy, medium and small vessel vasculitis (predominantly over skin and CNS), recurrent fever, hematologic abnormality, hypogammaglobulinemia. Anti-TNFα therapy, replacement of immunoglobulin and hematopoietic stem cell transplantation are the treatment options.

Deficiency of IL-36 receptor antagonist (DITRA): Fever and generalized pustular psoriasis are the main features. Palmoplantar pustules might appear in infancy along with nail and joint involvement. Anakinra, secukinumab, ustekinumab, and anti-TNFα therapy are the available therapeutic options [25].

H syndrome: Features include hyperpigmentation, hypertrichosis, progressive sclerotic skin lesions, heart abnormalities, hypogonadism, hearing loss, hepatosplenomegaly, and short stature. Glucocorticoids, colchicine, cytotoxic immunosuppressants, IFNα, anakinra, canakinumab, adalimumab, and radiotherapy have been used with inadequate response [26].

Vibratory urticaria: Localized pruritic urticaria, erythema, angioedema after repetitive friction or vibratory stimuli. Sometimes there might be systemic symptoms like fatigue, flushing, and headache.

AP1S3 and autoinflammatory psoriasis: Predominantly pustular psoriasis and arthritis.

Sideroblastic anemia, immunodeficiency, fevers, and developmental delay (SIFD): Children present with fragile hair, severe microcytic anemia, recurrent fever, developmental delay, neurological abnormality, multiorgan failure, and B-cell deficiency.

14.6 Autoinflammatory Diseases Without an Identified Monogenic Etiology

Systemic-onset juvenile idiopathic arthritis (SoJIA): **Skin rash (transient)**, recurrent fever, arthritis, serositis, and lymphadenopathy are the features of SoJIA. Treated with IL-1 and IL-6 blocking agents [27].

Idiopathic pericarditis: Intermittent episodes of pericarditis characterize this disease. NSAIDs are the drugs of choice.

14.7 Autoinflammatory Bone Disorders

CRMO: Children present with multifocal recurrent sterile osteomyelitis of long bones, fever, and other constitutional symptoms. NSAIDs, bisphosphonates (bone manifestation), and TNFα blocking agents are part of therapeutic armamentarium.

Majeed syndrome: Dyserythropoietic anemia with/without neutrophilic dermatoses, and sterile osteomyelitis. Neutrophilic skin lesions include Sweet's syndrome and pustulosis. IL-1 blocking agents are the treatment of choice [28].

DIRA: Pustular lesions over the body, osteitis, periostitis over long bones and vertebrae with usually no fever develop in the first few months of life. There is good response to anakinra.

Cherubism: Osteolytic lesions develop in the mandible around 2–5 years of age followed by fibrotic dysplastic soft tissue overgrowth in these areas leads to puffy cheeks of patients in cherubism. There may be involvement of ribs. Adalimumab and bisphosphonates have been used in the past [29].

In my short experience of 6 years in dermatology, I came across very few cases of pustulosis, pyoderma-gangrenosum-associated syndromes, and H-syndrome. In pyoderma gangrenosum-associated syndromes the response to conventional anti-inflammatory agents was found to be almost similar to classical pyoderma gangrenosum and hidradenitis suppurativa.

Also, I've personally seen only one suspected case of CANDLE syndrome, who developed annular erythematous indurated skin lesions in early infancy. The skin biopsy was suggestive of neutrophilic dermatosis. However, the patient was lost to follow-up, so the confirmation of diagnosis could not be done.

Autoinflammatory syndromes are difficult to diagnose and are difficult to treat because of long-term need of anti-inflammatory agents. They can lead to deadly complications like systemic amyloidosis. We as dermatologists should be aware of this group of disorders for proper evaluation and management of affected individuals. There is also a need for research in this field to explore some good clinical pointers, investigations for the diagnosis, and effective treatment.

In my humble opinion, autoinflammatory syndromes are quite rare and with a high chance of being missed because of non-specific or overlapping clinical manifestations. A high index of suspicion is necessary for their early diagnosis and proper management.

References

1. Cush JJ. Autoinflammatory syndromes. Dermatol Clin. 2013;31(3):471–80.
2. Ozkurede VU, Franchi L. Immunology in clinic review series; focus on autoinflammatory diseases: role of inflammasomes in autoinflammatory syndromes. Clin Exp Immunol. 2012;167(3):382–90.
3. Awad F, Assrawi E, Jumeau C, Georgin-Lavialle S, Cobret L, Duquesnoy P, et al. Impact of human monocyte and macrophage polarization on NLR expression and NLRP3 inflammasome activation. PLoS One. 2017;12(4):e0175336.
4. Willingham SB, Allen IC, Bergstralh DT, Brickey WJ, Huang MT-H, Taxman DJ, et al. NLRP3 (NALP3, Cryopyrin) facilitates in vivo Caspase-1 activation, necrosis, and HMGB1 release via Inflammasome-dependent and -independent pathways. J Immunol. 2009;183(3):2008–15.
5. Ostring GT, Singh-Grewal D. Periodic fevers and autoinflammatory syndromes in childhood. J Paediatr Child Health. 2016;52(9):865–71.

6. Krause K, Grattan CE, Bindslev-Jensen C, Gattorno M, Kallinich T, de Koning HD, et al. How not to miss autoinflammatory diseases masquerading as urticaria. Allergy. 2012;67(12):1465–74.
7. Nguyen TV, Cowen EW, Leslie KS. Autoinflammation: from monogenic syndromes to common skin diseases. J Am Acad Dermatol. 2013;68(5):834–53.
8. McGonagle D, McDermott MF. A proposed classification of the immunological diseases. PLoS Med. 2006;3(8):e297.
9. Marino A, Tirelli F, Giani T, Cimaz R. Periodic fever syndromes and the autoinflammatory diseases (AIDs). J Transl Autoimmun. 2020;3:100031.
10. Figueras-Nart I, Mascaró JM, Solanich X, Hernández-Rodríguez J. Dermatologic and Dermatopathologic features of monogenic autoinflammatory diseases. Front Immunol. 2019;10:2448.
11. Manthiram K, Zhou Q, Aksentijevich I, Kastner DL. The monogenic autoinflammatory diseases define new pathways in human innate immunity and inflammation. Nat Immunol. 2017;18(8):832–42.
12. Oldham J, Lachmann HJ. The systemic autoinflammatory disorders for dermatologists. Part 1: overview. Clin Exp Dermatol. 2020;45(8):962–6.
13. Broekaert SMC, Böer-Auer A, Kerl K, Herrgott I, Schulz X, Bonsmann G, et al. Neutrophilic Epitheliotropism is a histopathological clue to neutrophilic urticarial dermatosis. Am J Dermatopathol. 2016;38(1):39–49.
14. Kitamura A, Sasaki Y, Abe T, Kano H, Yasutomo K. An inherited mutation in NLRC4 causes autoinflammation in human and mice. J Exp Med. 2014;211(12):2385–96.
15. Masters SL, Lagou V, Jéru I, Baker PJ, Van Eyck L, Parry DA, et al. Familial autoinflammation with neutrophilic dermatosis reveals a regulatory mechanism of pyrin activation. Sci Transl Med. 2016;8(332):332ra45.
16. Standing ASI, Malinova D, Hong Y, Record J, Moulding D, Blundell MP, et al. Autoinflammatory periodic fever, immunodeficiency, and thrombocytopenia (PFIT) caused by mutation in actin-regulatory gene WDR1. J Exp Med. 2017;214(1):59–71.
17. Miceli-Richard C, Lesage S, Rybojad M, Prieur AM, Manouvrier-Hanu S, Häfner R, et al. CARD15 mutations in Blau syndrome. Nat Genet. 2001;29(1):19–20.
18. Schipp C, Nabhani S, Bienemann K, Simanovsky N, Kfir-Erenfeld S, Assayag-Asherie N, et al. Specific antibody deficiency and autoinflammatory disease extend the clinical and immunological spectrum of heterozygous NFKB1 loss-of-function mutations in humans. Haematologica. 2016;101(10):e392–6.
19. Blaydon DC, Biancheri P, Di W-L, Plagnol V, Cabral RM, Brooke MA, et al. Inflammatory skin and bowel disease linked to ADAM17 deletion. N Engl J Med. 2011;365(16):1502–8.
20. Boisson B, Laplantine E, Dobbs K, Cobat A, Tarantino N, Hazen M, et al. Human HOIP and LUBAC deficiency underlies autoinflammation, immunodeficiency, amylopectinosis, and lymphangiectasia. J Exp Med. 2015;212(6):939–51.
21. Boisson B, Laplantine E, Prando C, Giliani S, Israelsson E, Xu Z, et al. Immunodeficiency, autoinflammation and amylopectinosis in humans with inherited HOIL-1 and LUBAC deficiency. Nat Immunol. 2012;13(12):1178–86.
22. Damgaard RB, Walker JA, Marco-Casanova P, Morgan NV, Titheradge HL, Elliott PR, et al. The Deubiquitinase OTULIN is an essential negative regulator of inflammation and autoimmunity. Cell. 2016;166(5):1215–1230.e20.
23. McDermott A, Jacks J, Kessler M, Emanuel PD, Gao L. Proteasome-associated autoinflammatory syndromes: advances in pathogeneses, clinical presentations, diagnosis, and management. Int J Dermatol. 2015;54(2):121–9.
24. Ferreira CR, Crow YJ, Gahl WA, Gardner PJ, Goldbach-Mansky R, Hur S, et al. DDX58 and classic singleton-Merten syndrome. J Clin Immunol. 2019;39(1):75–80.
25. Marrakchi S, Guigue P, Renshaw BR, Puel A, Pei X-Y, Fraitag S, et al. Interleukin-36-receptor antagonist deficiency and generalized pustular psoriasis. N Engl J Med. 2011;365(7):620–8.
26. Molho-Pessach V, Ramot Y, Camille F, Doviner V, Babay S, Luis SJ, et al. H syndrome: the first 79 patients. J Am Acad Dermatol. 2014;70(1):80–8.

27. Cimaz R. Systemic-onset juvenile idiopathic arthritis. Autoimmun Rev. 2016;15(9):931–4.
28. Herlin T, Fiirgaard B, Bjerre M, Kerndrup G, Hasle H, Bing X, et al. Efficacy of anti-IL-1 treatment in Majeed syndrome. Ann Rheum Dis. 2013;72(3):410–3.
29. Morice A, Joly A, Ricquebourg M, Maruani G, Durand E, Galmiche L, et al. Cherubism as a systemic skeletal disease: evidence from an aggressive case. BMC Musculoskelet Disord. 2020;21:564.

Entangled: The New Era of Aggressive Dermatomycosis

15

Vishal Gaurav and Shukla Das

The word "dermatomycosis" is derived from the Greek word "derma," meaning skin, and "mykes," meaning "mushroom." It is an all-encompassing term that denotes fungal infection of the skin and its appendages. However, it has also been used in literature to denote cutaneous infection caused by non-dermatophytic molds (NDMs). The term "dermatophytosis" is only used when the infection is caused by a dermatophyte. However, these terms are often used interchangeably. Irrespective of the term used, there is no doubt that dermatophytosis has acquired an epidemic-like proportion in the Indian subcontinent [1–3]. The ever-increasing cases of recalcitrant (recurrent and chronic) dermatophytosis and therapeutic failure after first contact with general practitioners, needing a specialist's opinion, are alarming. Despite being such a prevalent dermatological disease, and causing so much morbidity, the quality and quantity of research in this field are inadequate because of the lack of support and funding for research into this perceived "harmless" disease. There is an urgent need to study the immunopathogenesis of dermatophytosis to understand and develop new drug targets. With a limited armamentarium of antifungals effective against dermatophytes, and recent studies showing resistance, antifungal susceptibility patterns of clinically isolated dermatophytes need to be continually measured and monitored to determine the level of resistance prevalent in the community and form the basis for good drug selection for a cure. The drug resistance mechanisms and their prevalence also need to be thoroughly documented to enable the development of mechanisms to circumvent drug resistance, as well as

V. Gaurav
Department of Dermatology and Venereology, All India Institute of Medical Sciences, Delhi, India

S. Das (✉)
Department of Microbiology, University College of Medical Sciences and Guru Teg Bahadur Hospital, Delhi, India

S. Gupta et al. (eds.), *Critical Thinking in Contemporary Dermatology: Cognitive Essays*, https://doi.org/10.1007/978-981-97-0411-8_15

to develop modalities that can enhance the effectiveness and longevity of the currently available antifungals.

The prevalence of superficial mycoses has been estimated to be around 20–25% of the global population [4]. Dermatophytoses are the most common skin infections globally [5]. The true data regarding the incidence and prevalence of dermatophytosis is lacking due to the absence of a robust system of data collection for superficial fungal infections [1]. The reported prevalence in India varies widely and ranges from 6.09%–61.5% in different hospital-based studies of 1–2 years duration [6, 7]. The assumption of higher prevalence in southern India based on climatic variations, with southern India being hotter and more humid, is not supported by studies. The incidence of chronic, relapsing, and recurring dermatophytosis is rising. Though there was a lack of a uniform definition for chronic, recurrent, relapsing, and recalcitrant dermatophytosis, before ECTODERM India (2018), the reported data estimated that 62.5 to 65.3% of infections were chronic (disease duration >3 months) while 9.3 to 60% infections were recurrent [8–12]. Similar trends have been reported from the neighboring countries of Pakistan and Sri Lanka, as well as from other countries like Africa [13–15].

While all forms of dermatophytosis are common in middle-aged to elderly, with the exception of tinea capitis, the incidence of all of them has increased in children. Children, including infants and toddlers, presenting with tinea corporis or faciei is not infrequent (Fig. 15.1) [16, 17]. Erythrodermic dermatophytosis is also being reported in children (Fig. 15.2). This could be happening due to an increase in the

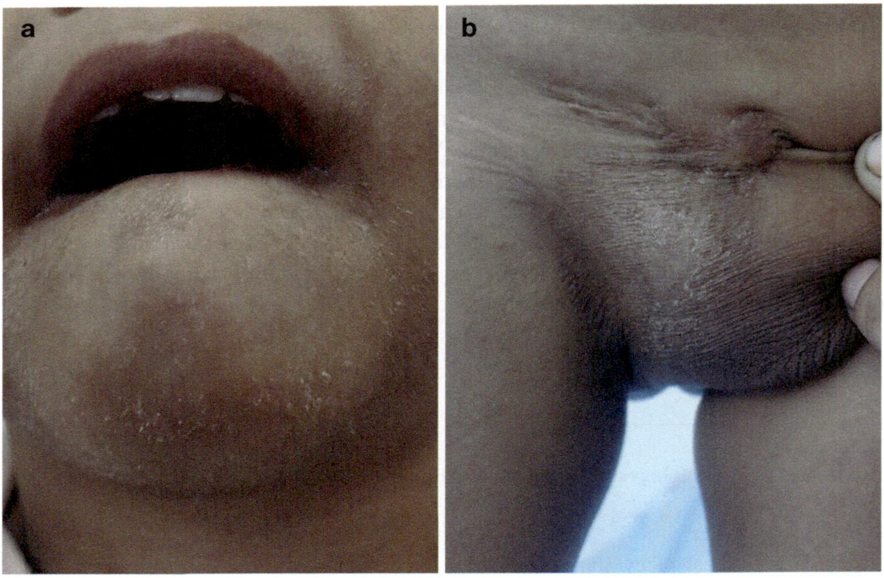

Fig. 15.1 Dermatophytosis in children (**a**) Tinea faciei in an 8-year-old boy. (**b**) Tinea cruris in 4-year-old boy

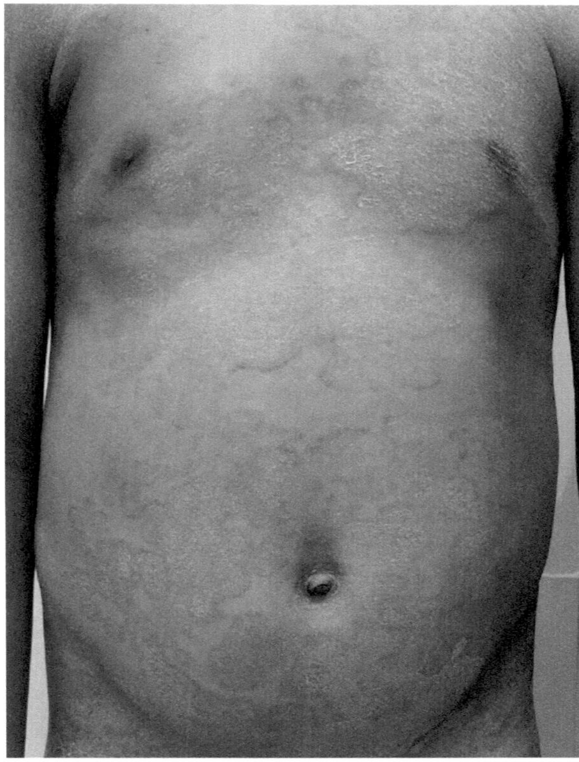

Fig. 15.2 Erythrodermic dermatophytosis in an 8-year-old boy

use of antifungal-steroid combination creams, increased virulence of the organism, or acquisition from an infected family member (s). Chronic dermatophytosis is commoner in late middle-aged adults (fifth decade onwards), which coincides with the onset of lifestyle disorders (including diabetes) and waning immunity [18]. However, the incidence has been increasing in young adults as well [18].

Dermatophytosis, including tinea cruris, tinea pedis, and tinea unguium is commoner in men compared to women due to the increased frequency of outdoor work predisposing them to hot and humid environments favorable for the growth of dermatophytes. However, the male-to-female ratio has decreased in the last 3–4 years (from 3–5:1 to < 2:1) [19]. The increasing incidence in women can be attributed to the increase in the number of employed women with a proportionate increase in women working outdoors, and hence exposure to the same working environment as men. The concomitant change in clothing patterns (western/jeans over clothes that allow ventilation) in women and the increased incidence of lifestyle disorders may be contributory.

Different ethnic groups seem more commonly affected by different types of dermatophytic infections. Scalp dermatophytic infections are more common in Negroids than Caucasians and nail infections are more common in Caucasians [20]. Tinea imbricata caused by *Trichophyton concentricum* is endemic in South Pacific islands (Polynesia and Melanesia), South Asia, and some specific areas of South America [21].

Like many other infectious diseases, dermatophytosis is more common in people belonging to lower socioeconomic groups. This can be attributed to poor living conditions, overcrowding, unhygienic practices, and poor nutrition [16].

Tinea pedis occurs at an increased frequency in miners and butchers, possibly due to the use of rubber boots which cause occlusion. Similarly, artificial nails are associated with an increased risk of onychomycosis. Earlier reports relating farming, swimming pools, and beach sand relating to dermatophytosis need to be studied further [22].

Dermatophytosis has a worldwide distribution but geographical variations do occur. The tropical climate is more humid, and causes excessive sweating, which is compounded by occlusive clothing, socks, and footwear. This predisposes to dermatophytosis.

Recently, two additional risk factors were identified to increase the risk of chronic relapsing dermatophytosis; the family history of tinea, and exposure to hot environments as a result of cooking food. The same study concluded that wearing jeans, frequency of washing clothes or taking baths, excessive sweating, pets in the home, and body mass index do not increase the risk of chronic or chronic-relapsing dermatophytosis [9].

The incidence of dermatophytosis has increased in school-going children and students in general due to prolonged use of tight-fitting footwear and clothes as well as increased sweating due to physical activity [23].

The presence of similar infections in numerous family members raises questions about the influence of genetic factors, a subject that remains incompletely understood. Initially, a genetic connection was hypothesized in Tinea imbricata, with an autosomal dominant pattern of inheritance and incomplete penetrance. Similarly, susceptibility to persistent *T. rubrum* infection is inherited through an autosomal dominant mode. Approximately 50% of parents with children affected by onychomycosis also exhibit onychomycosis. Several factors contribute to an increased susceptibility to chronic and resistant infections in the host. These factors include a single nucleotide polymorphism in the Dectin-1 receptor gene, deficiency in CARD-9 (caspase recruitment domain–containing protein 9), HLA-DR8, elevated levels of CD4 + CD25+ regulatory T cells, a decreased count of DEFB4 genes, and heightened serum levels of human β-defensin and IL-22. Interestingly, HLA-DR8 has been identified as a protective factor [24]. Additionally, primary immunodeficiencies such as chronic mucocutaneous candidiasis have been linked to recurrent and resistant dermatophytosis [25, 26].

An important social factor spearheading this rise of chronic recalcitrant infections is the misuse of steroids, both topical and oral, by patients. It is not uncommon for patients to use the steroid and steroid-combinations creams, available over-the-counter, for years together at the suggestion of the pharmacist, family, friends, or general physicians. Treatment-naïve tinea is a rarity as most of the patients have used topical steroid-antifungal combination as well as systemic steroids (oral/injectable) for tinea [9, 27]. The frequency of topical steroid use has been reported to be as high as 81% [28]. The initial fast symptomatic relief due to an anti-inflammatory effect of steroids leads to continuous usage which over time leads to immunosuppression and chronic and recalcitrant infections.

Identification of the etiologic agent and subsequent assessment of antifungal resistance is one of the ways to tackle this increasing prevalence of recalcitrant infections. *Trichophyton mentagrophytes* is at the center stage of the current epidemic of dermatophytosis, contributing as high as 97.2% of the cases [18]. Originally a zoophilic species, *T. mentagrophytes* has undergone anthropization making it capable of human-to-human transmission. Environmental factors (humidity, temperature, trauma), host factors (host–parasite relationship, host susceptibility), and immunological factors as well as the increased virulence of this species have been implicated in this epidemiological shift [28]. The rapid growth of *T. mentagrophytes* compared to other dermatophytes manifests as inflammatory and extensive lesions. *T. mentagrophytes complex* is further subclassified into genotypes based on Ribosomal DNA (rDNA) sequencing including ITS1, ITS2, and 5.8S regions along with translation elongation factor (TEF)-1αgene. This process led to the description of 10 genotypes, type I and II for *T. interdigitale* (anthropophilic) and types III, III*, IV, V, VI, VII, VIII, and IX* for *T. mentagrophytes* (zoophilic), which are associated with the geographic origin as well as the source of infection [29]. *T. mentagrophytes* genotype VIII has been found to be the cause of the ongoing epidemic, and harbors a unique topoisomerase 2 (TOP2) sequence [30].

A reanalysis of ITS sequences submitted from India, where *T. intergitale* was reported as the cause of the ongoing epidemic, showed that these species were *T. mentagrophytes* genotype VIII and not *T. interdigitale* [31]. Few authors have proposed it to be a separate species named *T. indotineae*, which is controversial as *T. mentagrophytes* genotype VIII is another variety within the *T. mentagrophytes* complex [32]. Human-to-human transmission of a zoophilic species like *T. mentagrophytes* can be explained by the concept of "anthropization," which refers to the adaptation of geophilic or zoophilic dermatophytes to human skin. The anthropization of a geophilic dermatophyte, *T. rubrum*, has also been described previously [28].

Another explanation for the increased prevalence can be the multiple virulence factors that have increased the pathogenicity of dermatophytes. These include endoproteases (e.g., subtilisin-like protease, fungalysin-like metalloprotease), exoproteases (leucine aminopeptidase, dipeptidyl peptidase), cysteine dioxygenases, hydrophobins, extracellular vesicles, heat shock proteins, and other hydrolases. The role of C-type lectin receptors as well as NLRP3 inflammasome and IL-1β has also been emphasized [33].

The infection follows a relatively uncomplicated two-step process. Initially, arthrospores adhere to keratinized surfaces (skin), and subsequently, invasion takes place. In the presence of keratin, there is an upregulation of proteolytic enzyme release [34]. In vitro, this process is completed within approximately 2 h of contact, leading to spore germination and penetration of keratinocytes. Evidence of indentation in keratinocyte layers beneath growing hyphae may be a result of enzymatic action [35]. *Trichophyton rubrum* attaches to epithelial cells using carbohydrate-specific adhesins on the microconidia surface, while *T. mentagrophytes* develops fibrillar projections during the adherence phase [36]. At the skin surface, long, sparse fibrils connect fungal arthroconidia to keratinocytes and each other. Newly formed arthroconidia initially exhibit thin, short appendices covering their entire surface, gradually disappearing as a substantial contact area is established between conidia and skin tissue [37]. Fungal adherence to host cells is facilitated by fungal adhesins and their interactions with host receptors. Unlike other fungal species, sialic acids are absent from the cell surface of these fungi and are thus not implicated in the pathogenesis [38].

The subsequent phase, invasion, is facilitated by trauma and maceration. Specific proteases, lipases, and ceramidases play a crucial role in this process, and their digestive byproducts also function as nutrients for the fungi [39]. Mannans, integral components of fungal cell walls, exhibit inhibitory effects on keratinocyte proliferation and cell-mediated immunity [40]. Dermatophytes genetically regulate the production of keratin-specific proteases. In vitro, non-keratin substances extracted from keratinized tissues support dermatophyte growth. These fungi produce proteolytic enzymes that operate effectively in acidic, alkaline, and neutral environments. Certain dermatophytes induce keratinase activity in response to low-molecular-weight peptides released from the epidermis by the action of other fungal proteinases [41]. Additional enzymes, including sulfur transporters, are also involved. In *Microsporum canis*, at least three genes—SUB1, SUB2, and SUB3—encode the synthesis of metalloproteases associated with infection. Once established, spores must germinate and penetrate the stratum corneum at a rate faster than desquamation [42]. Dermatophytes secrete multiple serine-subtilisins and metallo-endoproteases (fungalysins), formerly known as keratinases, which are predominantly found in dermatophytes (Fig. 15.3) [39]. However, limited information is available about hydrolases such as lipases and a ceramidase produced by

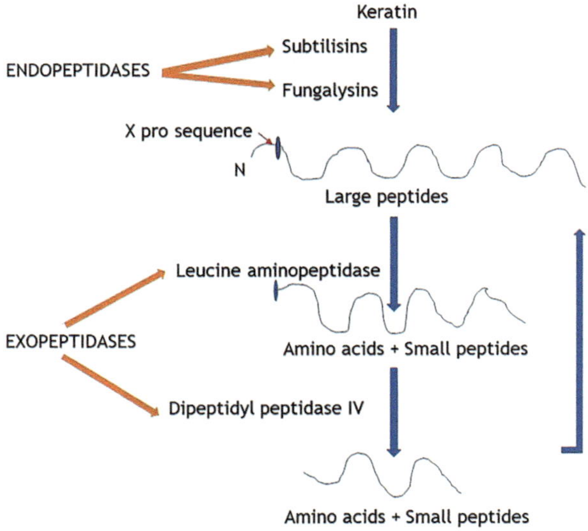

Fig. 15.3 Enzymatic pathway of keratin degradation by dermatophytic exo- and endopepitidases

these fungi. The mechanism by which mucolytic enzymes, aiding in penetration, also serve as nutrition for the fungi remains unknown. These dermatophytic keratinolytic proteases are inactive until disulfide bridges within the dense protein network of keratinized tissues are reduced. Sulfur molecules are transported out of the cell through a sulfite efflux pump encoded by the SSU1 gene. The excretion of sulfite by this transporter enables sulfitolysis of proteins, making them accessible for proteases, while concurrently functioning as a potential detoxification pathway—a prospective target for novel antifungal treatments (Fig. 15.4) [43].

The role of biofilms in recalcitrance to treatment is well documented for dermatophytoma, a form of tinea unguium [44]. Nail, being an immune-privileged site, favors biofilm formation. Other factors contributing to the nail being a preferred site for biofilm formation include nail trauma, dryness of the nail from aging, removal of nail cuticle, removal of protective lipids by soaking, external damage by mycotoxins, and minor defects in the normal nail architecture [45].

Biofilms are microbial colonies cemented in an extracellular matrix secreted by the resident organisms. The nature of the extracellular matrix allows the biofilm to be metabolically active even in adverse conditions. The different stages of biofilm formation are depicted in Fig. 15.5. The biofilms provide the resident organisms with multiple mechanisms to evade the antifungals [46]. Biofilms also harbor persisters. Once the drug levels are high in the surrounding environment, the organism hides in the biofilm and comes out after the drug levels have lowered [47]. The electron microscopic examination of the biofilm has revealed the presence of extracellular material adhered to the hyphae at multiple sites [48]. Crystal violet binds nonspecifically to negatively charged surface molecules such as polysaccharides and eDNA in

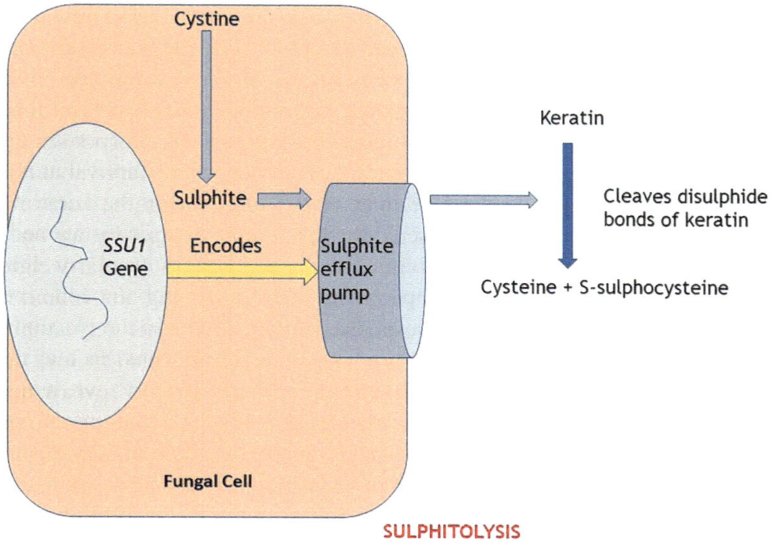

Fig. 15.4 Mechanism of sulphite efflux and sulphitolysis by fungal cell

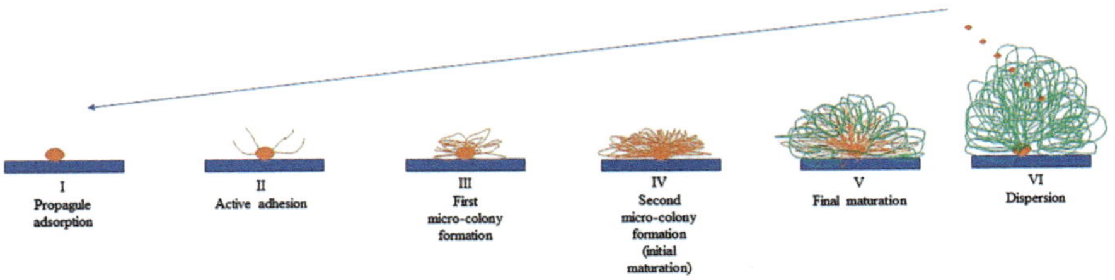

Fig. 15.5 Stages of biofilm formation in dermatophytes

the extracellular matrix [49]. Because it binds cells as well as matrix components, it is generally used to evaluate biofilm biomass in toto [50]. Biofilm antifungal susceptibility assay of dermatophytes shows a 100- to 1000-fold increase in minimum inhibitory concentrations of antifungals compared to planktonic forms [51, 52].

The human body initiates a variety of host responses against dermatophytes through several nonspecific mechanisms, including fungistatic fatty acids [51]. Among these defense mechanisms, keratinocytes serve as the first line of living cells to confront invading fungal elements, undertaking various functions to thwart infection. These functions include increased shedding, the secretion of antimicrobial peptides like human β-defensin-221, and the release of pro-inflammatory cytokines (IFN-α, TNFα, IL-1β, 8, 16, and 17). As the infection progresses to deeper layers of the epidermis, additional nonspecific defenses, such as competition for iron facilitated by unsaturated transferrin, come into play [51].

The subsequent line of defense involves cell-mediated immunity, leading to a specific delayed-type hypersensitivity. The inflammatory response associated with this hypersensitivity is linked to clinical resolution. Contrary to the Th2 response, which does not seem to offer protection, patients exhibiting elevated fungal antigen antibody titers often display extensive dermatophyte infections. Recent findings suggest a potential role for the Th17 response in dermatophyte infections, indicated by the discovery of hyphal elements binding to Dectin-2, a C-type lectin pattern recognition receptor on dendritic cells crucial for inducing Th17 responses [52].

Immunologic and inflammatory responses that restrict fungal survival and spread are pivotal in controlling dermatophyte infections. Fungi within the keratin layers release substances that reach the viable epidermis, inducing contact-irritant and allergic contact dermatitis. Additionally, the organisms release low-molecular-weight chemotactic factors and directly fix complement, both enhancing the inflammatory response, particularly the neutrophilic response. In 25% of chronic dermatophytosis cases, antibodies are present, with *T. rubrum*-specific IgE detected in low titers in most cases. Skin testing in patients with chronic dermatophytosis reveals multiple sensitivities and elevated serum IgE levels, indicating a probable atopic condition [53].

Moreover, in vitro lymphocyte reactivity is generally positive in patients with chronic dermatophytosis, despite negative skin tests. These findings suggest a potential interference with or blockage of cellular immunity by IgE-specific antibodies in patients with chronic dermatophytosis, leading to an increased tendency to produce specific IgE antibodies. Dermatophytosis does not exhibit an elevated frequency in patients with immunologic defects limited to immunoglobulin production, emphasizing the crucial role of cell-mediated immunity in managing dermatophyte infections [53].

Another factor for the recurrence of infection may be the persistent infection of vellus hair follicles on glabrous skin and subclinical infection of nails may be acting as a reservoir of infection. Vellus hair involvement has been seen using dermoscopy of glabrous tinea lesions [54–56].

Lastly, there seems to have been a shift in the clinical spectrum of superficial dermatophytosis. Tinea corporis et cruris is the commonest presentation. However, the incidence of tinea faciei has been increasing due to the rampant use of topical steroids as fairness creams or in combination with hydroquinone and retinoids as part of depigmenting therapy. The clinical behavior is aggressive, with acute onset and rapidly progressive (within days) lesions. However, the inflammatory response is very variable resulting in non-erythematous plaques with profuse powdery white scales ("noninflammatory") when the inflammation is less and pustular/bullous lesions when the inflammation is high. Both types of lesions (inflammatory as well as noninflammatory) can be encountered in the same individual, at different sites.

The characteristic annular plaque with central clearing and pustulation with scaling (Fig. 15.6) at the margin is a rarity rather than a commonality as most of the

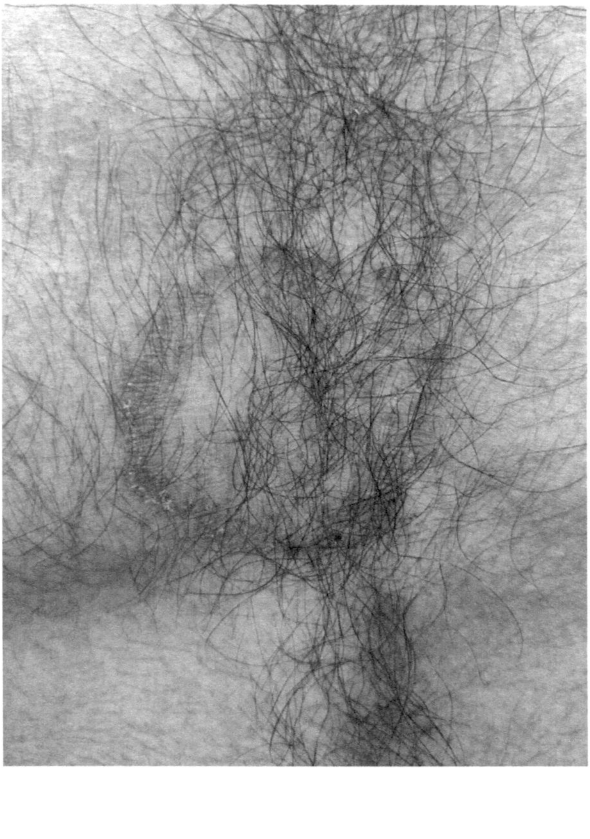

Fig. 15.6 Characteristic annular plaque of dermatophytosis with central clearing and scaling at the margin

patients have already taken some treatment (either from general physicians or self-medication) before consulting a dermatologist. Tinea incognita/tinea incognito, more appropriately termed "steroid-modified tinea" (Fig. 15.7) is frequently encountered in clinical practice. Clinical variants like Majocchi's granuloma (Fig. 15.8), which used to be rare, are not uncommon now. Apart from the classical granuloma trichophyticum, cystic granuloma trichophyticum has also been reported [57]. Dumbbell-shaped, arcuate, horse-shoe shaped, bizarre-shaped geographic lesions formed due to the coalescence of multiple lesions are not uncommon. Erythrodermic dermatophytosis (Fig. 15.2) is being encountered not only in patients with immunosuppression but in immunocompetent individuals as well [58]. It is not uncommon to encounter tinea lesions which clinically appear eczematous, psoriasiform, or lichenified (Fig. 15.9). Impetigo-like (Fig. 15.10), lupus erythematosus-like, molluscum-like, scutula-like, rosacea-like, erythema multiforme-like, granuloma annulare-like, pityriasis rosea-like (Fig. 15.11), nummular eczema-like (Fig. 15.12), pustular psoriasis-like (Fig. 15.13), Sweet's syndrome-like, annular secondary syphilis-like, bullous pemphigoid-like lesions have been described. Purpuric, bullous, pustular, ulcerative (Fig. 15.14), and pseudomembranous morphologies have also been described [17, 59]. The varying clinical presentations depend on the frequency, duration, and strength of the topical steroid which

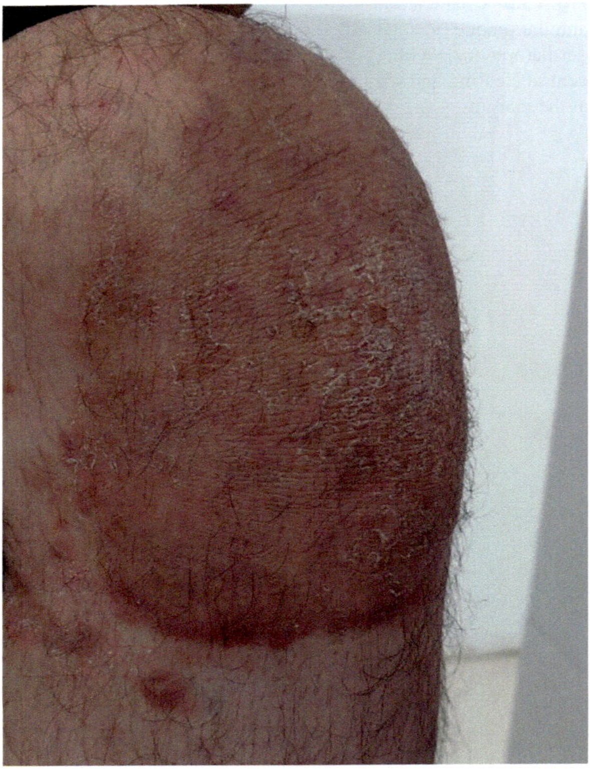

Fig. 15.7 Steroid modified tinea (4 weeks after application of clobetasol propionate 0.05% cream)

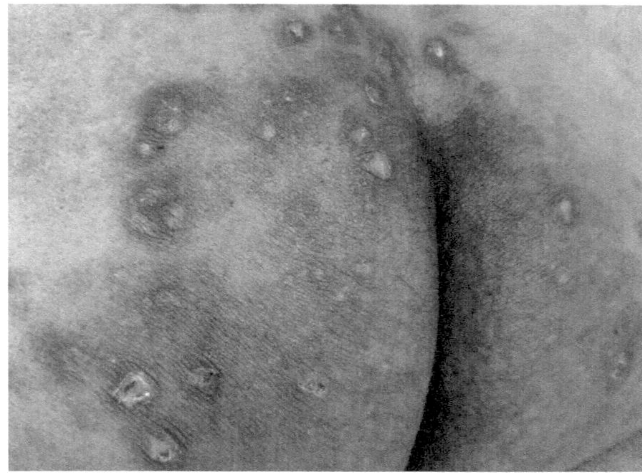

Fig. 15.8 Majocchi's granuloma over buttocks presenting as follicular papules and nodules

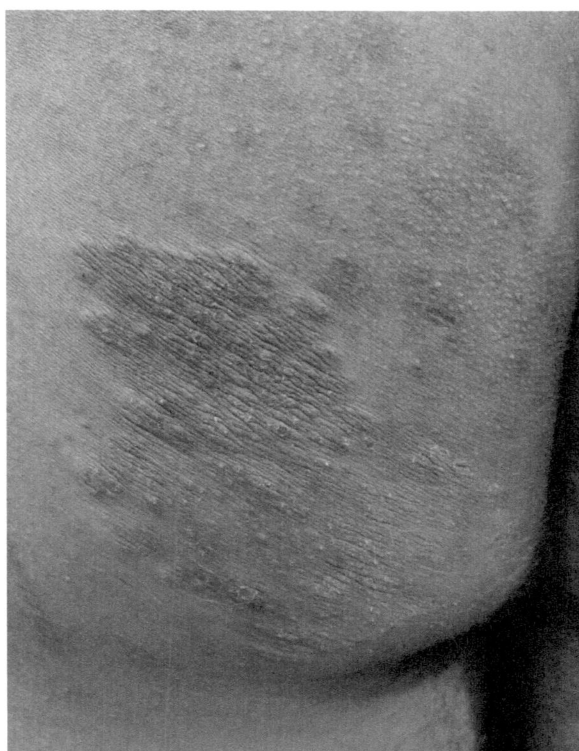

Fig. 15.9 Lichenified tinea lesion over left buttock

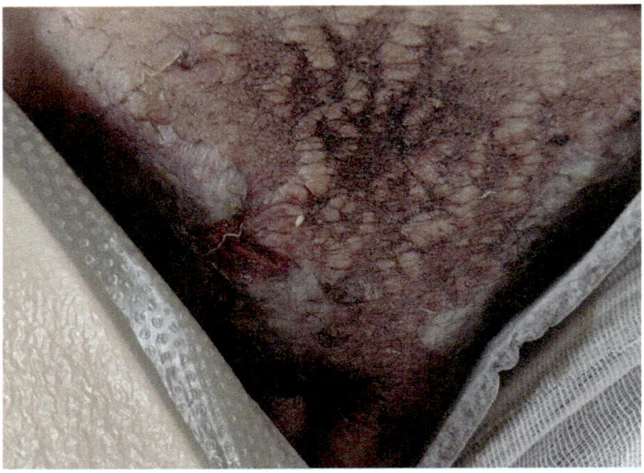

Fig. 15.10 Bullous impetigo-like tinea cruris

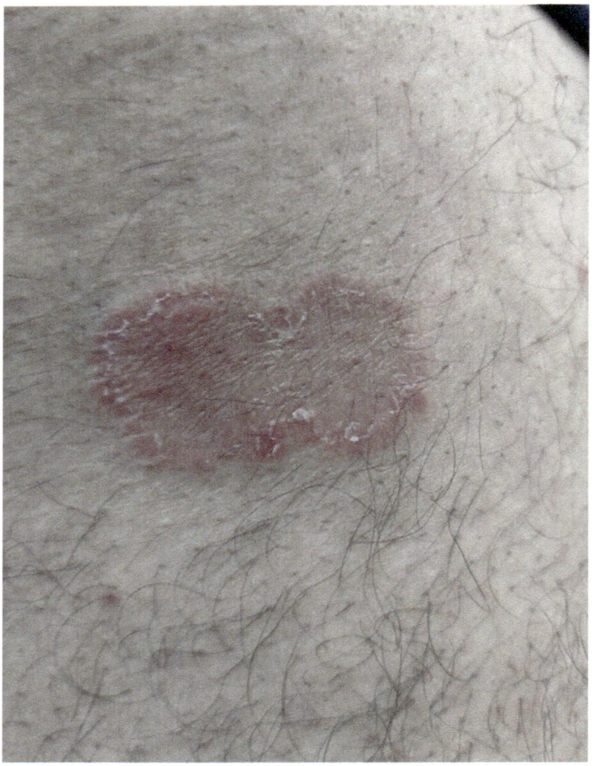

Fig. 15.11 Pityriasis rosea-like tinea corporis

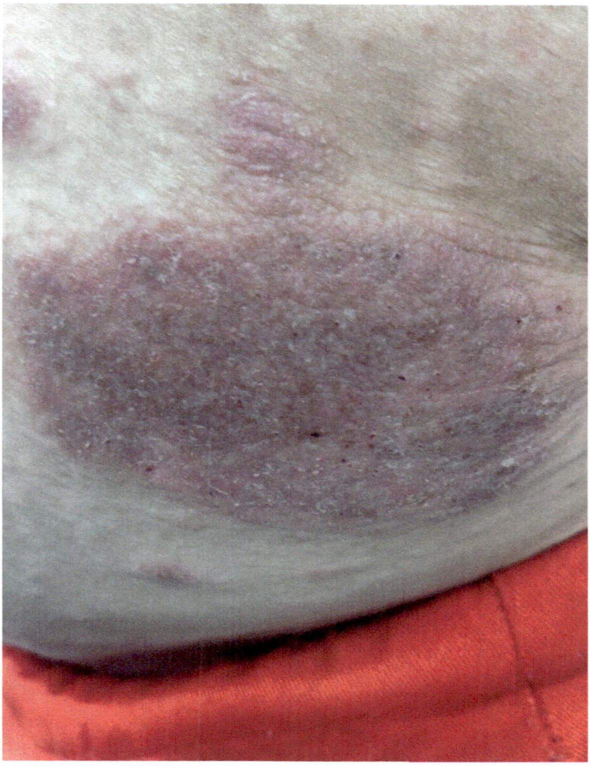

Fig. 15.12 Nummular eczema-like tinea corporis

manipulates the cutaneous immunity with interspersed steroid-free intervals. This also leads to presentations like "tinea pseudoimbricata" and "double-edged" tinea (Fig. 15.15) [60]. Similarly, tinea lesions with "pseudoporokeratotic" edges have also been described [17]. Tinea recidivans is yet another rare presentation where new lesions appear at the periphery of a healed lesion (Fig. 15.16). This could be happening due to a state of relative anergy in the surrounding skin induced by dermatophytes. By virtue of this anergy, this area becomes an immunocompromised zone favoring reinfection/recurrence. Vitiligo, lichen planus, varicella, and herpes zoster have been seen at sites of previous tinea lesions [61]. Amputation stump, surgical incisions, and tattoo sites are also recognized as immunocompromised districts (of Ruocco), which explains the occurrence of tinea lesions on these sites [62].

Involvement of unusual sites, not reported to be infected by dermatophytes earlier, is being reported. These include tinea auricularis (dermatophytosis of the ear), tinea genitalis (dermatophytosis of genitalia) and tinea pubogenitalis (tinea cruris et genitalis) (Fig. 15.17), tinea of glabrous scalp, tinea labialis (dermatophytosis of lips), and tinea blepharociliaris (dermatophytosis of eyelids and eyelashes) [17, 59].

It is not uncommon for steroid-modified tinea lesions to feature hypo- or depigmentation, striae, atrophy, telangiectasia, and ulceration. Secondary bacterial infection is also seen. Severe irritant contact dermatitis induced by dithranol, salicylic

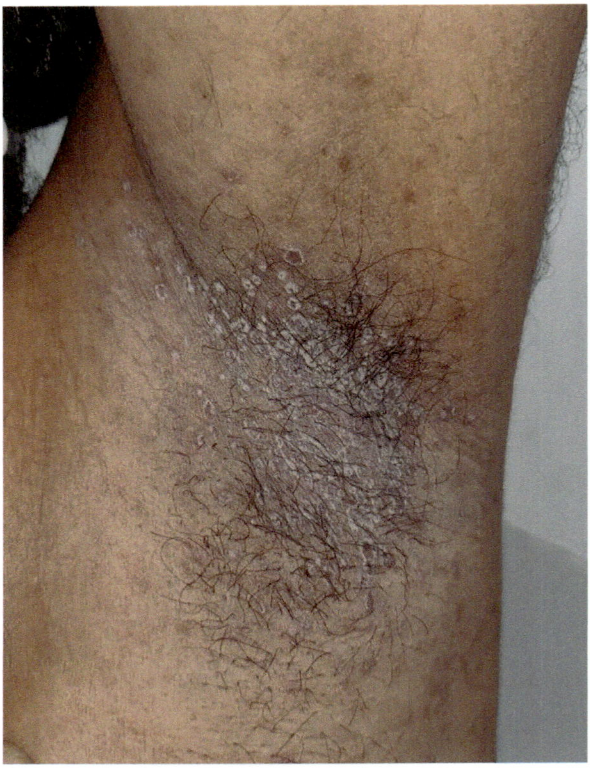

Fig. 15.13 Pustular psoriasis-like tinea cruris

acid, anthralin, sulfur, etc., especially in groins, is not infrequent. Iatrogenic Cushing's syndrome due to prolonged application of super-potent steroids and injectable steroids is also seen [27].

Pruritus is the most common symptom of dermatophytosis of glabrous skin. The pruritus is most severe at night and is increased by heat and sweating, and may be associated with a burning sensation. Few patients complain of persistent itching even after resolution; this is likely due to xerosis secondary to topical steroid use or impaired skin barrier due to scratching. The itch is severe enough to disturb sleep and significantly impairs quality of life.

Evaluation of a patient of superficial dermatophytosis begins with a direct visual examination. Dermoscopy is useful in the rapid diagnosis of tinea capitis by visualization of comma, corkscrew, pigtail, and morse code hairs. The utility of dermoscopy in the diagnosis of tinea of glabrous skin is limited due to the presence of nonspecific features. Vellus hair involvement at presentation, even if the body surface involvement is less, or at follow-up after topical antifungal therapy has been proposed as an indicator of chronicity, necessitating systemic antifungal therapy [63]. Translucent hairs, morse code/barcode hairs, follicular micropustules, brown spots surrounded by a white-yellowish halo, perifollicular scales, and reddish-brown or black globules are seen. The most characteristic dermoscopic feature of

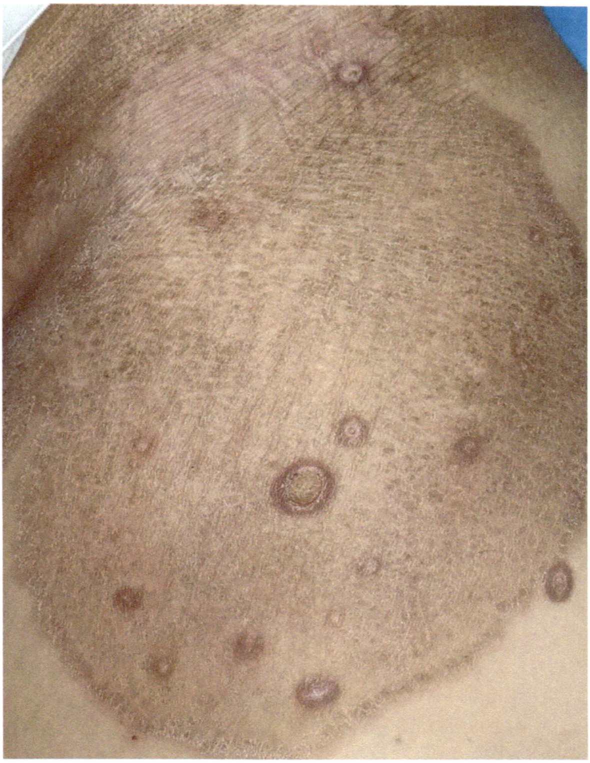

Fig. 15.14 Ulcerated tinea corporis

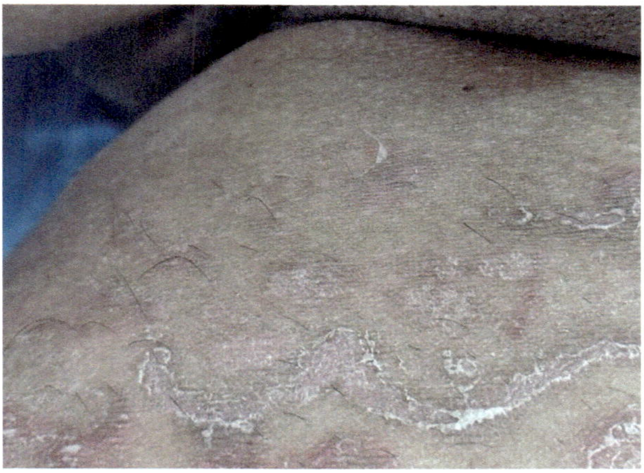

Fig. 15.15 Double-edged tinea cruris

dermatophytosis is the presence of reddish-brown and black globules with white scales which can be used for monitoring. Completion of therapy is indicated by the disappearance of dermoscopic patterns [64]. The dermoscopic features of topical

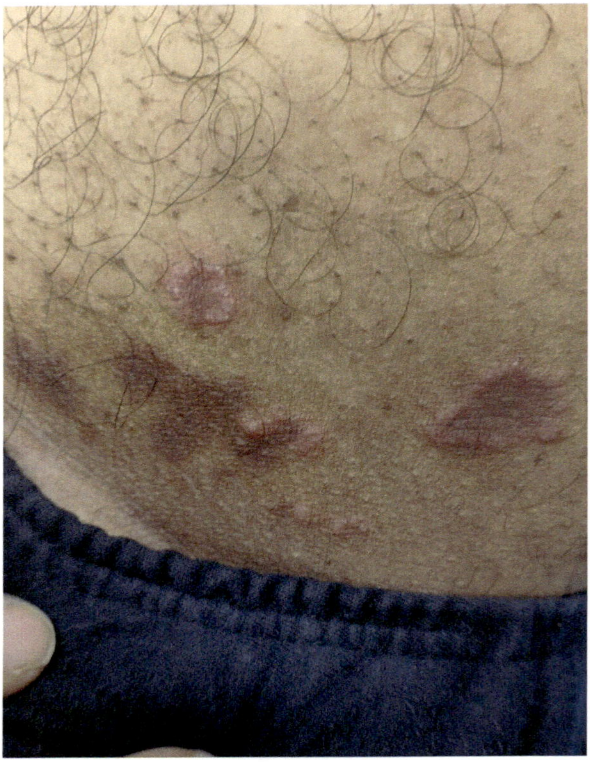

Fig. 15.16 Tinea recidivans presenting as annular plaque adjacent to post-inflammatory hyperpigmentation of resolved tinea lesion

steroid abuse, including erythematous background with telangiectasia, can be frequently seen concomitantly.

Trichophytin antigen elicits an immune response in most patients. The immediate hypersensitivity (IH) response to trichophytin is mediated by IgE and IgG4 antibodies indicating the involvement of Th2 limb of the acquired immunity (Fig. 15.18). High IgE antibodies may deplete the antigen, either by combining with it or by forming complexes that could block the receptors on the antigen presenting cells (APCs) and blocking the synthesis and release of cytokines and chemokines involved in activation of the cell-mediated immune (CMI) response [65].

The prolonged antigen exposure, in the recalcitrant dermatophytosis group, can be implicated in the downregulation of or ineffective CMI, due to the induction of anergy (immunologic unresponsiveness). Fungi produce prostaglandins and leukotrienes from arachidonic acid by elaborating phospholipases. While prostaglandins have been implicated in immunosuppression of the host, leukotrienes initiate a pro-inflammatory response [66].

Chitin (a component of the fungal cell wall) is degraded into chitin particles by the action of chitinases released from neutrophils and macrophages. Upon binding to the mannose receptors, chitin particles induce IL-10 secretion by activating the NOD2 and TLR9 pathways in APCs and macrophages [67]. IL-10, an

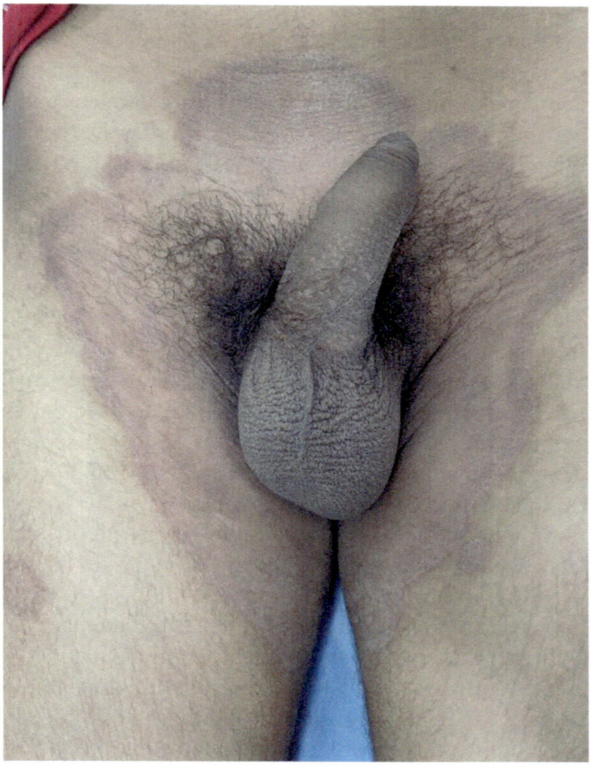

Fig. 15.17 Tinea pubogenitalis (Tinea cruris et genitalis)

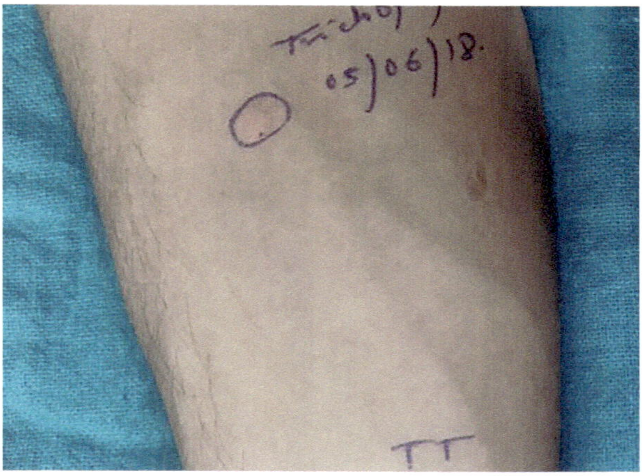

Fig. 15.18 Immediate hypersensitivity to intradermal trichophytin test

anti-inflammatory cytokine, downregulates the production of pro-inflammatory cytokines and induces tolerance. It also encourages the development of immunosuppressive CD4+ CD25+ T regulatory response, which plays a crucial role in dampening immune responses against pathogens and in maintaining self-tolerance and immune surveillance utilizing suppressive cytokines, IL-10 and TGF-β, and inhibiting the function of many cells including NK cells, NK/T cells, DCs, macrophages, and B cells [68].

Potassium hydroxide (KOH) mount for fungal elements is a cost-effective, rapid point-of-care test for confirmation of dermatophytic infections (Fig. 15.19). However, its sensitivity is low compared to Calcofluor or Blankophor preparations. The sample is usually collected from the advancing edge of lesions by scraping from the center to edge, crossing the margins using the blunt end of a sterile blade after cleaning with 70% alcohol or normal saline. The microscopic tests lack specificity due to their inability to differentiate different dermatophyte species. Fungal culture can provide this information. The skin scrapings are plated on Sabouraud dextrose agar with gentamicin (0.0025%) and/or chloramphenicol (0.005%) & cycloheximide (0.04%) or Sabouraud peptone-glucose agar (Emmons' modification) with cycloheximide to inhibit the growth of saprophytes. The media is inoculated with the material and incubated at 22–33 °C for 1–6 weeks. Dermatophytes usually show growth and sporulation within 7–10 days. The growth is differentiated into dermatophytes, yeasts, or molds based on macroscopic characteristics (obverse and reverse side of colonies as well as pigmentation). Dermatophytes exhibit white, cottony growth on the obverse with or without wine-red pigment on the reverse. The cultures of *T. mentagrophytes* genotype VIII are flat, white, fast-growing, and expanding colonies with hyphae bundles in the periphery and slight yellowish-to-beige pigmentation in the center (Fig. 15.20a and b).

Lactophenol cotton blue (LPCB) tease mounts are examined under the microscope to visualize the macroconidia, microconidia, and hyphae. LPCB mount from cultures of *T. mentagrophytes* complex show small and large round microconidia

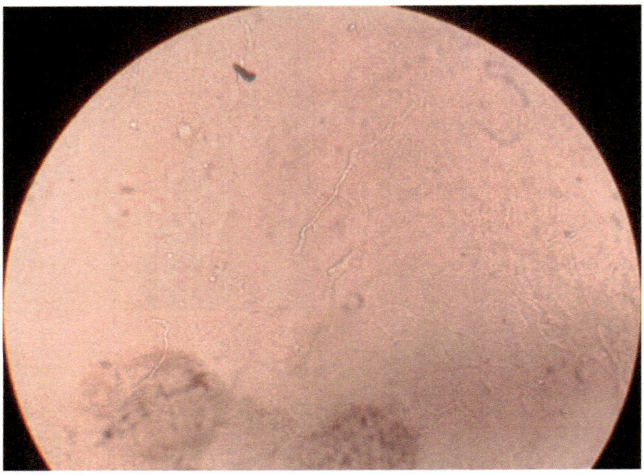

Fig. 15.19 Potassium hydroxide (KOH) mount showing refractile hyphae (40X)

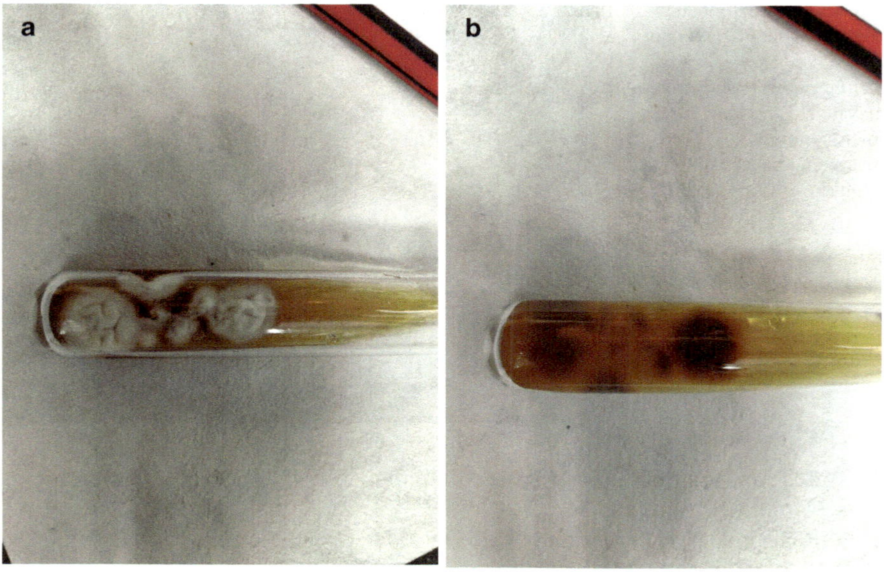

Fig. 15.20 Culture morphology (**a**) Flat, white, fast-growing and expanding colonies of *T. mentagrophytes* genotype VIII with hyphae bundles in the periphery and slight yellowish-to-beige pigmentation in the centre. (**b**) Orange pigmentation on reverse

together with chlamydospores of different sizes and cigar-shaped macroconidia (Fig. 15.21). Older cultures show spiral hyphae. Special media like Christensen urea agar (for urea hydrolysis) or enriched media like vitamin and amino acid-supplemented Trichophyton agars are utilized for species identification. In vitro hair perforation test is characteristic of *T. mentagrophytes* complex. Cultures frequently exhibit limited sensitivity and consume significant time, particularly for molds, which may take 7–28 days. The identification of filamentous fungi at the species level based on morphological characteristics demands expertise from skilled personnel. In instances where the identification of dermatophyte isolates is challenging in primary cultures, additional subcultures on specialized media, such as potato dextrose agar and cornmeal agar, are often required to induce conidiation and/or pigment production [2].

With recent advances in molecular techniques, direct detection of fungal organisms from the sample is quick and reproducible. Due to ongoing taxonomic revisions within the fungal kingdom relying largely on DNA profiles and pathogenicity rather than conventional morphological features, molecular methods detecting DNA signatures provide higher diagnostic advantage. Genotyping methods available for detection of dermatophytes, based on ITS 1 & 4, are as follows:

- PCR—polymerase chain reaction.
  - PCR—fingerprinting.
  - Random amplification of polymorphic DNA.

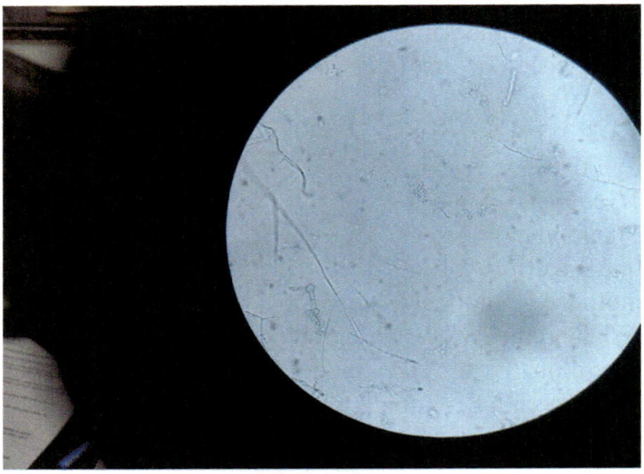

Fig. 15.21 Lactophenol cotton blue (LPCB) mount of *Trichophyton mentagrophytes* showing clavate to spherical microconidia, macroconidia and spiral hyphae (40X)

  - PCR and restriction fragment length polymorphism analysis.
  - Arbitrarily primed PCR.
  - Real-time PCR for dermatophyte DNA detection.
- MALDI-TOF-MS—Matrix-Assisted Laser Desorption/Ionization—Time of Flight—Mass Spectrometry.

To guide the selection of an appropriate antifungal agent, the Clinical and Laboratory Standards Institute (CLSI)(M38-A2) has introduced guidelines for the antifungal susceptibility testing (AFST) for dermatophytes. Clinical breakpoints (CBPs), which are based on information derived from clinical outcome, pharmacokinetics, and pharmacodynamics of the drug, may help in predicting response to treatment. In view of lack of CBPs, either the epidemiological cut-off values (ECVs or ECOFFs) or the upper limit of wild-type minimum inhibitory concentration (MIC) (UL-WT) may be useful to differentiate wild-type (WT) and non-wild-type (NWT) isolates, as these depend only on the MIC [69].

Antifungal resistance has emerged as an intense and distressing issue with a rise in clinical as well as mycological resistance. Cultures with high MIC predict low susceptibility to the antifungal, which may either be intrinsic or extrinsic (acquired due to prior exposure to antifungal). Drug resistance in dermatophytes is not a recent phenomenon; the resistant phenotype is not always sharply defined as it may co-exist with drug-sensitive ones. Despite the extensive use of antifungals, resistance was rarely reported in dermatophytes previously. The rising trend of resistance among dermatophytes leading to poor response and frequent relapses is of serious concern and has been attributed to inappropriate treatments with steroid combination creams, improper dosages of antifungals, and lifestyle changes. Self-medication, easy availability, and irrational use may be some of the other factors contributing to terbinafine and fluconazole resistance [70]. There is paucity of data regarding development of drug resistance in dermatophytes or correlation between in vitro and in vivo activities of antimycotic agents against dermatophytes.

Sometimes, AFST may produce erroneous results due to interference of ingredients of culture media. Also, the absence of clinical break-point makes it difficult to identify the microbiological resistant strains as per European Committee on Antimicrobial Susceptibility Testing (EUCAST) and CLSI. Though studies reported a very high level of terbinafine-resistance based on AFST, the genotypic identification of squalene epoxidase gene are more precise tools to declare resistance to this drug. Using this, a novel species Trichophyton indotineae was described in December 2020, isolated from patients from India and Nepal [69, 71].

Griseofulvin exhibits a broad MIC range and is currently regarded as an alternative medication for resistant tinea. To aid clinicians in determining appropriate therapy, antifungal susceptibility testing, coupled with accurate fungal identification, can be valuable [70]. Reports indicate that repetitive exposure to azole antifungals may contribute to the development of azole resistance in dermatophytes. Prolonged exposure to sub-inhibitory concentrations of azoles, amorolfine, and terbinafine can lead to the development of resistance in T. rubrum, resulting in treatment failures and contributing to persistence and chronicity. Global instances of azole resistance in dermatophytes are increasing [72, 73]. Given the rising drug resistance in dermatophytes, conducting antifungal drug susceptibility tests is essential, particularly in cases of chronic/recurrent dermatophytosis or instances of treatment failure/relapse.

The management of dermatophytosis has become challenging, as clinicians are often treating infection alone but the steroid-damaged skin as well. General measure which are helpful, include wearing loose-fitting breathable cotton garments to avoid undue friction and sweating, thorough cleansing bath with a syndet soap [74]. Bathing twice daily can be helpful in patients who are involved in vigorous physical activity or work in an environment which predisposes them to excessive sweating. The clothes should preferably be washed with hot water and detergent as arthrospores of dermatophytes die above 60 °C for 30 min. Sun drying is preferred over ironing [75].

Transmission to family members can be prevented by avoiding close contact and sharing of clothes. Consort or conjugal cases are also reported, and *T. mentagrophytes* genotype VII (Thai variant) is considered a sexually transmitted infection due to its association with genital dermatophytosis [76]. Also, all family members who are affected should be treated simultaneously. Special focus should be on elimination of reservoirs of infection (nails, glabrous skin) before discontinuing antifungals.

Topical therapy is generally indicated for localized infection involving a small area of the body. They are also used in situations where systemic therapy is contraindicated or unsafe, e.g., infants and pregnant females. It is also used along with oral anti-fungal therapy as it offers the advantages of increased local concentration, additional anti-inflammatory and antibiotic action, and increased patient satisfaction.

The general principles to be followed, while prescribing topical therapy, include application of antifungals over and 2 cm beyond the active margin, prescription of topical and oral antifungals of different classes and continuation of the topical antifungals for 2 weeks after clinical cure (as mycological cure occurs after clinical cure) [8].

The role of topical keratolytic is controversial [77, 78]. The use of short-contact ketoconazole or ciclopirox olamine lotion lacks sufficient evidence. There are no significant differences between effectiveness of different topical antifungals; however, few studies have shown sertaconazole to be superior to amorolfine and terbinafine [77–81].

Oral antifungal therapy is indicated in case of failure of topical therapy, extensive disease, disease involving multiple anatomical sites, chronic, recurrent, and recalcitrant dermatophytosis, steroid-modified tinea, and Majocchi's granuloma [8].

Itraconazole is the most favored agent for oral therapy owing to increasing resistance to terbinafine and slower response with longer treatment duration of griseofulvin and fluconazole. Itraconazole is used at a dose of 100 mg twice daily for a minimum of 2–4 weeks in naïve cases and 4 weeks in recalcitrant cases [8]. The role of pellet number and size, drug-polymer ratio all have been emphasized while choosing an appropriate brand of itraconazole. Dermoscopy and dissolution at acidic pH has been suggested as office-based methods to assess different itraconazole brands. However, the evidence is not very strong [82, 83]. To circumvent this problem of pH-dependent ionization of itraconazole resulting in reduced absorption in patients on antacids, super-bioavailable itraconazole was launched. It shows less variability than conventional itraconazole and hence the absorption is not affected by fasted or fed state [84].

The role of oral isotretinoin and topical salicylic acid is controversial [78, 85].

Utilizing a combination of two oral antifungals, each operating through distinct mechanisms, can be advantageous for individuals experiencing irregular treatment or recurrent episodes within a span of six months. Recommended combinations in such cases involve fluconazole/itraconazole paired with terbinafine, griseofulvin combined with terbinafine, or griseofulvin combined with fluconazole/itraconazole. This approach is particularly considered in patients dealing with chronic dermatophytosis or resistant dermatophytosis, especially when a satisfactory response is not achieved after three weeks of conventional therapy. However, it is important to note that combining antifungals may increase the risk of adverse effects, underscoring the importance of baseline and frequent monitoring of liver function tests [86].

More research into immunopathogenesis of chronic dermatophytosis is essential to understand the disease and to develop newer drugs. Enlorofim, a new antifungal in the pipeline has shown activity against *Trichophyton* spp. [87]. Antibiofilm agents, like rhamnolipid, may be used in the future to damage biofilm microstructure and enhance drug penetration [88, 89]. Chronic dermatophytosis should no longer be treated just as an infection but as a multifactorial disease. Targeting the fungus with antifungals is not enough; a multipronged approach is often required. Immunological tests like intradermal trichophytin test can be helpful in predicting patients at risk of chronic and recurrent dermatophytosis. Activation of the immune system by immunotherapy, including auto-implantation therapy, is being used to treat extensive and recalcitrant infections [90]. There is a need for development of vaccines for prophylaxis and treatment of recurrent and chronic dermatophytosis [91].

References

1. Verma S, Madhu R. The great Indian epidemic of superficial Dermatophytosis: an appraisal. Indian J Dermatol. 2017;62:227.
2. Verma SB, Panda S, Nenoff P, Singal A, Rudramurthy SM, Uhrlass S, et al. The unprecedented epidemic-like scenario of dermatophytosis in India: II. Diagnostic methods and taxonomical aspects. Indian J Dermatol Venereol Leprol. 2021;87:326–32.
3. Panda S, Verma S. The menace of dermatophytosis in India: the evidence that we need. Indian J Dermatol Venereol Leprol. 2017;83(3):281–4.
4. Teklebirhan G, Bitew A. Prevalence of Dermatophytic infection and the Spectrum of dermatophytes in patients attending a tertiary Hospital in Addis Ababa. Ethiopia Int J Microbiol. 2015;2015:653419.
5. Maraki S, Mavromanolaki VE. Epidemiology of Dermatophytoses in Crete. Greece Med Mycol J. 2016;57:e69–75.
6. Kaur R, Panda PS, Sardana K, Khan S. Mycological pattern of dermatomycoses in a tertiary care hospital. J Trop Med. 2015;2015:157828.
7. Hanumanthappa H, Sarojini K, Shilpashree P, Muddapur SB. Clinicomycological study of 150 cases of dermatophytosis in a tertiary care hospital in South India. Indian J Dermatol. 2012;57:322–3.
8. Rajagopalan M, Inamadar A, Mittal A, Miskeen AK, Srinivas CR, Sardana K, et al. Expert consensus on the Management of Dermatophytosis in India (ECTODERM India). BMC Dermatol. 2018;18:6.
9. Singh S, Verma P, Chandra U, Tiwary NK. Risk factors for chronic and chronic-relapsing tinea corporis, tinea cruris and tinea faciei: results of a case-control study. Indian J Dermatol Venereol Leprol. 2019;85:197–200.
10. Rudramurthy SM, Shankarnarayan SA, Dogra S, Shaw D, Mushtaq K, Paul RA, et al. Mutation in the squalene epoxidase gene of *Trichophyton interdigitale* and *Trichophyton rubrum* associated with allylamine resistance. Antimicrob Agents Chemother. 2018;62:e02522–17.
11. Pathania S, Rudramurthy SM, Narang T, Saikia UN, Dogra S. A prospective study of the epidemiological and clinical patterns of recurrent dermatophytosis at a tertiary care hospital in India. Indian J Dermatol Venereol Leprol. 2018;84:678–84.
12. Agarwal US, Saran J, Agarwal P. Clinico-mycological study of dermatophytes in a tertiary care Centre in Northwest India. Indian J Dermatol Venereol Leprol. 2014;80:194.
13. Coulibaly O, L'Ollivier C, Piarroux R, Ranque S. Epidemiology of human dermatophytoses in Africa. Med Mycol. 2018;56:145–61.
14. Madarasingha NP, Eriyagama S. An emerging threat of recalcitrant dermatophytosis in Sri Lanka—are we ready to tackle? Int J Dermatol. 2022;61:e2–3.
15. Usman B, Rehman A, Naz I, Anees M. Prevalence and antifungal drug resistance of dermatophytes in the clinical samples from Pakistan. Acta Microbiol Immunol Hung. 2021;68:291–6.
16. Noronha T, Tophakhane R, Nadiger S. Clinico-microbiological study of dermatophytosis in a tertiary-care hospital in North Karnataka. Indian Dermatol Online J. 2016;7:264.
17. Verma SB, Panda S, Nenoff P, Singal A, Rudramuruthy SM, Uhrlass S, et al. The unprecedented epidemic-like scenario of dermatophytosis in India: I. Epidemiology, risk factors and clinical features. Indian J Dermatol Venereol Leprol. 2021;87:154–75.
18. Tigga RA, Das S, Bhattacharya SN, Saha R, Pandhi D, Datt S, et al. Burden of chronic dermatophytosis in a tertiary care hospital: interaction of fungal virulence and host immunity. Mycopathologia. 2018;183:951–9.
19. Patro N, Panda M, Jena A. The menace of superficial Dermatophytosis on the quality of life of patients attending referral Hospital in Eastern India: a cross-sectional observational study. Indian Dermatol Online J. 2019;10:262.
20. Blank F, Mann SJ, Reale RA. Distribution of dermatophytosis according to age, ethnic group and sex. Sabouraudia. 1974;12:352–61.

21. Bonifaz A, Vázquez-González D. Tinea imbricata in the Americas. Curr Opin Infect Dis. 2011;24:106–11.
22. Segal E, Frenkel M. Dermatophyte infections in environmental contexts. Res Microbiol. 2015;166:564–9.
23. Poluri LV, Indugula JP, Kondapaneni SL. Clinicomycological study of Dermatophytosis in South India. J Lab Physicians. 2015;7:084–9.
24. García-Romero MT, Arenas R. New insights into genes, immunity, and the occurrence of dermatophytosis. J Invest Dermatol. 2015;135:655–7.
25. Humbert L, Cornu M, Proust-Lemoine E, Bayry J, Wemeau JL, Vantyghem MC, et al. Chronic mucocutaneous candidiasis in autoimmune polyendocrine syndrome type 1. Front Immunol. 2018;9:2570.
26. Lanternier F, Cypowyj S, Picard C, Bustamante J, Lortholary O, Casanova JL, et al. Primary immunodeficiencies underlying fungal infections. Curr Opin Pediatr. 2013;25:736.
27. Thakran P, Agrawal S, Singal A, Verma S, Madhu SV. Iatrogenic Cushing's syndrome in patients with superficial Dermatophytosis. Indian Dermatol Online J. 2021;12:237–43.
28. Nenoff P, Verma SB, Vasani R, Burmester A, Hipler UC, Wittig F, et al. The current Indian epidemic of superficial dermatophytosis due to Trichophyton mentagrophytes-a molecular study. Mycoses. 2019;62:336–56.
29. Tang C, Kong X, Ahmed SA, Thakur R, Chowdhary A, Nenoff P, et al. Taxonomy of the *Trichophyton mentagrophytes/T. Interdigitale* species complex harboring the highly virulent, multiresistant genotype *T. Indotineae*. Mycopathologia. 2021;186:315–26.
30. Shamsizadeh F, Pchelin IM, Makimura K, Alshahni MM, Satoh K, Katiraee F, et al. DNA topoisomerase 2 gene polymorphism in dermatophytes. Mycoses. 2020;63:694–703.
31. Nenoff P, Verma SB, Uhrlaß S, Burmester A, Gräser Y. A clarion call for preventing taxonomical errors of dermatophytes using the example of the novel Trichophyton mentagrophytes genotype VIII uniformly isolated in the Indian epidemic of superficial dermatophytosis. Mycoses. 2019;62:6–10.
32. Kano R, Kimura U, Kakurai M, Hiruma J, Kamata H, Suga Y, et al. Trichophyton indotineae sp. nov.: a new highly terbinafine-resistant anthropophilic dermatophyte species. Mycopathologia. 2020;185:947–58.
33. Burstein VL, Beccacece I, Guasconi L, Mena CJ, Cervi L, Chiapello LS. Skin immunity to dermatophytes: from experimental infection models to human disease. Front Immunol. 2020;11:3143.
34. Baldo A, Monod M, Mathy A, Cambier L, Bagut ET, Defaweux V, et al. Mechanisms of skin adherence and invasion by dermatophytes. Mycoses. 2012;55:218–23.
35. Esquenazi D, de Souza W, Alviano CS, Rozental S. The role of surface carbohydrates on the interaction of microconidia of *Trichophyton mentagrophytes* with epithelial cells. FEMS Immunol Med Microbiol. 2003;35:113–23.
36. Esquenazi D, Alviano CS, de Souza W, Rozental S. The influence of surface carbohydrates during in vitro infection of mammalian cells by the dermatophyte *Trichophyton rubrum*. Res Microbiol. 2004;155:144–53.
37. Aljabre SH, Richardson MD, Scott EM, Shankland GS. Germination of *Trichophyton mentagrophytes* on human stratum corneum in vitro. J Med Vet Mycol. 1992;30:145–52.
38. Esquenazi D, Rozental S, Alviano CS, Travassos LR, Schauer R. Sialic acids are absent from the dermatophytes *Trichophyton mentagrophytes* and *Trichophyton rubrum*. Mycoses. 2003;46:197–202.
39. Vermout S, Tabart J, Baldo A, Mathy A, Losson B, Mignon B. Pathogenesis of Dermatophytosis. Mycopathologia. 2008;166:267–75.
40. Dahl MV. Dermatophytosis and the immune response. J Am Acad Dermatol. 1994;31:S34–41.
41. Samdani AJ. Dermatophyte growth and degradation of human stratum corneum in vitro (pathogenesis of dermatophytosis). J Ayub Med Coll Abbottabad. 2005;17:19–21.
42. Zhang X, Wang Y, Chi W, Shi Y, Chen S, Lin D, et al. Metalloprotease genes of *Trichophyton mentagrophytes* are important for pathogenicity. Med Mycol. 2013;52:1–10.
43. Tainwala R, Sharma Y. Pathogenesis of dermatophytoses. Indian J Dermatol. 2011;56:259–61.

44. Burkhart CN, Burkhart CG, Gupta AK. Dermatophytoma: recalcitrance to treatment because of existence of fungal biofilm. J Am Acad Dermatol. 2002;47:629–31.
45. Arrese JE, Goffin V, Piérard-Franchimont C, Piérard GE. Dirty nails and mycotoxins. Rev Med Liege. 2001;56:38–40.
46. Reichhardt C, Stevens DA, Cegelski L. Fungal biofilm composition and opportunities in drug discovery. Future Med Chem. 2016;8:1455–68.
47. Mah TF, O'Toole GA. Mechanisms of biofilm resistance to antimicrobial agents. Trends Microbiol. 2001;9:34–9.
48. Brilhante RSN, Correia EEM, GMM G, Pereira VS, Oliveira JS, Bandeira SP, et al. Quantitative and structural analyses of the in vitro and ex vivo biofilm-forming ability of dermatophytes. J Med Microbiol. 2017;66:1045–52.
49. Li X, Yan Z, Xu J. Quantitative variation of biofilms among strains in natural populations of *Candida albicans*. Microbiology. 2003;149:353–62.
50. Pitts B, Hamilton MA, Zelver N, Stewart PS. A microtiter-plate screening method for biofilm disinfection and removal. J Microbiol Methods. 2003;54:269–76.
51. Koga T. Fungal immunology in the skin: immune response to dermatophytes. Nippon Ishinkin Gakkai Zasshi. 2009;50:151–4.
52. Criado PR, de Oliveira CB, Dantas KC, Takiguti FA, Benini LV, Vasconcellos C. Superficial mycosis and the immune response elements. An Bras Dermatol. 2011;86:726–31.
53. Almeida SR. Immunology of Dermatophytosis. Mycopathologia. 2008;166:277–83.
54. Knöpfel N, Del Pozo LJ, Escudero MDM, Martín-Santiago A. Dermoscopic visualization of vellus hair involvement in tinea corporis: a criterion for systemic antifungal therapy? Pediatr Dermatol. 2015;32:e226–7.
55. Eksomtramage T, Aiempanakit K. Tinea of vellus hair: a diagnostic and therapeutic challenge. BMJ Case Rep. 2018;2018:223678.
56. Reddy A, Joseph NM, Khan PS, Bhat S. A mycological study of clinically normal nails and waistbands and their role as sources of infection in patients with tinea corporis. Int J Res Dermatol. 2019;5:239–42.
57. Castellanos J, Guillén-Flórez A, Valencia-Herrera A, Toledo-Bahena M, Ramírez-Cortés E, Toussaint-Caire S, et al. Unusual inflammatory tinea infections: Majocchi's granuloma and deep/systemic dermatophytosis. J Fungi. 2021;7:929.
58. Yousefian F, Crowley C, Skupsky H, Calame A, Cohen PR. Tinea corporis-associated erythroderma: case report and review of erythrodermic patients with chronic dermatophyte infection. Cureus. 2020;12:e7578.
59. Dogra S, Narang T. Emerging atypical and unusual presentations of dermatophytosis in India. Clin Dermatology Rev. 2017;1:12.
60. Bhagyashree M, Shilpashree P. A clinico mycological study of tinea pseudoimbricata. Indian Dermatol Online J. 2022;13:73–7.
61. Verma SB, Gupta S, Yadav A, Ruocco E. Varicella and herpes zoster appearing over sites of tinea corporis, hitherto unreported examples of immunocompromised districts: a case series. Int J Dermatol. 2020;59:758–9.
62. Verma S. Tinea confined to tattoo sites - an example of Ruocco's immunocompromised district. Indian Dermatol Online J. 2019;10:739.
63. Gómez-Moyano E, Crespo-Erchiga V. Tinea of vellus hair: an indication for systemic antifungal therapy. Br J Dermatol. 2010;163:603–6.
64. Ankad BS, Mukherjee SS, Nikam BP, Reshme AS, Sakhare PS, Mural PH. Dermoscopic characterization of dermatophytosis: a preliminary observation. Indian. Dermatol Online J. 2020;11:202.
65. Gupta C, Das S, Ramachandran VG, Saha R, Bhattacharya SN, Dar SA, et al. Possible role of trichophytin antigen in inducing impaired immunological clearance of fungus in onychomycosis. Mycopathologia. 2016;181:247–51.
66. Noverr MC, Toews GB, Huffnagle GB. Production of prostaglandins and leukotrienes by pathogenic fungi. Infect Immun. 2002;70:400–2.

67. Wagener J, Malireddi RKS, Lenardon MD, Köberle M, Vautier S, MacCallum DM, et al. Fungal chitin dampens inflammation through IL-10 induction mediated by NOD2 and TLR9 activation. PLoS Pathog. 2014;10:e1004050.
68. Kaya TI, Eskandari G, Guvenc U, Gunes G, Tursen U, Burak Cimen MY, et al. CD4+CD25+ Treg cells in patients with toenail onychomycosis. Arch Dermatol Res. 2009;301:725–9.
69. Shaw D, Singh S, Dogra S, Jayaraman J, Bhat R, Panda S, et al. MIC and upper limit of wild-type distribution for 13 antifungal agents against a *Trichophyton mentagrophytes-Trichophyton interdigitale* complex of Indian origin. Antimicrob Agents Chemother. 2020;64:e01964–19.
70. Gaurav V, Bhattacharya SN, Sharma N, Datt S, Kumar P, Rai G, et al. Terbinafine resistance in dermatophytes: time to revisit alternate antifungal therapy. J Mycol Med. 2021;31:101087.
71. Uhrla S, Verma SB, Gräser Y, Rezaei-Matehkolaei A, Hatami M, Schaller M, et al. Trichophyton indotineae-an emerging pathogen causing recalcitrant Dermatophytoses in India and world-wide-a multidimensional perspective. J Fungi (Basel). 2022;8(7):757.
72. Moreno-Sabater A, Normand AC, Bidaud AL, Cremer G, Foulet F, Brun S, et al. Terbinafine resistance in dermatophytes: a French multicenter prospective study. J Fungi. 2022;8:220.
73. Bhatia A, Kanish B, Badyal D, Kate P, Choudhary S. Efficacy of oral terbinafine versus itraconazole in treatment of dermatophytic infection of skin—a prospective, randomized comparative study. Indian J Pharmacol. 2019;51:116.
74. Verma SB, Panda S, Nenoff P, Singal A, Rudramurthy SM, Uhrlass S, et al. The unprecedented epidemic-like scenario of dermatophytosis in India: III. Antifungal resistance and treatment options. Indian J Dermatol Venereol Leprol. 2021;87:468–82.
75. Hammer TR, Mucha H, Hoefer D. Infection risk by dermatophytes during storage and after domestic laundry and their temperature-dependent inactivation. Mycopathologia. 2011;171:43–9.
76. Kupsch C, Czaika VA, Deutsch C, Gräser Y. Trichophyton mentagrophytes – a new genotype of zoophilic dermatophyte causes sexually transmitted infections. J der Dtsch Dermatologischen Gesellschaft. 2019;17:493–501.
77. Saoji V, Madke B. Efficacy of salicylic acid peel in dermatophytosis. Indian J Dermatol Venereol Leprol. 2021;87:671–5.
78. Das A, Kumar P, Sil A, Das A, Kumar P, Sil A. Salicylic acid peeling in dermatophytosis: an unjustifiable therapy. Indian J Dermatol Venereol Leprol. 2021;0:1–2.
79. Van Zuuren EJ, Fedorowicz Z, El-Gohary M. Evidence-based topical treatments for tinea cruris and tinea corporis: a summary of a Cochrane systematic review. Br J Dermatol. 2015;172:616–41.
80. Das A, Sil A, Sarkar TK, Sen A, Chakravorty S, Sengupta M, et al. A randomized, double-blind trial of amorolfine 0.25% cream and sertaconazole 2% cream in limited dermatophytosis. Indian J Dermatol Venereol Leprol. 2019;85:276–81.
81. Choudhary S, Bisati S, Singh A, Koley S. Efficacy and safety of terbinafine hydrochloride 1% cream vs. sertaconazole nitrate 2% cream in tinea corporis and tinea cruris: a comparative therapeutic trial. Indian J Dermatol. 2013;58:457–60.
82. Sonthalia S, Sardana K, Sharma P, Sehgal VN, Pandey A, Gupta KS. An office-based evaluation of various itraconazole brands. J Am Acad Dermatol. 2019;S0190-9622:32894.
83. Jakhar D, Kaur I, Mehta RK. Dissolution at acidic pH, and not dermatoscopy, is the preferred method to test the quality of itraconazole pellets. J Am Acad Dermatol. 2019;S0190-9622:32895–6.
84. Rauseo AM, Mazi P, Lewis P, Burnett B, Mudge S, Spec A. Bioavailability of single-dose SUBA-itraconazole compared to conventional itraconazole under fasted and fed conditions. Antimicrob Agents Chemother. 2021;65:e0013421.
85. Srivastava A, Kothiwala S. Isotretinoin may affect pharmacokinetics of itraconazole in the skin: is it rational to combine both for the treatment of dermatophytosis? Indian J Dermatol Venereol Leprol. 2017;83:68–9.
86. Rengasamy M, Chellam J, Ganapati S. Systemic therapy of dermatophytosis: practical and systematic approach. Clin Dermatology Rev. 2017;1:19.
87. McCarty TP, Pappas PG. Antifungal pipeline Front Cell Infect Microbiol. 2021;11:811.

88. Sen S, Borah SN, Bora A, Deka S. Rhamnolipid exhibits anti-biofilm activity against the dermatophytic fungi *Trichophyton rubrum* and *Trichophyton mentagrophytes*. Biotechnol reports. 2020;27:e00516.
89. Pereira FDO. A review of recent research on antifungal agents against dermatophyte biofilms. Med Mycol. 2021;59:313–26.
90. Kumar S, Kaur A, Kaur S. Autoimplantation therapy in extensive and recalcitrant dermatophytosis: a case series. J Clin Aesthet Dermatol. 2021;14:34.
91. Mignon B, Tabart J, Baldo A, Mathy A, Losson B, Vermout S. Immunization and dermatophytes. Curr Opin Infect Dis. 2008;21:134–40.

Skin Disease in Tropics: Impacted by Heat, Humidity, and Healthcare Neglect

16

Ananya Sharma and Somesh Gupta

The word 'tropic' comes from Ancient Greek τροπή (*tropē*), meaning 'to turn' or 'change direction'. Geographically, it refers to the equatorial zone between the Tropic of Cancer at 23° north, and the Tropic of Capricorn at 23° south. This region has a climate that is hot and humid throughout the year, and the word 'tropical' has now become synonymous with this warm and moist climate itself. Medical historians approach tropical dermatology differently. While some equate it primarily to the infectious diseases caused by vectors like mosquitoes, fleas, and sandflies that thrive in such an environment; others have included all skin conditions encountered in the tropics—from dermatoses caused or exacerbated by sweat to nutritional dermatoses and bite reactions [1].

These regions are exposed to the equatorial sun at noon all year round, leading to a greater average temperature (at least 18 °C in the coldest month), higher annual rainfall as well as less seasonal change [2]. Within the tropical zone, there is the wet equatorial climate (within 5° north and south of the equator), which is characterized by constant heat, rainfall, and humidity; dry tropical climate (between latitudes 15° and 30° north and south), which includes the hot arid desert areas of North Africa, Arabia, and Northwest India; and the alternately wet and dry tropical climate between 5° to 15° north and south in South America, West and Central Africa, and Australia.

Despite their rich natural resources as well as varied social and political backgrounds, almost all of the tropical countries remain under-developed. In 1992, GNP per capita in the tropical regions was 25% of that in the temperate-zone [3]. Agriculture was the earliest mode of economic progress, and tropical soil was of poor quality for it, containing a very thin layer of humus which was easily washed away by the first heavy rainfall. The rainfall itself was highly variable, being either

A. Sharma · S. Gupta (✉)
Department of Dermatology and Venereology, AIIMS, New Delhi, India
e-mail: someshgupta@aiims.edu

S. Gupta et al. (eds.), *Critical Thinking in Contemporary Dermatology: Cognitive Essays*, https://doi.org/10.1007/978-981-97-0411-8_16

too much or too little, with recurrent droughts. Though methods like shifting cultivation emerged, this meant that growth of a settled rather than nomadic community was not attained [4]. The hot and humid climate also serves to provide a suitable environment for continued reproduction of pests and insects throughout the year affecting crop produce, while in the temperate zone, the annual winter frost serves to knock back the insects each year leading to overall better outcomes for food crops [5]. These insects and arthropods also act as vectors, leading to a much higher burden of infectious diseases in the tropics. In the midst of over-population (the tropics were home to 40% of the world's population and 55% of children under 5 years of age in 2014; estimated to rise to 60% by 2050 [6]), standards of hygiene and healthcare are difficult to maintain, and a vicious cycle ensues that traps these countries in poverty.

Imperialism by the temperate zone on the tropical zone has been massive, with European nations controlling 67% of the world by 1878, and over 84% by 1914. With the occupancy of Africa and Asia emerged the need to invest in healthcare of primarily European troops and civilian populations in the tropics, and these medical investments and research emerged as tropical medicine [7]. However, insufficient resources are devoted to research in this area, with many opinions emphasizing mismanagement of globalization. While the technology for handling temperate zone disease from the developed countries could be incorporated, the different ecological zones and their requirements were not addressed [8]. Medical education in these countries was also often largely focussed on the Western model, with inadequate emphasis on the prevailing diseases in the community. Many of the international agencies like World Trade Organization and International Monetary Fund are largely undemocratic and focus on capitalism, leaving the interests of the impoverished unaddressed. Some authors go as far as to say that in modern times, perhaps terrorism has succeeded in promoting Western engagement with poverty! At the same time, counter-terrorism and corporate colonialism have become modern forms of imperialism [8].

Contemporary tropical medicine thus becomes not only about recognizing the exotic dermatoses of this region but also about learning to practice good medicine in a poor situation. Dr. Larry W. Laughlin, a US Naval Medical research officer and an expert in tropical medicine, equated the circumstances to 'not having drugs available to treat dying infants while reading an MRI scan on a healthy foreign diplomat'. [9] The emergence of the Global Fund revitalized the resources available for international attempts to control TB, malaria, and HIV; with 12 billion US dollars allocated for 2020-22. Meanwhile, many neglected parasitic and bacterial diseases were among some of the most common infections in the estimated 2.7 billion people who live on less than $2 per day [10], causing approximately 2 lakh deaths and loss of 19 million DALYs (disability adjusted life years) annually [11]. Experts argued that re-allocation of a segment of these funds would be an effective way 'to make poverty history'. These have only recently gained recognition and international attention in 2015, with the Sustainable Development Goals (SDG target 3.3). The story of leprosy exemplifies that of tropical diseases, wherein a treatable disease was a great cause of stigma and permanent deformities for years before political focus and public health interventions led to its elimination in all but a few countries.

In 2020, even though life expectancy has increased, Neglected Tropical Diseases (NTDs) (a group of 20 diseases listed by the World Health Organization (WHO) that affect more than 1 billion people each year, predominantly in the tropics) continue to cause widespread disability and a substantial burden of disease [12].

16.1 Dermatoses Directly Due to the Tropical Climate

More common than the striking infections that spring to mind when we talk of tropical skin diseases, are the mundane group of dermatoses that arises as a combination of heat, moisture and friction on various body sites. Skin is the organ most exposed to environmental variations and thus tends to have a high sensitivity to the climate. While cold and dry climates are associated with greater trans-epidermal water loss and an altered skin barrier leading to conditions like xerosis, pruritus, atopic dermatitis, and psoriasis [13]; in the tropics, overhydration of the skin and increased ambient heat leads to excessive sweating as well as obstruction of the eccrine duct, leading to miliaria and secondary anhidrosis. Factors like friction or occlusive clothing further precipitate this obstruction [1].

Miliaria, commonly known as 'prickly heat', occurs when the eccrine duct is blocked at various levels in the epidermis. The clinical spectrum ranges from tiny 1-2 mm superficial, fragile and punctate vesicles called miliaria crystallina when blocked at the level of stratum corneum (Fig. 16.1); to deeper obstruction leading to itchy erythematous or flesh-coloured papules. The sweat is refluxed back into the epidermis or dermis, leading to an inflammatory reaction. Superficial infection of miliaria is called periporitis staphylogenes, a peculiar presentation in children of tropical regions which is not extensively described in Western literature. When miliaria affects large areas, ineffective thermoregulation may even lead to secondary anhidrosis and heat exhaustion.

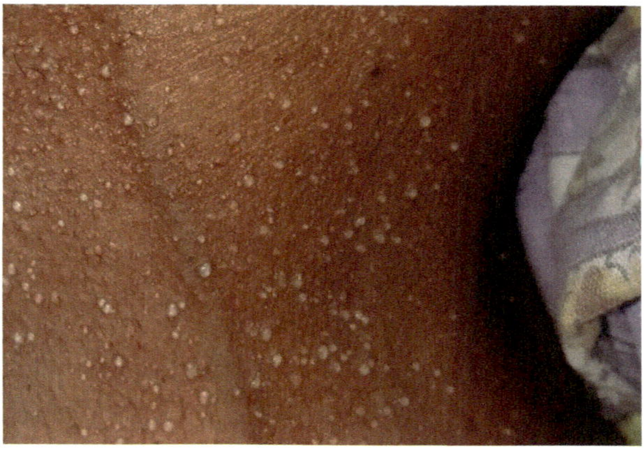

Fig. 16.1 *Miliaria crystallina*: Superficial, fragile vesicles occurring on the neck due to blocking of the eccrine duct at the level of stratum corneum (Credits: Dr. Prashant Bharti)

Perspiration may act as an irritant, causing hyperpigmented, fissured, wrinkled plaques localized to sites of friction, especially seen during the summer months. This is known as *sweat dermatitis,* and it affects both the convex surfaces of the body in contact with clothing and the folds where sweat accumulates, associated with a stinging sensation (Fig. 16.2). Various hypothesis include cumulative damage by water and removal of natural moisturizing factors from the skin, proteolytic enzymes in sweat as well as a high concentration of sodium chloride [14]. A similar warm and moist climate is simulated in babies of diaper dermatitis, which predisposes to irritant contact dermatitis by excreta. Sebum secretion tends to be greater in warmer climates as well, with half the patients with acne reporting seasonal variation, most of them exacerbating in the summer and rainy season [15, 16].

The simulation of such an environment all over the world is exemplified in the present era of COVID-19 in which many studies document that long hours (more than 6 h/day) of wearing occlusive personal protective equipment led to adverse dermatological effects in as many as 97% of health care workers in some studies [17]. Irritant contact dermatitis, frictional dermatitis, sweat dermatitis, facial acne, folliculitis, and flares of eczema were the most common problems [18, 19], reflecting well the common skin diseases in the tropics, being an exaggerated version of the same!

In contrast, the prevalence of atopic dermatitis has been found to have a positive correlation with latitude and negative correlation with mean outdoor temperature and indoor relative humidity [20]. Relative humidity depends on temperature, and

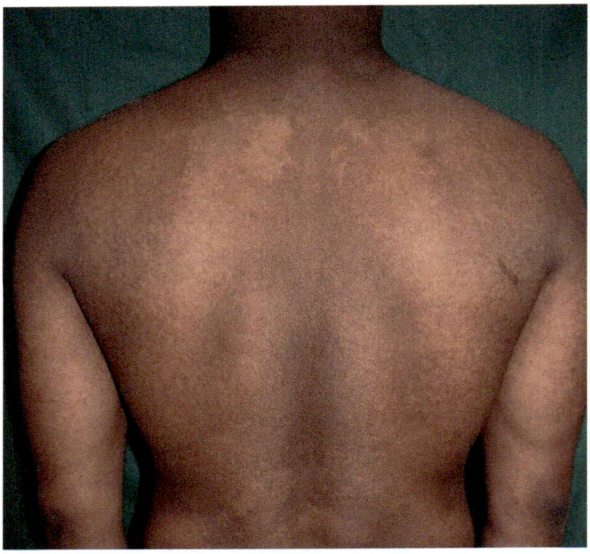

Fig. 16.2 *Sweat dermatitis*: Hyperpigmented, wrinkled plaques at sites of contact with clothing (Credits: Dr. Prashant Bharti)

warm air can hold more water than cold air. When cold air is heated as done in indoor heating systems, the relative humidity drops. The effect of humidity has been investigated in mouse models, wherein mice that were transferred from a humid environment (relative humidity≥80%) to a dry environment (relative humidity ≤10%) developed a rougher and drier skin surface, increased transepidermal water loss (TEWL), as well as reduced filaggrin expression after 2 weeks. Human skin also shows a decrease in stratum corneum lipids during the winter season, and skin complaints during winter (simulating cold and dry climate) are well described, including more tendency for itch and increased reaction to skin irritants [21]. In addition, according to the archaic concept of 'hygiene hypothesis', higher exposure to viral and bacterial pathogens in the tropics would lead to an obligatory stimulation and development of the immune system; leading to a lower incidence of autoimmune and atopic diseases. This has however been subsequently challenged, with convincing evidence for an inverse relationship between helminth infections and atopic dermatitis, but no other pathogens [22].

The epidemiology of psoriasis also shows a contrast, ranging from a prevalence of 0.7–2.9% in the temperate zone, to <0.5% in Africa, Asia, and Latin America [23]. This is hypothesized to be correlated to geographical UV distribution, the immunomodulatory effects of which are well-established in decreased the hyperresponsiveness of antigen presenting cells and autoreactive dermal T-cells for the treatment of psoriasis.

16.2 Infections

In outpatient or community studies conducted in the tropics, cutaneous infections were either the most common dermatological condition encountered or second only to eczema in some studies, ranging from 10% to 47.15% of patients with skin lesions [24–26]. The most common of them include pyoderma, superficial fungal infections, scabies, and pediculosis, which are also often quickly resolved. Mycobacteria, however, have a special significance in the tropics, with both tuberculosis and leprosy being important preventable and treatable causes of chronic suffering in these areas. The reasons for these high rates of cutaneous infections are numerous, yet all interconnected, including low levels of hygiene, overcrowding, lack of proper water supply, dissemination by insects, and a trend of self-medication and often scientifically unfounded cultural practices. Due to the high number of untrained caregivers and lack of effective regulation, even persons who present to local health facilities may be inadequately or incorrectly treated, the most common example being the menace of topical steroids prescribed for dermatophytosis. Allopathic doctors were estimated to comprise only one-third (30.6%) of all health workers in India, and more than half (57.3%) of Indian 'allopathic' practitioners are estimated to lack a medical qualification [27]. It is important to note that tropical infections may also be seen in tourists, migrants, or soldiers who return from tropical areas of the world, the diagnosis often being missed when a proper travel history is not elicited.

16.2.1 Microbiota of the Skin

The human microbiome includes microorganisms and their collective genome residing in an anatomical niche. Most frequently studied in the gut, skin, and vagina; four phyla comprise the major bacteria residing on the skin: *Firmicutes*, *Bacteroidetes*, *Proteobacteria*, and *Actinobacteria*. These organisms help to prevent skin infections by providing ecologic competition with pathogenic microorganisms and by hydrolyzing lipids of sebum to produce free fatty acids, which are toxic to many pathogenic bacteria. Moreover, both innate and adaptive immune functions in the skin are influenced by the commensal skin microbiota. High-temperature and high-humidity are however associated with a change in the composition, including increased bacterial population on the back, axillary vault, and feet and higher number of gram negative bacilli and fungi as compared with moderate-temperature low-humidity conditions [28]. Increased hydration of the skin has been shown to increase staphylococci and micrococci in early stages and later lipophilic coryneforms [29]. This may form part of the reason why people in such climates are predisposed to these infections. On the other hand, ultraviolet (UV) light is a well-documented bactericidal treatment, and longitudinal and/or latitudinal variation in UV exposure may lead to geographical variability in skin microbiota [30].

16.2.2 Common Infections and Infestations

Although the term '*pyoderma*' encompasses a broad range of bacterial infections, it is most commonly used for staphylococcal and streptococcal disease, which comprise 77% and 3-7% of pyoderma isolates, respectively [31, 32]. Some authors also classify pyodermas as primary and secondary, the secondary ones occurring as a superimposed infection on diseases like scabies, dermatitis, or conditions of skin denudation such as pemphigus. The importance of the non-bullous form of impetigo (Fig. 16.3), caused by streptococci, lies in its strong association with post-streptococcal glomerulonephritis. In fact, 97% of the world's burden of post-streptococcal glomerulonephritis is estimated to be in developing countries because of the frequency of cutaneous infections [33].

The portal of entry for many of these agents is often through minor trauma or breaks in the skin such as those caused by insect bites, also common in these areas. Thus, localization is often at exposed sites such as lower legs. In poorer regions where antibiotics are not easily available or affordable, topical agents like 1% gentian violet lotion may be used, which have a bacteriostatic effect. Other antiseptics that have been used to prevent infections but do not have a clear role in treating them

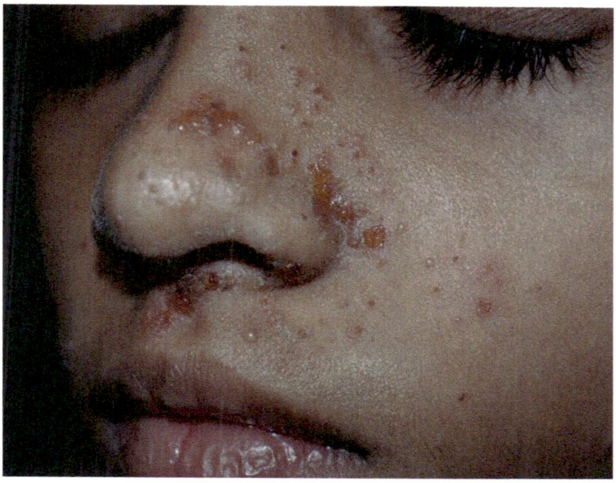

Fig. 16.3 *Impetigo contagiosa*: Periorificial tiny vesicles and superficial erosions with 'honey' coloured crusts in a young child (Credits: Dr. Prashant Bharti)

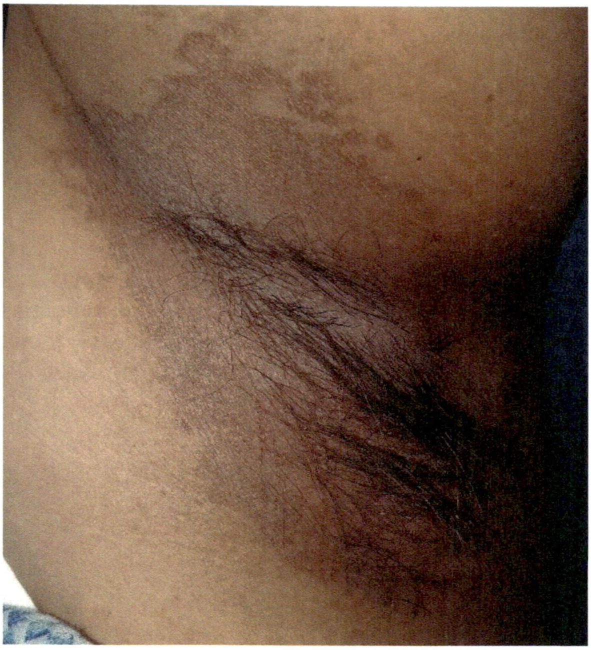

Fig. 16.4 *Erythrasma*: Hyperpigmented, non-inflammatory, and largely well-defined scaly plaques in the axilla (Credits: Dr. Prashant Bharti)

include potassium permanganate, burrow's solution, boric acid, and preparations like Castellani's paint. Acetic acid 1% soaks work well against pseudomonas infection.

The coryneform infections of the skin like erythrasma (Fig. 16.4), trichomycosis axillaris, and pitted keratolysis also tend to occur in conditions of occlusion and moisture; and are largely seen in the tropics.

Amongst infestations; *scabies* is endemic in the tropics, and is estimated to affect more than 130 million people worldwide at a given time [34]. Children and older people in low-resource regions are the most vulnerable groups, among whom the prevalence, morbidity, and secondary complications are greatest (Fig. 16.5). A study from the 1980s in Bangladesh reported a majority of pre-school children experiencing at least one infestation per year [35]; whereas the disease occurs sporadically in high-income countries, with reported outbreaks in various settings such as nursing homes, child day care centres, jails, psychiatric facilities, and homes for elderly; reflecting the disease to be an indirect reflection of poverty and overcrowding. The 3-day survival time of the mite outside the human host provides sufficient time to latch onto another one in these circumstances. In the Global Burden of Disease 2015 Study, scabies ranked 101 in age-standardized global DALYs, just ahead of atrial fibrillation or flutter (102) and acute lymphoid leukaemia (103), out of 246 conditions included [36]. In resource-limited regions, scabies-related impetigo is the principal cause of post-streptococcal glomerulonephritis as well as rheumatic fever and rheumatic heart disease, which account for at least 300,000 deaths worldwide every year [37]. *Pediculosis* is another menace, most commonly presenting as head lice caused by *Pediculus capitis*. Infestation results in distress, social stigma, and absence from school. Moreover, there is increasing resistance to pyrethroids and malathion, the most commonly used first-line topical agents [38].

The issue of antimicrobial resistance is one that initially emerged in association with hospital-based infections in the West, but is now reported in its highest rates from low- and middle-income countries (LMICs) in Asia, Africa, and the Middle East. More than 90% of the mortality currently attributable to antimicrobial resistance occurs in regions that are already disproportionately burdened with infectious diseases [39]. This is linked to the variable and empiric consumption of antimicrobials for human medicine and the food industry; as well as migration. Syndromic approach, over-the-counter availability and inadequate surveillance for resistance also contribute.

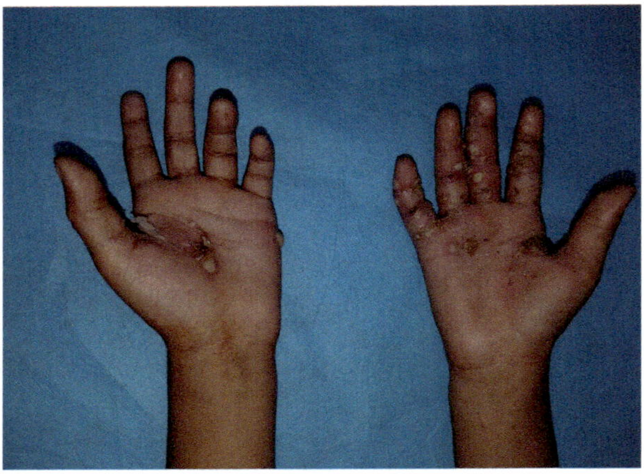

Fig. 16.5 *Scabies with secondary infection*: Itchy, acral vesiculo-pustules in a young child with secondary pyoderma

Amongst fungal infections, dermatophytes are the oldest group of fungi implicated with superficial infections affecting 20–25% of the general population throughout the world [40], making them the most frequent form of infection. Dermatophytes thrive at surface temperatures of 25–28 °C, and infection of human skin is supported by warm and humid conditions, leading to geographical and seasonal variability. What was once considered an innocuous, easy-to-treat infection of tropical and subtropical countries, mainly seen during the summer and rainy seasons, has now become a perennial and difficult-to-treat entity in many countries of Asia, including and especially in India, with prevalence rates between 36.6% and 78.4% [41]! So much so, that it requires a separate, deep insight as elaborated in another essay in this book. Tinea pedis is the one exception, with similar prevalence rates across countries, owing to more local factors like occlusive footwear [42]. However, the tropical environment has always been conducive to all sorts of fungi, reflected in the high rates of candidemia in tropical countries like Pakistan and Brazil, with the lowest rates in countries like Austria and Portugal [43]. The incidence of mucormycosis has been estimated at nearly 70 times the generally accepted rates in Western countries [44], though also influenced by the high rate of diabetes prevalence in India, at 9%. Trauma is a risk factor in 7.5–22% of mucormycosis cases in India, with majority of the patients presenting with cutaneous mucormycosis after trauma, burns, and nosocomial infections at the surgery or injection site [45]. This was recently highlighted and caused much public panic in context of the COVID-19 pandemic and the larger numbers of patients admitted in intensive care units, most suffering from comorbidities.

Pityriasis versicolor, tinea nigra, and white and black piedra are other classical superficial mycoses seen in the tropics; with minimal inflammation (Fig. 16.6) [45].

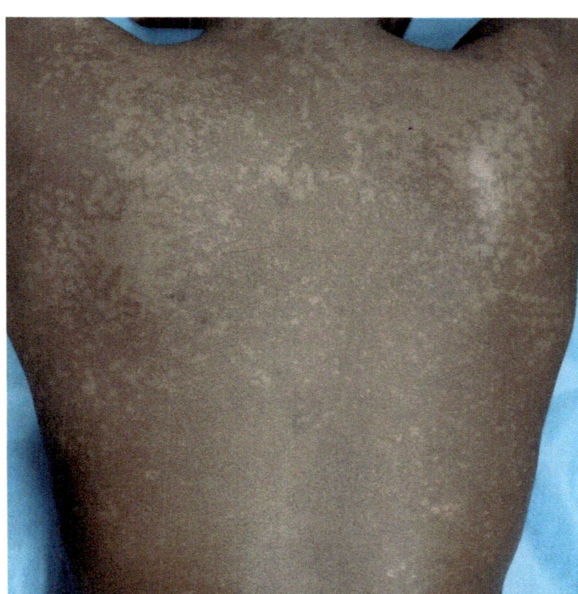

Fig. 16.6 *Pityriasis versicolor*: Hypopigmented, barely elevated plaques with fine scaling

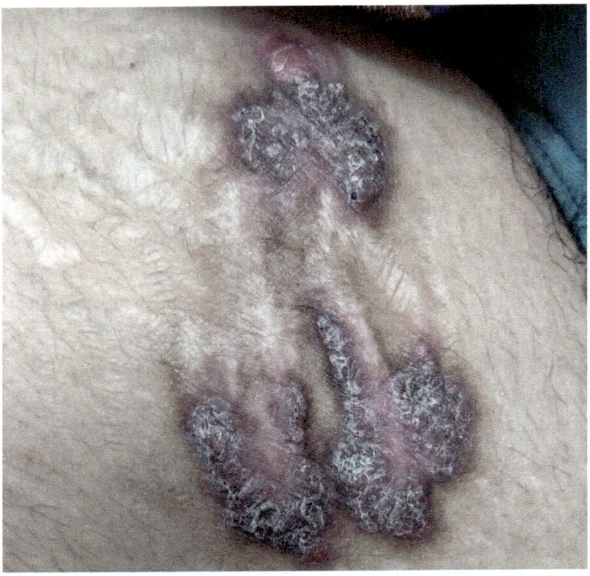

Fig. 16.7 *Lupus vulgaris*: Annular, erythematous scaly plaque with central clearing

Though merely a nuisance than a major illness, they comprise a large proportion of people seeking intervention.

Tuberculosis remains a formidable infection despite effective chemotherapy and strategic health programmes across various levels of care. In its cutaneous form, it comprises 1.5% of extrapulmonary tuberculosis; which is a considerable number considering that India reported an annual incidence of 2.64 million cases of tuberculosis [46]. The association of tuberculosis with tropics is one purely that of an opportunist of poverty, overcrowding, and malnutrition; little to do with the climate per se. Meanwhile, the incidence in sub-Saharan Africa has increased as a consequence of the HIV pandemic. Apart from the greater incidence, there are some peculiarities like the location of lupus vulgaris lesions on the buttocks of children rather than the face as typical in the West (Fig. 16.7), and tuberculosis verrucosa cutis on feet after trauma due to barefoot walking [47]. Scrofuloderma presenting in children and adolescents on the cervical and supraclavicular area remains the most common form. With tuberculosis in the community, tuberculids like lichen scrofulosorum, papulonecrotic tuberculid and erythema induratum are also seen.

16.2.3 Peculiar Infections of the Tropics

Some infections encountered in the tropics are neither run-of-the-mill nor have been highlighted as part of the global health initiatives, and thus receive little attention and education. *Tropical ulcer* is a prototype, a mixed synergistic bacterial infection caused by *Fusobacterium ulcerans*, spirochaetes, and other anaerobic bacteria, that is usually seen in children (5-15 years) in tropical and subtropical regions as acute, painful, malodorous necrotic ulcers on the lower limb with considerable slough. In the past, it has been referred to as 'ulcus tropics', 'tropical phagedenic ulcer', and Naga sore. A greater number of cases occur in the monsoon, which may be attributed to increased sweating, maceration, and scratching of the skin leading to inoculation of organisms. The role of overcrowding, poor hygiene, and poor nutrition has been hypothesized, though formal studies have not corroborated the same [48].

Rhinoscleroma is a chronic, granulomatous disease caused by *Klebsiella rhinoscleromatis,* involving the upper respiratory tract, especially the nasopharynx. It is endemic to Egypt, Central America, Central Africa, India, Indonesia, and the Middle East [49]. It progresses from a non-specific rhinitis to infiltrative granulomatous stage with granulation tissue filling the nasal fossa and eventually scarring, and may cause massive facial deformities with delayed treatment, ever so common in these areas.

Cutaneous anthrax and *erysipeloid* are both uncommon diseases that are transmitted through contact with infected animals, and hence often encountered on the exposed sites (e.g. dorsum of hand, face) of people who work with them. Their occurrence is often associated with a lack of standard simple protective equipment such as gloves, or lack of regulations to use the same, in the poorer tropical countries. The cultural proximity and rearing of animals also results in a greater incidence of nematode infestations, with sandy, warm, moist, shaded areas being favourable. The infection is usually acquired by walking barefoot on ground contaminated with animal faeces containing larvae, but the buttock or other body sites can become infected via contact with contaminated soil or sand. The larva penetrates the skin using enzymes, including proteases and hyaluronidase; and then creeps within the skin in serpiginous paths, at the rate of ~3 mm/day (hence denoted *cutaneous larva migrans*). The lesions are intensely itchy, sometimes producing a burning sensation.

Insects and their larvae also abound in the tropics as elucidated earlier, leading to occurrence of myiasis, most commonly as wound myiasis when larvae are deposited on open wounds. A lack of hygiene and poor socioeconomic status, the elderly and debilitated, psychiatric patients, alcoholics, and other patients with either loss of sensation or inability to discourage flies from depositing eggs are predisposed [44]. Meanwhile, migratory or creeping myiasis caused by the larvae of horse and cattle bot flies simulate helminthic cutaneous larva migrans, but can be differentiated by a longer duration and slower movement. In a study that looked at the frequency of dermatoses associated with travel to tropical countries, the most common conditions were in fact cutaneous larva migrans in one-fourth, pyodermas in 18%, pruritic arthropod-reactive dermatitis in 10%, followed by myiasis (9%) and tungiasis (6%) [50]. Tungiasis is another skin disease caused by epidermal penetration of female sand fleas (*Tunga penetrans*), which despite having all the merits of a neglected tropical disease (NTD) is not specifically included in WHO's list of NTDs. It is endemic in Latin America, the Caribbean, and sub-Saharan Africa, and causes a local infestation of the feet, and may lead to severe secondary complications such as loss of toenails and auto-amputations of digits, tetanus, sepsis, lymphedema, and gangrene [51]. The neglect is such that health-seeking behaviour amongst severely affected patients remains poor as it is considered a nuisance rather a serious infection, as well as associated stigma. There has not been any thorough investigation of the ecology associated with the ectoparasite, nor till very recently, a systematic review of its complications and treatment modalities. The treatment recommended by WHO in endemic areas is surgical removal of fleas, which unfortunately is frequently done using unsafe practices in resource-poor communities, further leading to bacterial superinfections and possible transmission of pathogens like HIV, Hepatitis B, or Hepatitis C [52].

16.2.4 Neglected Tropical Diseases

Neglected tropical diseases (NTDs) are enlisted by the WHO as 20 communicable diseases that affect more than 1.5 billion people in the rural poor and remote communities, with devastating health, social, and economic impact. For effective and efficient control, the WHO recommends that affected countries implement integrated control interventions that take into account the different co-endemic NTDs in the same community.

Skin NTDs are diseases that present with lesions on the skin surface which may, in turn, provide not only practical clues to the diagnosis but also a greater understanding of disease through investigations. The skin NTDs include Buruli ulcer, cutaneous leishmaniasis, post-kala-azar dermal leishmaniasis, leprosy, lymphatic filariasis (lymphoedema and hydrocele), mycetoma, onchocerciasis, scabies, yaws, and fungal diseases.

The majority of these diseases have decreased in prevalence in the past decade, with the biggest declines for dracunculiasis (Guinea worm) (decreased 99%) and African trypanosomiasis (decreased 72.5%). In contrast, the prevalence of dengue (up 74.7%) and cutaneous leishmaniasis (up 28.6%) increased during the past decade [53]. According to the WHO, *cutaneous leishmaniasis* is the most common form of leishmaniasis (the others being mucocutaneous leishmaniasis and visceral leishmaniasis) (Fig. 16.8). It presents mainly as ulcers or crusted plaques on the exposed sites of the body, which resolve themselves with scars and are associated with serious disability and stigma. About 95% of cutaneous leishmaniasis cases occur in the Americas, the Mediterranean basin, the Middle East, and Central Asia [54]. Mucocutaneous leishmaniasis, meanwhile, leads to partial or total destruction of mucous membranes of the nose, mouth, and throat. Over 90% of mucocutaneous leishmaniasis cases occur in Bolivia, Brazil, Ethiopia, and Peru. India forms a large part of the burden of visceral leishmaniasis, comprising, along with Bangladesh and Sudan, of 90% of total cases worldwide [54]. This also marks the regions where post kala-azar dermal leishmaniasis (PKDL) is found. PKDL usually appears 6 months to one or more years after apparent cure of VL, but it may occur earlier or even concurrently with VL, especially in Sudan. PKDL heals spontaneously in most cases in Africa but rarely in patients in India.

Phlebotomus spp., the main vector of the causative agent of leishmaniasis, occurs predominantly in warm, humid, tropical climates, and semi-desert vegetation

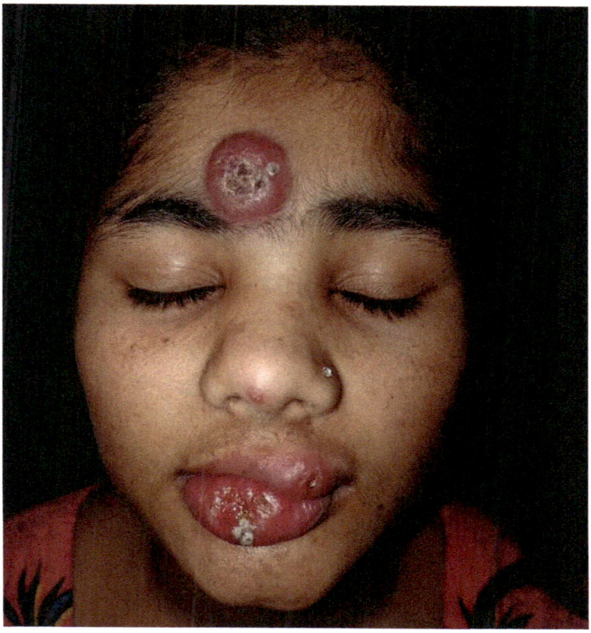

Fig. 16.8 *Cutaneous leishmaniasis*: Crusted erythematous, edematous plaques on the face in a young girl from Nepal

habitats, although a few species occur in temperate zones. They are able to colonize rural, peri-urban, and urban areas. The general conditions that favour transmission of leishmaniasis are rural areas that are less than 600 m above sea level; a heavy annual rainfall; a mean humidity above 70%; a maximum temperature of 38 °C and a minimum temperature of 15 °C, with a diurnal variation of less than 7 °C; and abundant vegetation and subsoil water [55]. Leishmaniasis occurs in agricultural villages where houses are constructed with mud walls and earthen floors, and cattle and other livestock are kept close to humans. Human behaviour, such as sleeping outside or on the ground, which is prevalent culturally (and economically!) in many of these countries, may increase the risk of infection. Risk factors for visceral leishmaniasis include living in the same household as someone who has an active case of the disease or of PKDL and poverty-related factors, such as poor nutrition and housing conditions. Apart from this, travel of both skilled and unskilled workers from endemic areas in the Middle East and the growing global warming and climate change may be a reason for infection in non-endemic regions.

Although considerable progress has been made in the development of safe, effective, and easily administered therapeutic agents, most patients still have little or no access to care. Cutaneous leishmaniasis is often not easily recognized in the peripheral healthcare setup; and even if it is, the existing drugs that are safe and convenient for treatment are simply unavailable in the government supply or in the commercial market. The latter is caused by a lack of coordination, willingness, and interest of pharmaceutical manufacturers and the international community, despite considerable advocation by WHO and NGOs [56]. Most drugs for leishmaniasis are produced by only a single manufacturer. These manufacturers require yearly forecasts of needs to avoid irregular production, shortage, or over-production and subsequent destruction of drugs, which would cause them financial damage. Such forecasts need to be made in a collaboration between manufacturers, countries, WHO and NGOs. Buffer stocks should be supported to aid control measures. Moreover, drug quality is an issue; with counterfeit miltefosine distributed in control programmes in Bangladesh, and in several instances, antimonial drugs of inferior quality leading to unacceptable toxicity and death in India and South America. Drug affordability is another issue to be tackled.

The story of *leprosy* spans many decades, drug regimens, and programmes, and much has been written about it. The introduction of dapsone therapy in the late 1940s was the first effective treatment for leprosy, and this was followed by the move to short course multidrug therapy (MDT) in 1981. The World Health Assembly Resolution in 1991 to 'eliminate leprosy as a public health problem by 2000' galvanized extraordinary international support including that by WHO, national governments and organizations like the Nippon Foundation, Novartis and the International Federation of Anti-Leprosy Organizations (ILEP). This led to a fall in the point prevalence of patients registered for treatment of leprosy by over 90% to less than 1 in 10,000 at the global level, fulfilling the definition of elimination [57]. Since then, the focus has moved from prevalence of leprosy to incidence as measured by reported new case detection, to sustain the achievements and to reduce the burden of disease; particularly reduction and prevention of disability associated with leprosy, and rehabilitation of those facing the long-term consequences of the disease. However, there has been a reduction in planned case detection, that has allowed the numbers of new cases to stabilize and, in some areas, to increase. Several countries such as India and Brazil are still reporting substantial case numbers.

Mycetoma is an implantation subcutaneous mycosis, characterized by a triad of tumefaction (swelling), sinus, and grain discharge (Fig. 16.9). It usually occurs within 15° south to 30° north of the equator including Mexico, Senegal, Sudan, and India, where the climate is appropriate for the germination and growth of fungi. It can be caused by diverse microorganisms, both of filamentous bacterial (actinomycetoma) and fungal origin (eumycetoma). The most common causative

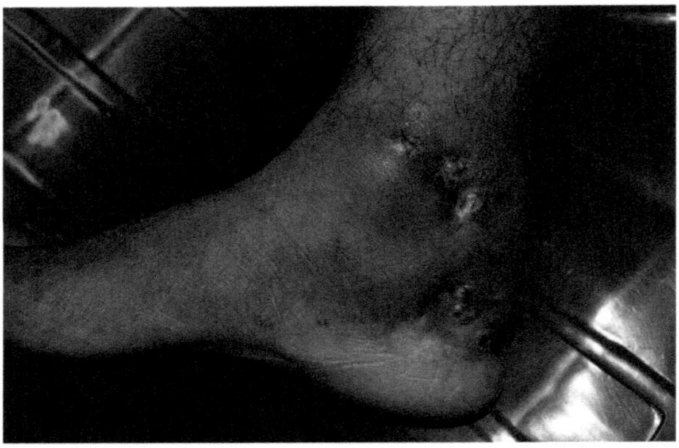

Fig. 16.9 *Mycetoma on the foot*: Showing a diffuse swelling studded with numerous sinuses (Credits: Dr. Akash P. Mustari)

agents include the fungus *Madurella mycetomatis* and the actinomycetes *Nocardia brasiliensis, Actinomadura madurae, Streptomyces somaliensis*, and *Actinomadura pelletieri*. More males than females are affected, and it commonly occurs in field labourers and cultivators whose occupation involves direct contact with the soil, but its true prevalence and incidence are not well defined. Studies range from 3.49 cases per 100,000 inhabitants in Mauritania to <0.01 cases per 100,000 inhabitants in many other countries [58]. Meanwhile, a field survey from West Nile State of Sudan, a country uniquely believed to be the most endemic in the world, yielded a prevalence of 14.5/1000 population in 2010. If not detected and managed early, it results in gruesome deformity of the limbs, severe disability, premature termination of occupation, difficulty in finding jobs and partners among young adults, and accelerates the rate of dropouts from school in children [59].

A variety of other 'exotic' fungal infections, including subcutaneous and systemic mycoses may be encountered in the tropics, and it is paramount that the diseases be recognized or at least thought of clinically. Mycoses with subcutaneous involvement include mycetomas, lobomycosis, chromoblastomycosis, entomophthoromycosis, and sporotrichosis. Geographically restricted mycoses with systemic dissemination are illustrated by paracoccidioidomycosis. Other systemic mycoses, such as histoplasmosis and cryptococcosis, are not restricted to tropical areas and affect patients all over the world [60].

Sporothrix spp. live in vegetation, plants, or plant debris in the soil, and therefore infections are more common in agricultural workers and people working in open areas. Sporotrichosis is considered an occupational disease in forest wardens, gardeners or people who work in farms. Patients affected with chromoblastomycosis often give history of a traumatic injury involving wood or vegetation, and over 80% are rural workers in Africa, Asia, and South America who tend to walk barefoot [61]. *Lacazia loboi,* the causative agent of lobomycosis; also has a similar mode of entry. Entomophthoromycosis is one of the least recognized fungal infections, characterized by the appearance of a hard, progressive mass that affects the subcutaneous tissues (Fig. 16.10). It is low endemic in southern India. There are two variants. The first is caused by *Basidiobolus ranarum*, occurs around the pelvic girdle and buttocks and is more common in children. The second variant is caused by *Conidiobolus coronatus* and affects the face of adults, causing an indurated swelling and severe deformation of the nose, lips, and cheeks. These infections may occur in immunocompetent patients. Fungi are still underappreciated as major pathogens by both the public and public health officials, while diseases caused by protozoa, bacteria, and viruses have been recognized as important public health issues for centuries. A shift has been brought about by an increase in the number of immunosuppressed individuals; by virtue of diseases like HIV and diabetes mellitus and iatrogenic during treatment of other diseases.

Lymphatic filariasis, commonly known as elephantiasis, occurs when filarial parasites are transmitted to humans through mosquitoes (Fig. 16.11). Infection is usually acquired in childhood causing covert damage to the lymphatic system 63% of the population at risk of lymphatic filariasis and 50% of the people infected worldwide live in Southeast Asia. India alone harbours 40% of the world's burden

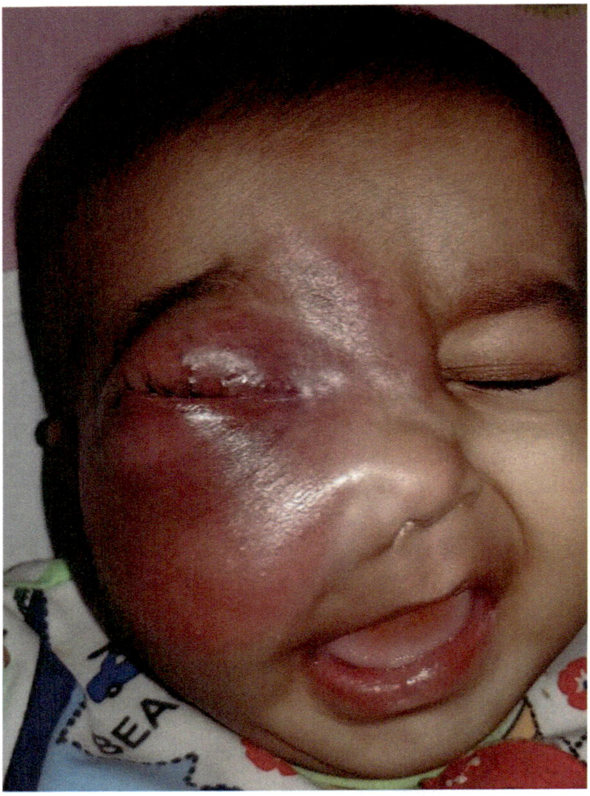

Fig. 16.10 *Entomophthoromycosis*: Woody hard indurated plaque over the face in a young child, causing significant facial deformity

of disease [62]. The WHO-recommended preventive chemotherapy strategy for lymphatic filariasis elimination is mass drug administration (MDA); the composition of which (albendazole/ivermectin/diethylcarbamazine) depends on the co-endemicity with other filarial diseases, predominantly onchocerciasis. Morbidity management and vector control are important supplementary activities. Onchocerciasis predominantly affects the eyes ('river blindness'), but also causes a wide range of cutaneous manifestations including acute papular onchodermatitis, lichenified onchodermatitis, onchocercal atrophy, and the classical 'leopard skin' representing onchocercal depigmentation. Skin snips are used for diagnosis.

The endemic treponematoses, which comprise yaws, endemic syphilis (bejel), and pinta, are a group of chronic bacterial infections caused by *Treponema pallidum pertenue*, *Treponema pallidum endemicum*, and *Treponema pallidum carateum* respectively. Yaws, the most common, presents with papillomas and ulcers in children aged less than 15 years, with sometimes disfiguring lesions of the skin, cartilage, face, soft tissue of the mouth, and bones. It is found primarily in poor rural

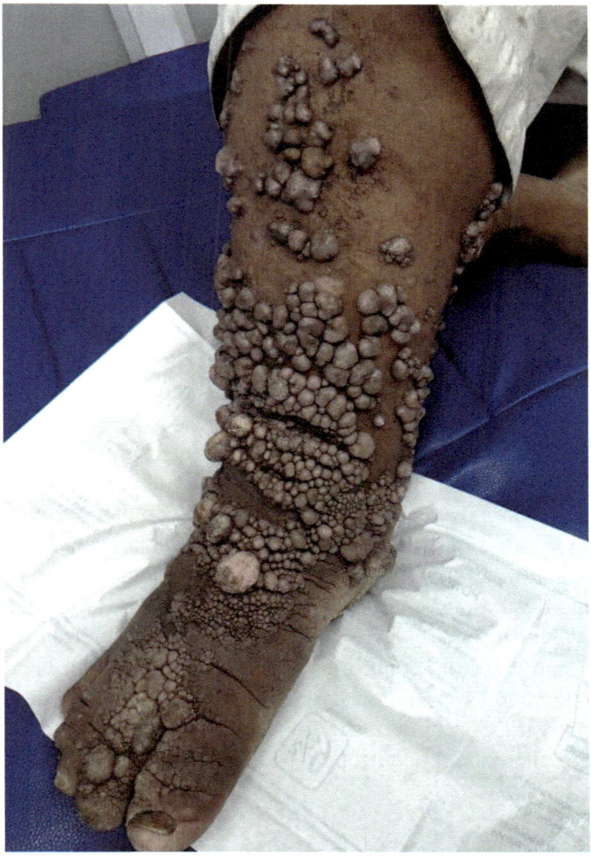

Fig. 16.11 Elephantiasis verrucose nostras developing on post-filarial lymphedema limb

communities in warm, humid, and tropical forest areas of Africa, Asia, Latin America, and the Pacific and is now targeted for eradication. Meanwhile, no disability or complication occurs with pinta; hypopigmented skin is the only main residual effect of the disease.

16.3 Others

Beyond infections, there are some peculiar occurrences in the tropics such as the development of contact irritant lymphedema to red clay soil, known as *podoconiosis,* largely preventable simply by wearing protective footwear, maintaining foot hygiene, and covering housing floors. Most of the epidemiological studies have been in Africa, touting around four million cases [63]. There is no single diagnostic test and it remains largely clinical; to be differentiated from other important forms of lymphedema including filariasis. Although high prevalence of podoconiosis has been reported intermittently across a range of settings, it has never been prioritized either in intervention or research programmes.

Endemic pemphigus foliaceous {*fogo selvagem* (FS)}, which means 'wildfire' in the Portuguese language), though synonymous with Brazil, also occurs in other South American countries. It has a higher occurrence in children and young adults and occurs in rural areas with familial cases. Intimately related to the tropical forest, it is an autoimmune bullous disease that occurs due to the production of autoantibodies to the protein antigen LJM11 of the salivary glands of the phlebotomine or sandfly (*Lutzomyia longipalpis*) followed by conformational molecular mimicry to Desmoglein 1.

The equatorial and tropical zones are subject to greater UV-B radiation because light travels a lesser distance through the atmosphere at these latitudes. Photodermatoses are among the most common skin disorders in tropical countries. Some important skin diseases caused or aggravated by sun exposure in these regions include actinic prurigo (most of afflicted patients live in tropical Latin America), phytophotodermatitis (a common occupational and recreational disease), and pellagra (largely a nutritional disease exacerbated by photo-exposure and still a common cause of disease in underdeveloped tropical countries) [64]. Polymorphic light eruption, especially the pinpoint and papular variants as well as actinic lichen planus are more common in people with a dark skin [65].

Nutritional disorders, per se, are also common in the tropics, with poverty being a major factor. Conditions typical of both protein-energy malnutrition and vitamin deficiencies are commonly seen, often present concurrently. Flaky paint dermatosis, pellagra, phrynoderma, acrodermatitis enteropathica, cheilitis, and magenta tongue are of frequent occurrence [66].

16.3.1 Tropical Skin Diseases beyond the Tropics

Because of modern travel and migration patterns, tropical diseases are now seen throughout the world. An entire segment of medicine now deals with diseases in travellers returning from the tropics, in migrants, and the military, as recognition of these cases needs to be emphasized in a medical community not used to seeing them. In an international study concerning 17,353 returning travellers, dermatologic disorders were the third most common cause of health problems after systemic febrile illness and acute diarrhoea. The most common causes of dermatologic problems were insect bites (with or without secondary infection), cutaneous larva migrans, allergic reactions, and skin abscesses [67]. Many of the earliest descriptions of tropical diseases have, in fact, been through military medicine.

To conclude, skin diseases in the tropics are caused and perpetuated by a multitude of intertwined factors, and it is no surprise that it begets a branch unto itself as tropical medicine. These biodiverse and culturally rich areas, which show the highest burden of preventable and controllable diseases and the extremes of poverty, also offer the most heart-warming results when simple health measures are implemented and political initiative taken. WHO has now developed an NTD road map for

2021-2030, '*Ending the neglect to attain the Sustainable Development Goals*.' The road map sets global targets and milestones to prevent, control, eliminate, or eradicate the 20 neglected tropical diseases and disease groups, as well as overarching and cross-cutting targets aligned with the Sustainable Development Goals. Apart from international aid, the tropics must prioritize health care—a health care of their own, which needs to rise above Western models and embrace its communities in all their glory.

References

1. Arenas R. Estrada R. Landes Bioscience: Tropical dermatology; 2001.
2. Beck H. Tropical ecology. In: Encyclopedia of ecology; 2018. p. 671–8.
3. Sachs JD. Tropical underdevelopment; 2001.
4. Kamarck AM. Climate and economic development: is the location of many developing countries in the tropics a cause of their poverty? Fin Dev. 1973;0010:50.
5. Gallup JL, Sachs JD. Agriculture, climate, and technology: why are the tropics falling behind? Am J Agric Econ. 2000;82(3):731–7. https://doi.org/10.1111/0002-9092.00071.
6. Harding S, Mccomiskie R, Wolff M, Trewin D, Hunter S, Edelman A, et al. State of the tropics [2014 report]; 2014.
7. Chakrabarti P. Medicine and empire. Macmillan Education: UK; 2014.
8. Editorial. Tropical medicine: a brittle tool of the new imperialism. Lancet. 2004;363(9415):1087. https://doi.org/10.1016/S0140-6736(04)15928-X.
9. Ryan TJ. A brief history of tropical dermatology. Clin Dermatol. 2009;27(3):248–51. https://doi.org/10.1016/j.clindermatol.2008.10.004.
10. Hotez PJ, Molyneux DH, Fenwick A, Kumaresan J, Sachs SE, Sachs JD, et al. Control of neglected tropical diseases. N Engl J Med. 2007;357(10):1018–27. https://doi.org/10.1056/NEJMra064142.
11. World Health Organization. Neglected tropical diseases. 2021.
12. Harding S, Penny A, Ann R, Templeman S, Mckenzie M, Toral DT, et al. State of the tropics [2020 report]; 2020.
13. Balato N, Megna M, Ayala F, Balato A, Napolitano M, Patruno C. Effects of climate changes on skin diseases. Expert Rev Anti-Infect Ther. 2014;12(2):171–81. https://doi.org/10.1586/14787210.2014.875855.
14. Gopinath H, Karthiga R, Karthikeyan K. A cross-sectional study of sweat-induced dermatitis during a south Indian summer: a glimpse of sweat gland-mediated cutaneous inflammation. Int J Dermatol. 2019;58(1):86–90. https://doi.org/10.1111/ijd.14088.
15. Youn SW, Na JI, Choi SY, Huh CH, Park KC. Regional and seasonal variations in facial sebum secretions: a proposal for the definition of combination skin type. Skin Res Technol. 2005;11(3):189–95. https://doi.org/10.1111/j.1600-0846.2005.00119.x.
16. Narang I, Sardana K, Bajpai R, Garg VK. Seasonal aggravation of acne in summers and the effect of temperature and humidity in a study in a tropical setting. J Cosmet Dermatol. 2019;18(4):1098–104. https://doi.org/10.1111/jocd.12777.
17. Lan J, Song Z, Miao X, Li H, Li Y, Dong L, et al. Skin damage among health care workers managing coronavirus disease-2019. J Am Acad Dermatol. 2020;82(5):1215–6. https://doi.org/10.1016/j.jaad.2020.03.014.
18. Singh M, Pawar M, Bothra A, Maheshwari A, Dubey V, Tiwari A, et al. Personal protective equipment induced facial dermatoses in healthcare workers managing coronavirus disease 2019. J Eur Acad Dermatol Venereol. 2020;34(8):e378–80. https://doi.org/10.1111/jdv.16628.
19. Uthayakumar AK, Panagou E, Manam S, Schauer A, Veraitch O, Walker S, et al. PPE-associated dermatoses: effect on work and wellbeing. Future Healthc J Vol. 2021;8(11):e67–9.

20. Weiland SK, Hüsing A, Strachan DP, Rzehak P, Pearce N, Phase I, et al. Climate and the prevalence of symptoms of asthma, allergic rhinitis, and atopic eczema in children. Occup Environ Med. 2004;61(7):609–15. https://doi.org/10.1136/oem.2002.006809.
21. Rogers J, Harding C, Mayo A, Banks J, Rawlings A. Stratum corneum lipids: the effect of ageing and the seasons. Arch Dermatol Res. 1996;288(12):765–70. https://doi.org/10.1007/BF02505294.
22. Flohr C, Yeo L. Atopic dermatitis and the hygiene hypothesis revisited. Curr Probl Dermatol. 2011;41:1–34. https://doi.org/10.1159/000323290.
23. Parisi R, Symmons DPM, Griffiths CEM, Ashcroft DM. Identification and Management of Psoriasis and Associated ComorbidiTy (IMPACT) project team. Global epidemiology of psoriasis: a systematic review of incidence and prevalence. J Invest Dermatol. 2013;133(2):377–85. https://doi.org/10.1038/jid.2012.339.
24. Jain S, Barambhe M, Jain J, Jajoo U, Pandey N. Prevalence of skin diseases in rural Central India: a community-based, cross-sectional, observational study. J Mahatma Gandhi Inst Med Sci. 2016;21(2):111. https://doi.org/10.4103/0971-9903.189537.
25. Sardana K, Mahajan S, Sarkar R, Mendiratta V, Bhushan P, Koranne RV, Garg VK. The spectrum of skin disease among Indian children. Pediatr Dermatol. 2009;26:6–13.
26. Mahell A, Prua A, Konatk M, Lobin P. Skin Dis Child Mali Public Health Problem. 1995;89:467–70.
27. Anand S, Fan V, WHO. The health workforce in India, WHO 16; 2001.
28. Prescott SL, Larcombe DL, Logan AC, West C, Burks W, Caraballo L, et al. The skin microbiome: impact of modern environments on skin ecology, barrier integrity, and systemic immune programming. World Allergy Organ J. 2017;10(1):29. https://doi.org/10.1186/s40413-017-0160-5.
29. Bibel DJ, LeBrun JR. Changes in cutaneous flora after wet occlusion. Can J Microbiol. 1975;21(4):496–500. https://doi.org/10.1139/m75-070.
30. Grice EA, Segre JA. The skin microbiome. Nat Rev Microbiol. 2011;9(4):244–53. https://doi.org/10.1038/nrmicro2537.
31. Gandhi S, Ojha AK, Ranjan KP, Neelima. Clinical and bacteriological aspects of pyoderma. N. Am J Med Sci. 2012;4(10):492–5. https://doi.org/10.4103/1947-2714.101997.
32. Sadhiqua V, Joe EA, Dhanasekaran A. Bacteriological profile of pyoderma in paediatric age group (0-12 years) attending dermatology OPD in a tertiary care hospital. J Clin Diagn Res. 2020;14:DC19–23.
33. World Health Organization. The current evidence for the burden of group a streptococcal diseases department of child and adolescent health and development. World health Organization; 2005.
34. Romani L, Koroivueta J, Steer AC, Kama M, Kaldor JM, Wand H, et al. Scabies and impetigo prevalence and risk factors in Fiji: a national survey. PLoS Negl Trop Dis. 2015;9(3):e0003452. https://doi.org/10.1371/journal.pntd.0003452.
35. Karim SA, Anwar KS, Khan MAH, Mollah MAH, Nahar N, Rahman HEMR, et al. Socio-demographic characteristics of children infested with scabies in densely populated communities of residential madrashas (Islamic education institutes) in Dhaka. Bangladesh Public Health. 2007;121(12):923–34. https://doi.org/10.1016/j.puhe.2006.10.019.
36. Karimkhani C, Colombara DV, Drucker AM, Norton SA, Hay R, Engelman D, et al. The global burden of scabies: a cross-sectional analysis from the global burden of disease study 2015. Lancet Infect Dis. 2017;17(12):1247–54. https://doi.org/10.1016/S1473-3099(17)30483-8.
37. Carapetis JR, Steer AC, Mulholland EK, Weber M. The global burden of group a streptococcal diseases. Lancet Infect Dis. 2005;5(11):685–94. https://doi.org/10.1016/S1473-3099(05)70267-X.
38. Coscione S, Kositz C, Marks MM. Head lice: an under-recognized tropical problem. Am J Trop Med Hyg. 2017;97(6):1636–7. https://doi.org/10.4269/ajtmh.17-0656.
39. WHO. Antimicrobial resistance: global report on surveillance; 2014.
40. Havlickova B, Czaika VA, Friedrich M. Epidemiological trends in skin mycoses worldwide. Mycoses. 2008;51(Suppl 4):2–15. https://doi.org/10.1111/j.1439-0507.2008.01606.x.

41. Naglot A, Shrimali DD, Nath BK, Gogoi HK, Veer V, Chander J, et al. Recent trends of dermatophytosis in Northeast India (Assam) and interpretation with published studies. Int J Curr Microbiol Appl Sci. 2015;4:111–20.
42. Rudramurthy SM, Shaw D. Clinical practice of medical mycology in Asia. 1st ed. Springer Nature Singapore Pte Ltd; 2021.
43. Bongomin F, Gago S, Oladele RO, Denning DW. Global and multi-national prevalence of fungal diseases-estimate precision. J Fungi (Basel). 2017;3(4):57. https://doi.org/10.3390/jof3040057.
44. Fernandes LF, Pimenta FC, Fernandes FF. First report of human myiasis in GoiáS state, Brazil: frequency of different types of myiasis, their various etiological agents, and associated factors. J Parasitol. 2009;95(1):32–8. https://doi.org/10.1645/GE-1103.1.
45. Prakash H, Chakrabarti A. Epidemiology of mucormycosis in India. Microorganisms. 2021;9(3):1–12. https://doi.org/10.3390/microorganisms9030523.
46. WHO. Tuberculosis fact sheet. 2021.
47. Khadka P, Koirala S, Thapaliya J. Cutaneous tuberculosis: clinicopathologic arrays and diagnostic challenges. Dermatol Res Pract. 2018;2018:7201973. https://doi.org/10.1155/2018/7201973.
48. Mendiratta V. Tropical ulcer. In: Irvine AD, Hoeger PH, Yan AC, editors. Harper's textbook of paediatric dermatology. Blackwell Publishing Inc; 2011. p. 66.1–6.
49. Umphress B, Raparia K. Rhinoscleroma. Arch Pathol Lab Med. 2018;142(12):1533–6. https://doi.org/10.5858/arpa.2018-0073-RA.
50. Caumes E, Carrière J, Guermonprez G, Bricaire F, Danis M, Gentilini M. Dermatoses associated with travel to tropical countries: a prospective study of the diagnosis and management of 269 patients presenting to a tropical disease unit. Clin Infect Dis. 1995;20(3):542–8. https://doi.org/10.1093/clinids/20.3.542.
51. Heukelbach J, de Oliveira FA, Hesse G, Feldmeier H. Tungiasis: a neglected health problem of poor communities. Trop Med Int Health. 2001;6(4):267–72. https://doi.org/10.1046/j.1365-3156.2001.00716.x.
52. Abrha S, Heukelbach J, Peterson GM, Christenson JK, Carroll S, Kosari S, et al. Clinical interventions for tungiasis (sand flea disease): a systematic review. Lancet Infect Dis. 2021;21(8):e234–45. https://doi.org/10.1016/S1473-3099(20)30853-7.
53. Reed SL, McKerrow JH. Why funding for neglected tropical diseases should be a global priority. Clin Infect Dis. 2018;67(3):323–6. https://doi.org/10.1093/cid/ciy349.
54. WHO. Leishmaniasis. 2021.
55. Rather S, Wani M, Shah FY, Bashir S, Yaseen A, Giri FA, et al. Clinical and epidemiological study of cutaneous leishmaniasis in two tertiary care hospitals of Jammu and Kashmir: an emerging disease in North India. Int J Infect Dis. 2021;103:138–45. https://doi.org/10.1016/j.ijid.2020.11.002.
56. Den Boer M, Argaw D, Jannin J, Alvar J. Leishmaniasis impact and treatment access. Clin Microbiol Infect. 2011;17(10):1471–7. https://doi.org/10.1111/j.1469-0691.2011.03635.x.
57. Smith WC, van Brakel W, Gillis T, Saunderson P, Richardus JH. The missing millions: a threat to the elimination of leprosy. PLoS Negl Trop Dis. 2015;9(4):e0003658. https://doi.org/10.1371/journal.pntd.0003658.
58. van de Sande WWJ, Maghoub ES, Fahal AH, Goodfellow M, Welsh O, Zijlstra E. The mycetoma knowledge gap: identification of research priorities. PLoS Negl Trop Dis. 2014;8(3):e2667. https://doi.org/10.1371/journal.pntd.0002667.
59. Zijlstra EE, van de Sande WWJ, Welsh O, Mahgoub ES, Goodfellow M, Fahal AH. Mycetoma: a unique neglected tropical disease. Lancet Infect Dis. 2016;16(1):100–12. https://doi.org/10.1016/S1473-3099(15)00359-X.
60. Lupi O, Tyring SK, McGinnis MR. Tropical dermatology: fungal tropical diseases. J Am Acad Dermatol. 2005;53(6):931–51. https://doi.org/10.1016/j.jaad.2004.10.883.
61. Carrasco-Zuber JE, Navarrete-Dechent C, Bonifaz A, Fich F, Vial-Letelier V, Berroeta-Mauriziano D. Cutaneous involvement in the deep mycoses: a literature review. Part I—sub-

cutaneous mycoses. Actas Dermo Sifiliogr. 2016;107(10):806–15. https://doi.org/10.1016/j.ad.2016.05.017.
62. Specht S, Suma TK, Pedrique B, Hoerauf A. Neglected tropical diseases in South Asia: elimination of lymphatic filariasis in South East Asia. BMJ. 2019;364:k5198.
63. Deribe K, Cano J, Trueba ML, Newport MJ, Davey G. Global epidemiology of podoconiosis: a systematic review. PLoS Negl Trop Dis. 2018;12(3):e0006324. https://doi.org/10.1371/journal.pntd.0006324.
64. Domínguez L, Domínguez-Soto D, Maria Y, Hojyo-Tomoka T, Vega-Memije E, Cortés YR, et al. Photodermatoses in tropical countries; 1999.
65. Sharma VK, Sahni K, Wadhwani AR. Photodermatoses in pigmented skin. Photochem Photobiol Sci. 2012;121(12):65–77.
66. Mercy OY. Nutritional dermatoses in Nigeria. Int J Dermatol. 1995;34:11–6.
67. Freedman DO, Weld LH, Kozarsky PE, Fisk T, Robins R, von Sonnenburg F, et al. Spectrum of disease and relation to place of exposure among ill returned travelers. N Engl J Med. 2006;354(2):119–30. https://doi.org/10.1056/NEJMoa051331.

JAK-STAT Targeted Therapy for Autoimmune Diseases

17

Derek Ochi, Karmtej Singh Cheema,
Smriti K. Raychaudhuri, and Siba P. Raychaudhuri

Psoriatic disease was the first cutaneous condition for which JAK-STAT-directed therapies were investigated, along with its associated conditions, the spondyloarthropathies (SpA). The spondyloarthropathies are a heterogenous group of immune-mediated inflammatory conditions. The presentation of each of these autoimmune diseases varies depending on genetic predisposition, associated inflammatory cytokines, clinical features, spinal inflammation, radiological features, and comorbidities. Recent evidence suggests that the cytokine-induced JAK signaling system is important in the pathogenesis of an array of autoimmune diseases. Here we discuss the evidence for JAK cell signaling in the inflammatory and proliferative cascades of autoimmune diseases and opportunities for therapeutic intervention through inhibition of this pathway [1, 2]. Inflammation where ligaments and tendons are inserted on the bone surface is termed enthesitis. Enthesitis has long been considered a key event in the pathogenesis of spondyloarthropathy. However, increasing use of molecular imaging suggests that in addition to enthesitis, spondyloarthropathies are

D. Ochi · K. S. Cheema
School of Medicine, University of California, Davis, CA, USA
e-mail: dochi@ucdavis.edu; kasch@ucdavis.edu

S. K. Raychaudhuri
School of Medicine, University of California, Davis, CA, USA

Department of Veterans Affairs, VA Sacramento Medical Center, Northern California Health Care System, Mather, CA, USA

S. P. Raychaudhuri (✉)
School of Medicine, University of California, Davis, CA, USA

Department of Veterans Affairs, VA Sacramento Medical Center, Northern California Health Care System, Mather, CA, USA

Division of Rheumatology, Allergy and Clinical Immunology, Department of Medicine, Stanford University, Davis, CA, USA
e-mail: SRAYCHAUDHURI@UCADVIS.EDU

S. Gupta et al. (eds.), *Critical Thinking in Contemporary Dermatology: Cognitive Essays*, https://doi.org/10.1007/978-981-97-0411-8_17

characterized by more widespread inflammation that often spreads to adjacent soft tissue and bone [3].

It is hypothesized that enthesitis develops as a result of biomechanical stress and friction that results in chronic microscopic injury which in turn promotes inflammation and angiogenesis. This results in the homing of pathologic inflammatory cells that induce enthesitis and inflammation of the adjacent bone and synovium [1, 3]. Additional research is required to further elucidate how localized inflammation from mechanical stress results in a dysregulated systemic immune response.

Many times, connective tissue inflammation is the result of coordinated interactions between antigen-presenting cells and T-cell phenotypes [1, 2, 4, 5]. Activated T cells upregulate local inflammatory response and tissue damage through the release of inflammatory cytokines and activation of inflammatory cells with innate functions such as macrophages and neutrophils [1, 6–8]. It is also well known that cytokines released by T cells promote the development, differentiation, and regulation of both cellular and humoral adaptive immunity.

The JAK/STAT pathway is a mechanism for extracellular cytokines and growth factors to alter gene transcription. First, cytokines act on cell-surface receptors to induce conformational changes. Next, cytoplasmic kinase proteins are phosphorylated, resulting in STAT dimerization which promotes activation of the transcription factors and thus induction of signal transduction events (Fig. 17.1). A family of intracellular tyrosine kinases known as Janus kinases (JAKs) are involved with the signaling process of multiple cytokines associated with induction of inflammation (Fig. 17.2) [9, 10]. Because of the varied role of JAKs in the potentiation of pro-inflammatory signals, a new field has emerged to understand the role of JAKs in the pathogenesis of autoimmune disease and opportunities for therapeutic modulation of this pathway [1, 2, 10–12]. In this chapter, we will explore the functional significance of the JAK-STAT kinase cascades in the inflammatory-proliferative processes associated with autoimmune diseases. Our primary focus will be on its role in the pathogenesis of psoriatic diseases, encompassing conditions like spondyloarthritis (SpA) and various other autoimmune skin diseases. Additionally, we will delve into the potential application of oral synthetic JAK-STAT kinase inhibitors in addressing these conditions.

The Janus Kinase family comprises four members: JAK1, JAK2, JAK3, and tyrosine kinase 2 (TYK2). Simultaneously, the STAT family consists of seven members: STAT 1, STAT 2, STAT 3, STAT 4, STAT 5, STAT5a, and STAT6 [1, 9, 10]. The JAKs are associated with the intracellular domain of cytokine receptor subunits of class I and class II receptor superfamily. Various cytokines with an array of functions bind to type I and II receptors such as interferon (IFN)-like cytokines, IFNs, various growth factors/hormones and colony-stimulating factors (Fig. 17.2) [13].

The JAK-STAT pathway is one of the major cellular signaling pathways and is associated with cytokines that impact growth, apoptosis, as well as activation of T and B-lymphocytes, which suggests that it has an important role in the pathogenesis of autoimmune diseases (Fig. 17.2) [1, 9, 13–15].TYK2 and JAKs are recruited by multiple cytokines (Fig. 17.2), which in turn modulate T cells differentiation,

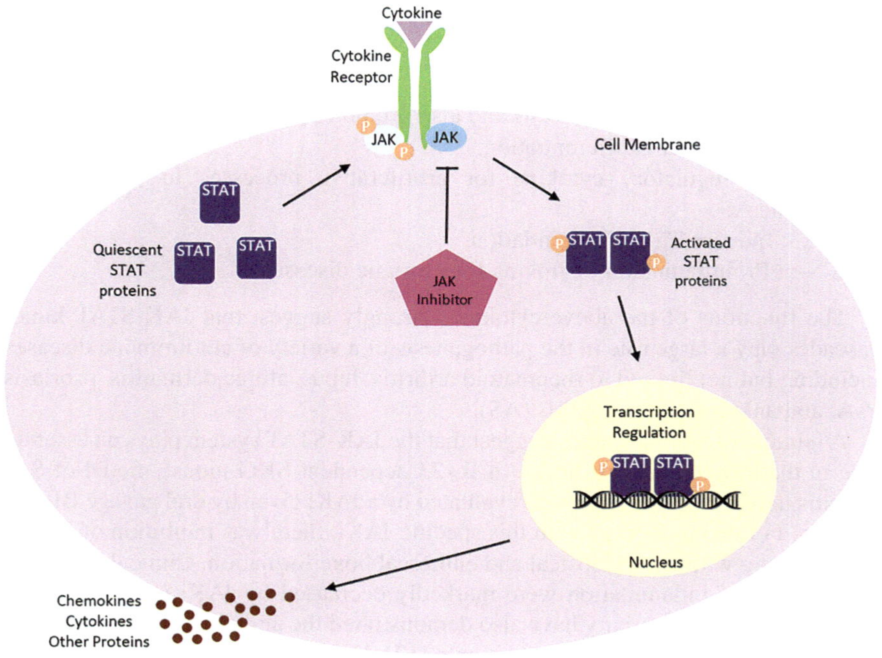

Fig. 17.1 Binding of cytokine and growth factors initiate JAK/STAT signaling transduction and immune-mediated inflammation. Binding of a cytokine to its receptor results in (1) conformational changes of the intracellular domain and (2) phosphorylation of the JAK proteins, (3) which helps to recruit the STATs via their SH2 domains (4) that leads to phosphorylation and dimerization of the STAT protein. The activated STAT homo/hetero dimers migrate to the nucleus and bind to specific DNA-binding sites and participate in gene transcriptions for an array of cytokines, chemokines, and growth factors which are required for the inflammatory and proliferative cascades of inflammatory diseases

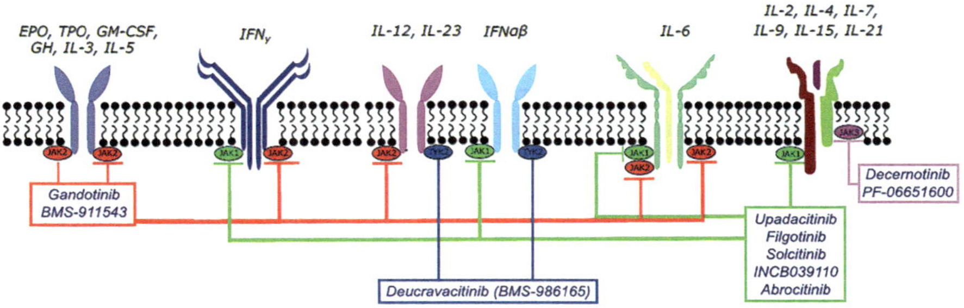

Fig. 17.2 This figure describes JAK-STAT signaling induction by the biologic agents that bind to type I and type II receptors such as interferons, interleukins, interferon-like cytokines, hormones, growth factors, and colony-stimulating factors and mechanisms of actions of new-generation JAK inhibitors. Binding of specific type I and type II cytokines to their representative receptor subunits results in activation of specific JAK pathways. It is important to notice that regulatory cytokines and growth factors associated in the pathogenesis of multiple autoimmune disease such as IL-2, IL-4, IL-6, IL-7, IL-9, IL-12, and IL-23 participate in JAK-STAT activation. Newer generation JAKi blocks a specific JAK molecule; here several new generation JAKi are mentioned along with their JAK targets

function, and cytokine release required for immune-mediated inflammation in autoimmune disease [4–10, 14, 15]:

- IL-2: A T cell growth factor.
- IL9: A growth factor for T cells and also promotes pannus formation.
- IL-12: Induces Th1 differentiation.
- IL-22: A regulatory cytokine for proliferative processes in psoriatic disease and AS.
- IL-23: Induces Th17 differentiation.
- IFN-γ: Proinflammatory cytokine for psoriatic disease.

The functions of the above cytokines strongly suggest that JAK-STAT kinase cascades play a large role in the pathogenesis of a variety of autoimmune diseases; including but not limited to rheumatoid arthritis, lupus, atopic dermatitis, psoriasis, PsA, and ankylosing spondylitis (AS).

A number of animal studies suggest that the JAK-STAT system plays an essential role in the development of SpA. An IL-23-dependent SKG mouse model of SpA arthritis induced with curdlan was evaluated by a JAKi given by oral gavage BID for 30 days. Following therapy with this specific JAKi, there was inhibition of inflammation along with less periosteal and entheseal bone formation. Clinical and histologic scores of inflammation were markedly decreased by JAKi ($p < 0.05$) [16]. JAKi of different selectivity have also demonstrated the ability to inhibit Th17 type responses in CD4+ T cells in AS patients [17]. Further, siRNA silencing of JAK1, JAK2, JAK3, and TYK2 in CD4+ T cells has been observed to result in a marked reduction of Th17 cytokines such as IL-17A, IL-17F, and IL-22 in CD4+ T cells [17].

Polymorphisms of the JAK-STAT kinases demonstrate the therapeutic potential of targeting specific proteins within the signaling pathway. Many single nucleotide polymorphisms (SNPs) associated with the TYK2 locus influence autoimmune diseases including AS. SNPs that reduce the function of TYK2 result in inhibition of inflammatory cytokine cell signaling without conferring immunodeficiency. Therefore, silencing of the TYK2 locus with novel therapeutics has the potential to confer protection without a significant rise in the rate of infections [18].

In an SKG mouse model of SpA, a specific TYK2 inhibitor (NDI-031407) has been reported to block disease progression supported by MRI imaging showing decreased joint space narrowing, bone marrow edema, and synovitis. The mechanism is likely through NDI-031407 medicated inhibition of TYK2 which is in turn thought to inhibit signaling of IL-23 19). In population studies, it has also been observed that the frequency of the loss-of-function TYK2 SNP (rs12720356) is inversely proportional to the rate of spinal fusion, suggesting that the presence of the loss-of-function TYK2 SNP is associated with less severe disease. Collectively, these data suggest that targeting TYK2 would likely be an effective therapeutic approach in the treatment for AS [19].

In addition to TYK2, there have been reports of JAK2 polymorphisms associated with ankylosing spondylitis (AS) [20]. Nucleotide polymorphisms within the JAK-STAT signaling system have also been observed in Crohn's disease [21], and STAT3 polymorphisms have been linked to psoriasis [22].

While JAK1, JAK2, and TYK2 exhibit ubiquitous expression in mammals, JAK3 is primarily expressed in hematopoietic/immune cells, associating specifically with the common γ-chain. Cytokines signaling through the common γ-chain, such as IL-2, IL-4, IL-7, IL-9, IL-15, and IL-21, play a crucial role in lymphocyte activation, proliferation, and differentiation. Tofacitinib, a small organic molecule, was initially designed to target JAK3 as a treatment for autoimmune arthritis, given its role in these cytokine pathways [23]. However, there are indications that tofacitinib also targets JAK1 and JAK2 with similar inhibitory concentration values to JAK3 [24].

The discovery that JAK1 and JAK2 are expressed not only in immune cells but also in non-immune cells, including joint synovial cells, has led to further exploration of potential cellular targets for JAK inhibitors. This includes regulating keratinocytes in psoriasis and synovial cells, specifically fibroblast-like synoviocytes (FLS), in conditions like psoriatic arthritis (PsA) and rheumatoid arthritis (RA) [25, 26].

Ex vivo studies focusing on PsA suggest that the JAK/STAT kinase pathway regulates pannus formation and the activation of Th17 cells in the synovium. In a co-culture study using synovial explants, tofacitinib demonstrated a reduction in JAK phosphoprotein expression in FLS, suggesting its inhibitory effect. In PsA explants, tofacitinib was found to inhibit JAK1/JAK2, thereby inhibiting FLS migration and the secretion of specific chemokines [27]. In PsA, the generation of the pathologic IL-17+ cells and their proliferation is regulated by IL23-induced JAK2/STAT3 signaling proteins, and tofacitinib inhibited IL-23-induced proliferation of these IL-17+ cells [28].

The development of numerous JAK inhibitors in recent years has progressed (Table 17.1), with the first-generation JAK inhibitors displaying pan-JAK activity, affecting three or all four members of the JAK family. The newer JAK inhibitors aim for increased selectivity against specific JAKs to minimize potential side effects.

First-generation JAKi act on multiple JAKs. They include ruxolitinib, tofacitinib, and baricitinib. Ruxolitinib is a JAK1 and JAK2 inhibitor, initially approved by the Food and Drug Administration (USA) for systemic use in the treatment of myelodysplastic syndrome and polycythemia vera [29]. More recently, it received FDA approval for chronic graft-versus-host disease and in its topical formation, for the treatment of mild to moderate atopic dermatitis [30]. To date, few studies have been done in SpA.

Tofacitinib stands as the pioneering JAK inhibitor (JAKi) approved for autoimmune disease treatment. It primarily inhibits JAK1/JAK3, displaying some activity against JAK2 and minimal activity towards TYK2 [31]. The therapeutic application of tofacitinib in spondyloarthritis (SpA) is discussed in the subsequent section. Another JAK inhibitor, Baricitinib, selectively targets JAK1/JAK2, and its efficacy in SpA is still under limited investigation [31].

The upcoming generation of JAK inhibitors is designed to selectively inhibit specific JAK pathways. While first-generation JAK inhibitors like tofacitinib have demonstrated clinical effectiveness in treating various autoimmune conditions such as rheumatoid arthritis (RA), psoriatic arthritis (PsA), and inflammatory bowel

Table 17.1 JAK-STAT inhibitors: The first-Generation and the next-generation JAK inhibitors (JAKi)

	JAK inhibitors	Target
First Generation (JAKi)	Baricitinib	JAK1/JAK2
	Ruxolitinib	JAK1/JAK2
	Tofacitinib	JAK1/JAK3
Next generation (JAKi)	Decernotinib (VX-509)	JAK3
	Upadacitinib (ABT494)	JAK1 > JAK2,JAK3
	Filgotinib GLPG0634	JAK1 > JAK2
	Peficitinib (ASP015K)	Pan-JAK
	Solcitinib (GSK2586184)	JAK1
	Deucravacitinib (BMS-986165)	TYK2
	Abrocitinib	JAK1
	INCB039110	JAK1 > JAK2
	STA-21	STAT3
	PF-06700841	TYK2/JAK1
	PF-06651600	JAK3
	PF-06263276	Pan-JAK

disease (IBD), their nonselective nature is associated with adverse effects. The development of next-generation JAK inhibitors with selective activity for a specific JAK aims to mitigate these adverse effects (Fig. 17.2, Table 17.1) [32]. In essence, these newer JAK inhibitors might be employed to address certain inflammatory disorders with lower doses and fewer adverse effects. Several biotechnology companies have succeeded in developing JAK inhibitors with the objective of creating molecules with high efficacy and minimal off-target effects (Table 17.1) [33].

Here we will discuss clinical trial data and indications of JAKi in systemic and cutaneous autoimmune diseases.

As previously mentioned, the JAK/STAT pathway plays a role in cytokine signaling in Psoriatic Arthritis (PsA), likely through the IL-23 and IL-17 cytokine axis [1, 28]. In a phase III trial, it was seen that tofacitinib, administered at doses of 5 mg or 10 mg twice daily to patients with PsA who may have had prior DMARD use, effectively alleviated the clinical burden of the disease across various domains. These include the reduction of arthritis, enthesitis, and dactylitis. The trial employed a double-blind, placebo-controlled design, with an active control arm treated with adalimumab. At the 3-month mark, the American College of Rheumatology 20% improvement criteria (ACR20) response rates were 30% in the placebo group, 50% in the 5 mg tofacitinib group, and 61% in the 10 mg tofacitinib group (significant difference compared to placebo for both the doses). The ACR20 response rate in the adalimumab group was 52%. However, by the 12-month follow-up, both the 5 mg and the 10 mg arms of the tofacitinib trial exhibited ACR20 response rates around 60% [34]. Recently published phase IV analysis provides efficacy data for 36 months and safety data for up to 48 months, representing the longest follow-up period for tofacitinib in active psoriatic arthritis. Rates of adverse events were similar to phase II analysis, suggesting that risk did not accumulate over time [35]. A phase-III trial demonstrated significant efficacy of upadacitinib in PsA. The primary endpoint was Assessment of Spondyloarthritis International Society 20% improvement (ASAS20) response rate at week 12 compared to placebo. ASAS20 response with upadacitinib 15 mg daily was 60% compared to 36% among the placebo group [36]. Previously FDA-approved for the treatment of rheumatoid arthritis, upadacitinib received FDA approval for the treatment of psoriatic arthritis in December of 2021 [37]. A phase II clinical trial of filgotinib has reported that at the 16th week 80% (52/65) achieved an ACR20 response in the filgotinib group compared to 33% (22/66) in the placebo group [38].

In Ankylosing spondylitis, a phase 2 trial demonstrated significant improvement in ASAS20 scores among patients randomized to receive tofacitinib 5 mg twice daily, at week 12. This trial examined three tofacitinib doses (2 mg, 5 mg, and 10 mg twice daily); however, improvement in patients receiving 2 mg and 10 mg was not significant compared to placebo [39]. The follow-up phase 3 study also showed encouraging results, with patients on 5 mg twice daily tofacitinib showing an ASAS20 response in 56.4% and ASAS 40% response in 40.6%, compared to 29.4% and 12.5% respectively, in the placebo group at 16 weeks follow-up period [40]. In December of 2021, Tofacitinib received FDA approval for the treatment of ankylosing spondylitis [41]. A phase-II placebo-controlled study of filgotinib demonstrated improved disease control compared to placebo after 4-8 weeks of therapy. In this 12-week study, filgotinib 200 mg once daily was noted to improve AS Disease Activity Score (ASDAS) in 33% of participants compared to 2% in the placebo group [42]. A follow-up analysis of this trial found a significant reduction in MRI-detected inflammation in ribs, transverse processes, spinous processes, soft-tissue inflammation, and postero-lateral vertebral body. As expected, given the short duration of the study, no difference was detected in erosions, and longer duration future studies are needed [43]. In a phase 2/3 trial, ASAS 40% response was seen in 52% NSAID-refractory patients on 15 mg daily upadacitinib compared to 26% patients on placebo after 14 weeks [44]. Even the secondary outcomes such as MRI-based assessment of sacroiliac joint inflammation were superior in the upadacitinib group [44].

Inflammatory bowel diseases is another group where JAK inhibitors have been found to be effective. Tofacitinib is FDA-approved for ulcerative colitis (UC), to be used when adult patients have failed a conventional or biologic agent therapy. Here, a dose of 10 m twice daily, higher than that used in PsA and RA is required [45]. A phase 2 trial examining the use of peficitinib in UC failed to demonstrate a dose response; however, a numerically greater number of patients receiving peficitinib therapy experienced clinical improvement and reduction in inflammatory markers [46]. Upadacitinib was found to induce remission as rapidly as within 2 weeks and demonstrate sustained clinical and endoscopic evidence of remission for the duration of the 52 week study [47]. In March 2022, upadacitinib received FDA approval for the treatment of ulcerative colitis.

No JAKi is currently approved for the treatment of Crohn's disease; however, upadacitinib is emerging as the front runner. A second phase 3 trial demonstrated a significant increase in clinical and endoscopic remission compared to placebo at week 12 [48]. In addition, filgoitinib may also be a promising candidate [49, 50].

Various JAK inhibitors (JAKi) and TYK2 inhibitors have undergone assessment for psoriasis treatment. Both tofacitinib and baricitinib have demonstrated clinical effectiveness, evidenced by a Psoriasis Area and Severity Index Improvement of 75% (PASI75) response, surpassing the placebo [51, 52]. The TYK2 inhibitor BMS-986165 has shown significant promise in treating psoriasis, achieving a PASI75 response rate of approximately 75% [53]. Ongoing trials with other JAK/STAT inhibitors are in progress, and it is anticipated that JAK/STAT inhibitors will emerge as a novel treatment option for psoriasis.

They are also potentially useful for atopic dermatitis, a chronic inflammatory skin disorder often associated with immense physical and mental patient burden. New topical JAK inhibitors such as ruxolitinib (JAK1/2 inhibitor) and delgocitinib (pan-JAK inhibitor) have provided a good option for the treatment of AD [54, 55].

The cream formulation of Ruxolitinib has met all primary and secondary endpoints in phase 3 clinical trials for mild-to-moderate AD with few adverse events and received FDA approval for treatment of AD in September 2021 [30]. Delgocitinib in the ointment formulation has been recently approved in Japan for pediatric and adult AD [55]. These topical preparations have demonstrated efficacy in the short-term management of AD and long-term safety data will be available with time. Several oral JAK inhibitors such as baricitinib (JAK1/2 inhibitor), abrocitinib (JAK1-selective), and upadacitinib (JAK1-selective) have shown clinical efficacy in AD [56–59]. All of these 3 drugs have met primary and secondary endpoints in multiple clinical trials.

JAK inhibitors also appear to induce hair growth in alopecia areata (AA). Though there are reports suggesting that topical formulations of tofacitinib and ruxolitinib are beneficial for AA [60], these agents are not currently approved for AA. Regrowth of hair in AA during treatment with tofacitinib has also been documented [61]. In addition to AD and AA, JAK inhibitors hold significant potential for a variety of dermatological conditions including but not limited to vitiligo and the dermatologic manifestations of lupus [62, 63].

An in-depth analysis of the safety profile of JAKi is not the purpose of this review; however, it is worth noting that the majority of pre-authorization clinical trials and subsequent meta-analyses suggest the overall rate of serious infections caused by FDA-approved JAKis is similar to conventional synthetic disease-modifying anti-rheumatic drugs (csDMARDS) and other bDMARD therapies, though post-authorization reports and comparison with TNFα-inhibitors have noted increased rates of certain adverse events as discussed below. Rates of serious infections among patients treated with JAKi have been found to be similar to that among patients treated with csDMARDs and bDMARDs from other classes, about 2.5 to 3.8 per 100 patient-years [64–68]. However, studies have consistently noted a greater risk of herpes zoster infection with tofacitinib, compared to bDMARDs from other classes; though herpes zoster in cases on tofacitinib is usually mild and limited to a single dermatome [69, 70].

In numerous pre-authorization clinical trials and long-term extension studies, JAK inhibitors (JAKi) have consistently demonstrated an overall acceptable safety profile. These findings might indicate that the use of JAK inhibitors does not entail a significantly increased risk of malignancy or deep vein thrombosis/pulmonary embolism (DVT/PE) [71–73]. However, some post-authorization studies have found a dose-response relationship between baricitinib and DVT/PE and comparisons between Tofacitinib and TNFα-inhibitors have noted differences such as increased rates of malignancy and major adverse cardiovascular event (MACE). The FDA and European Medicines Agency (EMA) identified a dose-response relationship between baricitinib and DVT/PE, with increased DVT/PE risk among patients receiving 4 mg as compared to 2 mg twice daily [74]. The EMA study identified a dose-response relationship at higher doses of tofacitinib, at 10 mg and 5 mg twice daily; after interim results demonstrating increased DVT/PE and all-cause mortality among patients treated with 10 mg daily, all patients were switched to 5 mg [75]. An open-label non-inferiority trial examining tofacitinib against TNFα inhibitors among patients with rheumatoid arthritis and at least one cardiovascular risk factor identified an elevated incidence of malignancy (4.2% vs. 2.9%) and major adverse cardiac events (MACE) (5.8% vs. 4.3%) among patients treated with tofacitinib for a median of 4 years without significant differences in clinical response [76]. Prior to this study, TNFα inhibitors had already been issued a black box warning regarding an elevated risk of cancer. Following this study, the FDA extended this warning to include tofacitinib, upadacitinib, and baricitinib. Moreover, the FDA refined the indications for tofacitinib and baricitinib, expanding from an incomplete response to methotrexate to also encompass an incomplete response to TNFα inhibitors in the treatment of rheumatoid arthritis [77]. Of note, this trial excluded non-melanoma skin cancers, a known risk associated with TNFα-inhibitors.

Further extended trials are necessary to gain a more comprehensive understanding of how the findings from this study translate into outcomes for patients; specifically, the burden of observed MACEs and cancers due to inflammation from rheumatoid arthritis and whether these findings can be applied to other conditions such as SpA.

17.1 Summary

The oral JAK inhibitors have provided a paradigm shift in the treatment of both cutaneous and systemic autoimmune diseases. The JAK-STAT signaling system plays an essential role for immune response and immune surveillance in humans. Intracellular JAK-STAT signaling system regulates effector memory T cells and its associated cytokines of various T-cell subgroups including regulation of Th1, Th2, Th9, Th17, and Th22 cells which play a pivotal role in the pathogenesis of systemic and cutaneous autoimmune diseases. Many JAKi have demonstrated good efficacy with reasonable safety in many different autoimmune diseases. Owing to their ability of blocking certain specific signaling protein, the new generation JAKi may have less adverse effects.

Financial Support and Sponsorship None

Conflicts of Interest No financial support or sponsorship for this article

References

1. Raychaudhuri SK, Raychaudhuri SP. Janus kinase/signal transducer and activator of transcription pathways in spondyloarthritis. Curr Opin Rheumatol. 2017;29(4):311–6. https://doi.org/10.1097/BOR.0000000000000399.
2. Nash P, Kerschbaumer A, Dörner T, Dougados M, Fleischmann RM, Geissler K, et al. Points to consider for the treatment of immune-mediated inflammatory diseases with Janus kinase inhibitors: a consensus statement. Ann Rheum Dis. 2021;80(1):71–87. https://doi.org/10.1136/annrheumdis-2020-218398.
3. Kehl AS, Corr M, Weisman MH. Review: Enthesitis: new insights into pathogenesis, diagnostic modalities, and treatment. Arthritis Rheumatol. 2016;68(2):312–22. https://doi.org/10.1002/art.39458.
4. Raychaudhuri SP, Raychaudhuri SK. IL-23/IL-17 axis in spondyloarthritis-bench to bedside. Clin Rheumatol. 2016;35(6):1437–41. https://doi.org/10.1007/s10067-016-3263-4.
5. Chudnovskiy A, Pasqual G, Victora GD. Studying interactions between dendritic cells and T cells in vivo. Curr Opin Immunol. 2019;58:24–30. https://doi.org/10.1016/j.coi.2019.02.002.
6. Raychaudhuri SK, Abria C, Raychaudhuri SP. Polyfunctional TEM cells in psoriatic arthritis synovium skewed towards Th17 cells. Ann Rheum Dis. 2022;81(1):e5. https://doi.org/10.1136/annrheumdis-2019-216658.
7. Raychaudhuri SP, Raychaudhuri SK. Mechanistic rationales for targeting interleukin-17A in spondyloarthritis. Arthritis Res Ther. 2017;19(1):51. https://doi.org/10.1186/s13075-017-1249-5.
8. Raychaudhuri SK, Abria C, Maverakis EM, Raychaudhuri SP. IL-9 receptor: regulatory role on FLS and pannus formation. Cytokine. 2018;111:58–62. https://doi.org/10.1016/j.cyto.2018.08.001.
9. Villarino AV, Gadina M, O'Shea JJ, Kanno Y. SnapShot: Jak-STAT Signaling II. Cell. 2020;181(7):1696–1696.e1. https://doi.org/10.1016/j.cell.2020.04.052.
10. Gadina M, Le MT, Schwartz DM, Silvennoinen O, Nakayamada S, Yamaoka K, et al. Janus kinases to jakinibs: from basic insights to clinical practice. Rheumatol (Oxf Engl). 2019;58(Suppl 1):i4–i16. https://doi.org/10.1093/rheumatology/key432.
11. Kerschbaumer A, Smolen JS, Nash P, Doerner T, Dougados M, Fleischmann R, et al. Points to consider for the treatment of immune-mediated inflammatory diseases with Janus kinase inhibitors: a systematic literature research. RMD Open. 2020;6(3):e001374. https://doi.org/10.1136/rmdopen-2020-001374.
12. Gerstenberger BS, Ambler C, Arnold EP, Banker ME, Brown MF, Clark JD, et al. Discovery of tyrosine kinase 2 (TYK2) inhibitor (PF-06826647) for the treatment of autoimmune diseases. J Med Chem. 2020;63(22):13561–77. https://doi.org/10.1021/acs.jmedchem.0c00948.
13. Clark JD, Flanagan ME, Telliez JB. Discovery and development of Janus kinase (JAK) inhibitors for inflammatory diseases. J Med Chem. 2014;57(12):5023–38. https://doi.org/10.1021/jm401490p.
14. Kundu-Raychaudhuri S, Abria C, Raychaudhuri SP. IL-9, a local growth factor for synovial T cells in inflammatory arthritis. Cytokine. 2016;79:45–51. https://doi.org/10.1016/j.cyto.2015.12.020.

15. Banerjee S, Biehl A, Gadina M, Hasni S, Schwartz DM. JAK-STAT signaling as a target for inflammatory and autoimmune diseases: current and future prospects. Drugs. 2017 Apr;77(5):521–46. https://doi.org/10.1007/s40265-017-0701-9.
16. Maeda Y, Huang T, Manning C, Shaughn B, Macoritto M, Hyland D, et al. Blockade of the JAK/STAT pathway inhibits inflammation and bone formation in two murine models of spondyloarthritis. Arthritis Rheumatol. 2018;70(Suppl):10.
17. Hammitzsch A, Chen L, de Wit J, Al-Mossawi MH, Ridley A, Sekine T, et al. Inhibiting ex-vivo Th17 responses in ankylosing spondylitis by targeting Janus kinases. Sci Rep. 2018;8(1):15645. https://doi.org/10.1038/s41598-018-34026-1.
18. Dendrou CA, Cortes A, Shipman L, Evans HG, Attfield KE, Jostins L, et al. Resolving TYK2 locus genotype-to-phenotype differences in autoimmunity. Sci Transl Med. 2016;8(363):363ra149. https://doi.org/10.1126/scitranslmed.aag1974.
19. Gracey E, Hromadová D, Lim M, Qaiyum Z, Zeng M, Yao Y, et al. TYK2 inhibition reduces type 3 immunity and modifies disease progression in murine spondyloarthritis. J Clin Invest. 2020;130(4):1863–78. https://doi.org/10.1172/JCI126567.
20. Chen C, Zhang X, Wang Y. Analysis of JAK2 and STAT3 polymorphisms in patients with ankylosing spondylitis in Chinese Han population. Clin Immunol. 2010;136(3):442–6. https://doi.org/10.1016/j.clim.2010.05.003.
21. Ferguson LR, Han DY, Fraser AG, Huebner C, Lam WJ, Morgan AR, et al. Genetic factors in chronic inflammation: single nucleotide polymorphisms in the STAT-JAK pathway, susceptibility to DNA damage and Crohn's disease in a New Zealand population. Mutat Res. 2010;690(1-2):108–15. https://doi.org/10.1016/j.mrfmmm.2010.01.017.
22. Ellinghaus D, Ellinghaus E, Nair RP, Stuart PE, Esko T, Metspalu A, et al. Combined analysis of genome-wide association studies for Crohn disease and psoriasis identifies seven shared susceptibility loci. Am J Hum Genet. 2012;90(4):636–47. https://doi.org/10.1016/j.ajhg.2012.02.020.
23. Pesu M, Candotti F, Husa M, Hofmann SR, Notarangelo LD, O'Shea JJ. JAK3, severe combined immunodeficiency, and a new class of immunosuppressive drugs. Immunol Rev. 2005;203:127–42. https://doi.org/10.1111/j.0105-2896.2005.00220.x.
24. Meyer DM, Jesson MI, Li X, Elrick MM, Funckes-Shippy CL, Warner JD, et al. Anti-inflammatory activity and neutrophil reductions mediated by the JAK1/JAK3 inhibitor, CP-690,550, in rat adjuvant-induced arthritis. J Inflamm (Lond). 2010;7:41. https://doi.org/10.1186/1476-9255-7-41.
25. Honma M, Minami-Hori M, Takahashi H, Iizuka H. Podoplanin expression in wound and hyperproliferative psoriatic epidermis: regulation by TGF-β and STAT-3 activating cytokines, IFN-γ, IL-6, and IL-22. J Dermatol Sci. 2012;65(2):134–40. https://doi.org/10.1016/j.jdermsci.2011.11.011.
26. Boyle DL, Soma K, Hodge J, Kavanaugh A, Mandel D, Mease P, et al. The JAK inhibitor tofacitinib suppresses synovial JAK1-STAT signalling in rheumatoid arthritis. Ann Rheum Dis. 2015;74(6):1311–6. https://doi.org/10.1136/annrheumdis-2014-206028.
27. Gao W, McGarry T, Orr C, McCormick J, Veale DJ, Fearon U. Tofacitinib regulates synovial inflammation in psoriatic arthritis, inhibiting STAT activation and induction of negative feedback inhibitors. Ann Rheum Dis. 2016;75(1):311–5. https://doi.org/10.1136/annrheumdis-2014-207201.
28. Raychaudhuri SK, Abria C, Raychaudhuri SP. Regulatory role of the JAK STAT kinase signalling system on the IL-23/IL-17 cytokine axis in psoriatic arthritis. Ann Rheum Dis. 2017;76(10):e36. https://doi.org/10.1136/annrheumdis-2016-211046.
29. Deisseroth AB, Kaminskas E, Grillo J, Chen W, Saber H, Lu HL, et al. U.S. Food and Drug Administration approval: ruxolitinib for the treatment of patients with intermediate and high-risk myelofibrosis. Clin Cancer Res. 2012;18(12):3212–7. https://doi.org/10.1158/1078-0432.CCR-12-0653.
30. Targum SL. NDA approval [letter]. 2021. https://www.accessdata.fda.gov/drugsatfda00ltr.pdf. Accessed 10 Jan 2021.

31. Choy EHS, Miceli-Richard C, González-Gay MA, Sinigaglia L, Schlichting DE, Meszaros G, et al. The effect of JAK1/JAK2 inhibition in rheumatoid arthritis: efficacy and safety of baricitinib. Clin Exp Rheumatol. 2019;37(4):694–704.
32. Virtanen T, Haikarainen T, Raivola J, Silvennoinen O. Selective JAKinibs: prospects in inflammatory and autoimmune diseases. BioDrugs. 2019;33(1):15–32. https://doi.org/10.1007/s40259-019-00333-w.
33. Raychaudhuri S, Cheema KS, Raychaudhuri SK, Raychaudhuri SP. Janus kinase-signal transducers and activators of transcription cell signaling in Spondyloarthritis: rationale and evidence for JAK inhibition. Curr Opin Rheumatol. 2021;33(4):348–55. https://doi.org/10.1097/BOR.0000000000000810.
34. Mease P, Hall S, FitzGerald O, van der Heijde D, Merola JF, Avila-Zapata F, et al. Tofacitinib or adalimumab versus placebo for psoriatic arthritis. N Engl J Med. 2017;377(16):1537–50. https://doi.org/10.1056/NEJMoa1615975.
35. Nash P, Coates LC, Kivitz AJ, Mease PJ, Gladman DD, Covarrubias-Cobos JA, et al. Safety and efficacy of tofacitinib in patients with active psoriatic arthritis: interim analysis of OPAL balance, an open-label, long-term extension study. Rheumatol Ther. 2020;7(3):553–80. https://doi.org/10.1007/s40744-020-00209-4.
36. McInnes IB, Anderson JK, Magrey M, Merola JF, Liu Y, Kishimoto M, et al. Trial of upadacitinib and adalimumab for psoriatic arthritis. N Engl J Med. 2021;384(13):1227–39. https://doi.org/10.1056/NEJMoa2022516.
37. Rinvoq (Upadacitinib). Full prescribing information. AbbVie. 2021. https://www.accessdata.fda.gov/drugsatfda_docs/label/2021/211675s002s005lbl.pdf.
38. Mease P, Coates LC, Helliwell PS, Stanislavchuk M, Rychlewska-Hanczewska A, Dudek A, et al. Efficacy and safety of filgotinib, a selective Janus kinase 1 inhibitor, in patients with active psoriatic arthritis (EQUATOR): results from a randomised, placebo-controlled, phase 2 trial. Lancet. 2018;392(10162):2367–77. https://doi.org/10.1016/S0140-6736(18)32483-8.
39. van der Heijde D, Deodhar A, Wei JC, Drescher E, Fleishaker D, Hendrikx T, et al. Tofacitinib in patients with ankylosing spondylitis: a phase II, 16-week, randomised, placebo-controlled, dose-ranging study. Ann Rheum Dis. 2017;76(8):1340–7. https://doi.org/10.1136/annrheumdis-2016-210322.
40. Deodhar A, Sliwinska-Stanczyk P, Xu H, Baraliakos X, Gensler L, Fleishaker D, et al. Tofacitinib for the treatment of adult patients with ankylosing spondylitis: primary analysis of a phase 3, randomized, double-blind, placebo-controlled study [abstract]. Arthritis Rheumatol. 2020;72(Suppl):10.
41. Xeljanz (Tofacitinib). Full prescribing information. Pfizer Labs. 2021. https://www.accessdata.fda.gov/drugsatfda_docs/label/2021/203214s028,208246s013,213082s003lbl.pdf.
42. van der Heijde D, Baraliakos X, Gensler LS, Maksymowych WP, Tseluyko V, Nadashkevich O, et al. Efficacy and safety of filgotinib, a selective Janus kinase 1 inhibitor, in patients with active ankylosing spondylitis (TORTUGA): results from a randomised, placebo-controlled, phase 2 trial. Lancet. 2018;392(10162):2378–87. https://doi.org/10.1016/S0140-6736(18)32463-2.
43. Baraliakos X, Østergaard M, Landewé RBM, Barchuk W, Liu K, Tasset C, et al. OP0141 effects of filgotinib on spinal lesions in ankylosing spondylitis: magnetic resonance imaging data from the Tortuga trial. Ann Rheum Dis. 2021;80(Suppl 1):83–4. https://doi.org/10.1136/annrheumdis-2021-eular.1797.
44. van der Heijde D, Song IH, Pangan AL, Deodhar A, van den Bosch F, Maksymowych WP, et al. Efficacy and safety of upadacitinib in patients with active ankylosing spondylitis (SELECT-AXIS 1): a multicentre, randomised, double-blind, placebo-controlled, phase 2/3 trial. Lancet. 2019;394(10214):2108–17. https://doi.org/10.1016/S0140-6736(19)32534-6.
45. Sandborn WJ, Ghosh S, Panes J, Vranic I, Su C, Rousell S, et al. Tofacitinib, an oral Janus kinase inhibitor, in active ulcerative colitis. N Engl J Med. 2012;367(7):616–24. https://doi.org/10.1056/NEJMoa1112168.
46. Sands BE, Sandborn WJ, Feagan BG, Lichtenstein GR, Zhang H, Strauss R, et al. Peficitinib, an oral Janus kinase inhibitor, in moderate-to- severe ulcerative colitis: results from a randomized, phase 2 study. J Crohns Colitis. 2018;12(10):1158–69. https://doi.org/10.1093/ecco-jcc/jjy085.

47. Sandborn WJ, Ghosh S, Panes J, et al. Efficacy and safety of upadacitinib as an induction therapy for patients with moderately to-severely active ulcerative colitis: data from the phase 2B study U-ACHIEVE. U Eur Gastroenterol J. 2018;6:A74.
48. Panés J, Sandborn WJ, Schreiber S, Sands BE, Vermeire S, D'Haens G, et al. Tofacitinib for induction and maintenance therapy of Crohn's disease: results of two phase IIb randomised placebo-controlled trials. Gut. 2017;66(6):1049–59. https://doi.org/10.1136/gutjnl-2016-312735.
49. Vermeire S, Schreiber S, Petryka R, Kuehbacher T, Hebuterne X, Roblin X, et al. Clinical remission in patients with moderate-to-severe Crohn's disease treated with filgotinib (the Fitzroy study): results from a phase 2, double-blind, randomised, placebo-controlled trial. Lancet. 2017;389(10066):266–75. https://doi.org/10.1016/S0140-6736(16)32537-5.
50. Ma C, Jairath V, Vande CN. Pharmacology, efficacy and safety of JAK inhibitors in Crohn's disease. Best Pract Res Clin Gastroenterol. 2019;38-39:101606. https://doi.org/10.1016/j.bpg.2019.03.002.
51. Strober BE, Gottlieb AB, van de Kerkhof PCM, Puig L, Bachelez H, Chouela E, et al. Benefit–risk profile of tofacitinib in patients with moderate-to-severe chronic plaque psoriasis: pooled analysis across six clinical trials. Br J Dermatol. 2019;180(1):67–75. https://doi.org/10.1111/bjd.17149.
52. Papp KA, Menter MA, Raman M, Disch D, Schlichting DE, Gaich C, et al. A randomized phase 2B trial of baricitinib, an oral Janus kinase (JAK) 1/JAK2 inhibitor, in patients with moderate-to-severe psoriasis. Br J Dermatol. 2016;174(6):1266–76. https://doi.org/10.1111/bjd.14403.
53. Papp K, Gordon K, Thaçi D, Morita A, Gooderham M, Foley P, et al. Phase 2 trial of selective tyrosine kinase 2 inhibition in psoriasis Ed 2018. N Engl J Med. 2018;379(14):1313–21. https://doi.org/10.1056/NEJMoa1806382.
54. Papp K, Szepietowski JC, Kircik L, Toth D, Eichenfield LF, Leung DYM, et al. Efficacy and safety of Ruxolitinib cream for the treatment of atopic dermatitis: results from 2 phase 3, randomized, double-blind studies. J Am Acad Dermatol. 2021;85(4):863–72. https://doi.org/10.1016/j.jaad.2021.04.085.
55. Dhillon S. Delgocitinib: first approval. Drugs. 2020 Apr;80(6):609–15. https://doi.org/10.1007/s40265-020-01291-2.
56. Bieber T, Simpson EL, Silverberg JI, Thaçi D, Paul C, Pink AE, et al. Abrocitinib versus placebo or Dupilumab for atopic dermatitis. N Engl J Med. 2021;384(12):1101–12. https://doi.org/10.1056/NEJMoa2019380.
57. Guttman-Yassky E, Teixeira HD, Simpson EL, Papp KA, Pangan AL, Blauvelt A, et al. Once-daily upadacitinib versus placebo in adolescents and adults with moderate-to-severe atopic dermatitis (measure up 1 and measure up 2): results from two replicate double-blind, randomised controlled phase 3 trials. Lancet. 2021;397(10290):2151–68. https://doi.org/10.1016/S0140-6736(21)00588-2.
58. Reich K, Teixeira HD, de Bruin-Weller M, Bieber T, Soong W, Kabashima K, et al. Safety and efficacy of upadacitinib in combination with topical corticosteroids in adolescents and adults with moderate-to-severe atopic dermatitis (AD UP): results from a randomised, double-blind, placebo-controlled, phase 3 trial. Lancet. 2021;397(10290):2169–81. https://doi.org/10.1016/S0140-6736(21)00589-4.
59. Simpson EL, Forman S, Silverberg JI, Zirwas M, Maverakis E, Han G, et al. Baricitinib in patients with moderate-to-severe atopic dermatitis: results from a randomized monotherapy phase 3 trial in the United States and Canada (BREEZE-AD5). J Am Acad Dermatol. 2021 Jul;85(1):62–70. https://doi.org/10.1016/j.jaad.2021.02.028.
60. Xing L, Dai Z, Jabbari A, Cerise JE, Higgins CA, Gong W, et al. Alopecia areata is driven by cytotoxic T lymphocytes and is reversed by JAK inhibition. Nat Med. 2014;20(9):1043–9. https://doi.org/10.1038/nm.3645.
61. Liu LY, Craiglow BG, Dai F, King BA. Tofacitinib for the treatment of severe alopecia areata and variants: a study of 90 patients. J Am Acad Dermatol. 2017;76(1):22–8. https://doi.org/10.1016/j.jaad.2016.09.007.

62. Chapman S, Kwa M, Gold LS, Lim HW. Janus kinase inhibitors in dermatology: part I. A comprehensive review. J Am Acad Dermatol. 2022;86(2):406–13. https://doi.org/10.1016/j.jaad.2021.07.002.
63. Chapman S, Gold LS, Lim HW. Janus kinase inhibitors in dermatology: part II. A comprehensive review. J Am Acad Dermatol. 2022;86(2):414–22. https://doi.org/10.1016/j.jaad.2021.06.873.
64. Smolen JS, Genovese MC, Takeuchi T, Hyslop DL, Macias WL, Rooney T, et al. Safety profile of Baricitinib in patients with active rheumatoid arthritis with over 2 years median time in treatment. J Rheumatol. 2019;46(1):7–18. https://doi.org/10.3899/jrheum.171361.
65. Sepriano A, Kerschbaumer A, Smolen JS, van der Heijde D, Dougados M, van Vollenhoven R, et al. Safety of synthetic and biological DMARDs: a systematic literature review informing the 2019 update of the EULAR recommendations for the management of rheumatoid arthritis. Ann Rheum Dis. 2020;79(6):760–70. https://doi.org/10.1136/annrheumdis-2019-216653.
66. Cohen SB, Tanaka Y, Mariette X, Curtis JR, Lee EB, Nash P, et al. Long-term safety of tofacitinib for the treatment of rheumatoid arthritis up to 8.5 years: integrated analysis of data from the global clinical trials. Ann Rheum Dis. 2017;76(7):1253–62. https://doi.org/10.1136/annrheumdis-2016-210457.
67. Genovese MC, Smolen J, Takeuchi T, Burmester GR, Deberdt W, Schlichting D, et al. FRI0123: safety profile of Baricitinib for the treatment of rheumatoid arthritis up to 8.4 years: an updated integrated safety analysis. Ann Rheum Dis. 2020;79(Suppl 1):638.
68. Cohen SB, van Vollenhoven R, Curtis JR, Calabrese L, Zerbini C, Tanaka Y, et al. THU0187: safety profile of Upadacitinib up to 3 years of exposure in patients with rheumatoid arthritis. Ann Rheum Dis. 2020;79(Suppl 1):315.
69. Curtis JR, Xie F, Yun H, Bernatsky S, Winthrop KL. Real-world comparative risks of herpes virus infections in tofacitinib and biologic-treated patients with rheumatoid arthritis. Ann Rheum Dis. 2016;75(10):1843–7. https://doi.org/10.1136/annrheumdis-2016-209131.
70. Curtis JR, Xie F, Yang S, Bernatsky S, Chen L, Yun H, et al. Risk for herpes zoster in tofacitinib-treated rheumatoid arthritis patients with and without concomitant methotrexate and glucocorticoids. Arthritis Care Res. 2019;71(9):1249–54. https://doi.org/10.1002/acr.23769.
71. Mease P, Charles-Schoeman C, Cohen S, Fallon L, Woolcott J, Yun H, et al. Incidence of venous and arterial thromboembolic events reported in the tofacitinib rheumatoid arthritis, psoriasis and psoriatic arthritis development programmes and from real-world data. Ann Rheum Dis. 2020;79(11):1400–13. https://doi.org/10.1136/annrheumdis-2019-216761.
72. Curtis JR, Lee EB, Kaplan IV, Kwok K, Geier J, Benda B, et al. Tofacitinib, an oral Janus kinase inhibitor: analysis of malignancies across the rheumatoid arthritis clinical development programme. Ann Rheum Dis. 2016;75(5):831–41. https://doi.org/10.1136/annrheumdis-2014-205847.
73. Desai RJ, Pawar A, Weinblatt ME, Kim SC. Comparative risk of venous thromboembolism in rheumatoid arthritis patients receiving tofacitinib versus those receiving tumor necrosis factor inhibitors: an observational cohort study. Arthritis Rheumatol. 2019;71(6):892–900. https://doi.org/10.1002/art.40798.
74. FDA briefing document arthritis advisory committee meeting. Vol. 2019; 2018. https://www.fda.gov/media/112372/download. Accessed 1 Feb 2021.
75. EMA confirms Xeljanz to be used with caution in patients at high risk of blood clots; 2019 [cited Feb 1, 2021]. https://www.ema.europa.eu/en/news/ema-confirms-xeljanz-be-used-caution-patients-high-riskblood-clots.
76. Ytterberg SR, Bhatt DL, Mikuls TR, Koch GG, Fleischmann R, Rivas JL, et al. Cardiovascular and cancer risk with tofacitinib in rheumatoid arthritis. N Engl J Med. 2022;386(4):316–26. https://doi.org/10.1056/NEJMoa2109927.
77. FDA requires warnings about increased risk of serious heart-related events, cancer, blood clots, and death for JAK inhibitors that treat certain chronic inflammatory conditions. US FDA drug safety and availability. Updated Dec 7, 2021. Published Sep 1, 2021. Accessed 10 Jan 2022.

The Placebo Effect in Dermatology: Managing Patients' Expectations

18

Nikhil Mehta and Somesh Gupta

18.1 Introduction

A placebo, which literally means "I shall please," pleases not just the patients, but doctors as well. Although initially coined as a somewhat derogatory term for hired funeral mourners in the fourteenth century, its use in medical literature is first documented in the late eighteenth century [1]. One of the first documented implementations of the use of placebo as a control was by John Haygarth in 1801, when he found out that wooden imitators of metallic rods (which were presumed to improve various diseases by electromagnetism) were similarly effective to relieve diseases [1]. Henry Beecher was one of the firsts to attempt to quantify the placebo effect in 1955 when he claimed that in 15 different trials of different diseases, 35% out of 1082 patients were satisfactorily relieved by a placebo alone. However, further re-analysis did not find this to be true, although this 35% figure has become entrenched in the literature [2].

Although the term "placebo" acquired its current medical sense in the late eighteenth century, placebos are ancient. Many therapies in medicine, including the alternative forms of medicine, before the advent of modern medicine and era of evidence-based medicine, can be considered to work through the placebo effect. Through a review of placebo-controlled homeopathy trials compared with placebo-controlled allopathy trials, it has been argued that the effects of homeopathy are likely placebo effects [3].

The use of placebo is widespread. In the Unites States, about half (46–58% depending on phrasing) of the rheumatologists and internists reported regular usage of placebos. They usually described them to patients as a potentially beneficial

N. Mehta · S. Gupta (✉)
Department of Dermatology and Venereology, All India Institute of Medical Sciences, New Delhi, India
e-mail: someshgupta@aiims.edu

S. Gupta et al. (eds.), *Critical Thinking in Contemporary Dermatology: Cognitive Essays*, https://doi.org/10.1007/978-981-97-0411-8_18

medicine or treatment not typically used for their condition. It was regarded as ethically permissible by them [4]. In another study from the United Kingdom, 97% general practitioners used placebos at least once in their career, and 77% used placebos at least once per week. Most participants regarded placebos as ethical in some circumstances [5]. Another meta-analysis revealed that 29–97% of general practitioners had used placebos once in their career, 46–95% in the last 1 year, and up to 15–89% use it at least once a month [6]. Looking at patients' perspective, majority (50–84%) of patients agreed that placebos should be used by clinicians, with percentage varying depending upon different indications [7].

The notion that if one believes that he/she will get better, then he/she will indeed get better, is undeniably romantic. It has been widely believed and demonstrated that mental stress affects the body. It can lead to reactivation of herpes and zoster [8, 9], "catching" a cold [10], and poor wound healing [11]. Similarly, stress worsens or leads to frequent exacerbations of psoriasis [12] and atopic dermatitis [13]. Some evidence also exists to support the opposite, 'healthy body due to a healthy mind' [14, 15]. Or a mind that expects to get healthy. Understanding the mind–body connection is fundamental to understand the workings of a placebo. Similarly, a mind that expects to get diseased will be more prone to the disease. Harmless leaves rubbed on patients 'known' to be hypersensitive to a Japanese lacquer/wax plant leaves have been shown to elicit actual physical urticarial rash if they have been told that the leaves are of the lacquer plant, while actual lacquer leaves did not cause rash as patients were told they were harmless. However, this often quoted 1962 study by Ikemi and Nakagawa has not been reported to be replicated [16]. Similarly, in another old 1970 study asthmatic patients showed constriction of airways when they were told that an inert substance they were inhaling was an allergen [17].

18.2 Definition-Placebo, the Placebo Effect, and the Placebo Response

A placebo is understood to be an inert substance or intervention which is thought to have no intrinsic therapeutic value for the targeted disease, but still impacts the patient. Placebo can make a patient feel better and alleviate the symptoms, but would not cure the disease or eliminate the cause of the symptoms. The therapeutic illusion/symbolic import of the treatment makes the placebo work through patients' expectancies. While the placebo effect is the beneficial psychological effect of the placebo in a patient. This simple understanding leads to many questions. It has an inherent paradox; why does a seemingly inert substance has a beneficial effect, and if it has a beneficial effect, why is it termed inert? Is multivitamin "supplementation" for oral aphthous ulcers a placebo or a therapy? In a patient taking a placebo, what component of the benefit is termed the placebo effect and what is not? Does a "no-treatment" third arm of a trial have a placebo effect?

Many researchers have tried to define placebo and placebo effect in a way that answers many of the above questions. The Society for Interdisciplinary Placebo Studies (SIPS) defines *placebo effects* as changes specifically attributable to placebo mechanisms, including the neurobiological and psychological mechanisms of expectations, whereas *placebo response* (also called "contextual effects") refers to all health changes resulting from administering an inactive treatment. They include the random fluctuation in the course of the disease, natural history of the disease, regression to the mean (where individual participants showing extreme responses at one observation time show fewer extreme responses during the second observation time), Hawthorne effect (in which participants' behavior changes when they know they are being observed) and response bias (which implies that participants in studies do not actually tell the responses that they feel) [18]. In fact, giving a placebo involves significant manipulation of the doctor–patient relationship which can lead to recording of a positive impact on the patient through several different interdependent ways, which are difficult to be defined and measured discreetly. As these factors are associated with the ritual of giving a treatment and patients' expectations rather than the treatment, these also contribute to the response to the studied active agent. So, putting in the form of a mathematical equation, response to an intervention in a trial = net benefit of the active ingredient + placebo contextual effects (placebo effect + effect of response bias + effect of Hawthorne effect + natural history/variation + regression to the mean + other factors). Using a "no-treatment" control group in addition of placebo can remove any benefit due to the natural history/variation of the disease and regression to the mean, but cannot remove the Hawthorne effect and response bias completely as even these unblinded patients are followed up, observed, and assessed for responses, so can change their behavior under observation and are prone to response biases. Hawthorne effect and response bias are also difficult to delineate clearly from each other [19].

The random fluctuation/natural history does not consistently accrue a better or worse response to placebo in a study comparing placebo with an unblinded "no-treatment" group. However, regression to the mean can lead to false overestimation of the effects of the placebo [20]. Hawthorne effect might tilt in favor of the placebo as patients are more likely to change their behavior when they think they are observed for responses to an active treatment. Response bias frequently entails that patients tell the answers which they feel are expected or desired by the doctor or investigator. For example, in a type of response bias participants may indicate a lower pain or itch score compared to what they feel in follow-up visits in response to an intervention, to please the doctor or investigator consciously or subconsciously [21]. In studies, it is often not possible to separate response bias from the true placebo effect and in general overestimates the placebo effect [21]. The excess relief in the pain score reported by participants of an experiment in the placebo group compared to participants of the no-treatment group might not be replicated in a clinical setting.

While defining the placebo effect, researchers have either used its narrow definition as mentioned above or used it in a broad sense indirectly meaning it to be equivalent to the placebo response. Various authors have considered different parts of the SIPS definition of the placebo response as constituents of the placebo effect. In general, studies done predominantly for finding the role of a placebo use a strict narrow definition of the placebo effect as mentioned above, while studies with only two arms of active intervention and placebo control group use the term "placebo effect" to mean the placebo response. While interpreting the placebo effect in a study, it is imperative to first know what the authors meant by the placebo effect.

Placebo effects can be positive or negative responses to the patient. While placebos are usually prescribed clinically for the benefit of the patient, they can lead to "adverse effects" or harmful effects similar to any active therapy. The term placebo effect is used to refer to the beneficial effects of the placebo, while nocebo effect refers to the harmful effects. Again, this definition is not consensus-based. The SIPS society ascribes any perceived harmful effect of a placebo as the nocebo effect, while some researchers necessarily require patient's expectation of a harmful effect (by being told by the clinician that the intervention given to them causes harmful effects) to ascribe something to the nocebo effect [18]. Negative effect even though the patient was told that the placebo is beneficial and the clinician thinks that patient's expectations are overtly positive, or negative expectations although patient was not told about any possible negative effects, or when patient was explicitly warned about negative effects—all three connotations have been variably used for the term "nocebo." Interestingly, in trials the adverse effects due to a placebo/nocebo are similar to the drug for which they serve as controls, as the patients in the placebo group expect and develop the same adverse drug profile they have been warned against.

In authors' opinion, the term "nocebo effect" should be used when negative effects develop due to conscious or unconscious negative expectations of patients, irrespective of whether these expectations are due to clinician's explicit description or not. A drug can simultaneously be both a placebo and nocebo. In a study comparing isotretinoin with placebo, a subset of patients on placebo may feel their acne to be improving but may complain of getting dry skin and lips. In this example these patients display both placebo and nocebo effects due to their expectations.

18.3 Classification of Placebos

Apart from the division of conventional placebos in research and clinical practice, there are some other types of distinctive placebo usage that have merited a distinctive adjective to be prefixed before the word placebo to imply a specific connotation.

18.3.1 Pure vs. Impure Placebos

A distinction is sometimes made for pure (which carry inert substances like saline/sugar pills) vs. impure (which may carry active ingredients which have pharmacological effects for other diseases but have no or uncertain effect on the pathology of the condition for which they are being used as placebos, like antibiotics for viral upper respiratory tract infections or multivitamins for aphthous ulcers) placebos. Impure placebos may not be considered as placebos by the general practitioners, as their use is more prevalent than pure placebos [22].

18.3.2 Open-Label Placebos

It is open to debate if "open-label" placebos, i.e., placebos without concealment or patient blinding, can be considered as true placebos. But what is not debatable is that they too work, as exemplified in a pilot study on irritable bowel syndrome, and subsequent controlled trials on chronic low back pain, knee pain, cancer-related fatigue, migraine headaches, and allergic rhinitis [23]. The usage in allergic rhinitis is significant to dermatologists as it motivates trials in other allergic conditions. In these trials patients were told that although they are getting inert substances they can still benefit, were educated about the placebo effect/mind–body connection, and they expected to get better. As patients benefitted from their expectations from a treatment, the essence of the placebo effect remains fulfilled despite lack of concealment, we opine that they indeed fulfil the criteria of placebos. They may lack some component of the placebo effect, but they have not been shown to be less effective than the conventional placebos. It is also not in doubt that open-label placebos are more ethical than the "conventional" blinded ones, as per SIPS [18] and as per interpretation of American Medical Association's (AMA's) ethical recommendations [23]. As per AMA's opinion, "physicians may use placebos for diagnosis or treatment only if the patient is informed of and agrees to its use. A placebo may still be effective if the patient knows it will be used but cannot identify it and does not know the precise timing of its use."

18.3.3 Dose-Extending Placebos

In contrast with the approach of giving a placebo in isolation, a dose-extending placebo (or "subclinical" dosage of an active drug as an impure placebo) is given in addition to or in rotation with an active treatment. This approach reduces the dose, cost, adverse effects, and dependence of the active agent. They are usually used for alleviating pain with/rotating with non-steroidal anti-inflammatory drugs and opioids. Studies have shown that giving placebos after repeated administration of active treatment agents demonstrates drug-like effects greater than those obtained through placebo alone. Conditioning and reinforcement learning principles are responsible for this boosting effect [24]. Again, they may be more ethical than the conventional placebos, and open-label placebos can be used for dose-extending purposes too.

18.4 Do Placebos Work?

With decades of clinical and experimental experience it is not a question of if placebos work, but in what proportion and how much (magnitude or effect size) do they work, in comparison to the active treatment, and in whom they work. Beecher's estimation and the belief that placebo works satisfactorily in a third of patients has been frequently questioned [2]. The trials which he analyzed did not report the magnitude of the placebo response to qualify labeling it satisfactorily, nor did they mention the proportion of patients who worsened while on placebos. They lacked adequate attempts to minimize extreme baseline readings/regression to the mean.

Hróbjartsson and Gøtzsche published multiple Cochrane meta-analyses to find out the impact of placebos compared to the "no-treatment" group by including studies which had both these groups [25]. Trials with a "no-treatment" arm obviously cannot be patient blinded. Due to participants' biases due to this lack of blinding, they argued that it is expected to observe some differences between the placebo vs. the "no-treatment" group even if placebos did not have any true effect. However, they found that the placebo group and "no-treatment" group did not have statistically significant difference in proportion achieving binary outcomes. The benefit of placebos over "no-treatment" group in continuous outcomes was modest and might not be clinically relevant overall.

However, there was a wide range in the effect size and in some individual studies, outcomes like pain and nausea were greatly impacted by placebo, compared to the "no-treatment" group. They concluded that different settings might impact the effect of placebo, and the benefit of the placebo effect could be clinically meaningful, especially when the outcome is patient-reported reduction in pain [25].

Using the same 186 trials as used by Hróbjartsson and Gøtzsche in their latest (2010) iteration of the meta-analysis, another meta-analysis by Christensen et al. found that on average nearly half (54%) of the overall treatment effect was attributable to contextual effects [26]. They used the ratio between improvement in the placebo group and the interventional group in different trials for this calculation. Similarly, another large meta-epidemiological study on 328 Cochrane systematic reviews found an overall proportion attributable to contextual effects as 65%, with a range of 40–95% [27].

18.5 Predicting Responders to Placebo

As individual placebo responses vary widely in trials, it is useful to know predictors of response to placebo. A wise clinician can usually judge quickly which patients will respond to placebo. Patient demographics, personality types, other psychological constructs, types of placebos, setting, and outcome studied all modify the placebo response and effect size [28]. In the meta-analysis by Hróbjartsson and Gøtzsche, it was also seen that larger effects of placebo were associated with physical placebo interventions like sham acupuncture, patient-involved outcomes including patient-reported outcomes such as pain, and in trials which did not inform patients that the trial involved placebos. The fact that the patient-reported outcomes show a greater response to placebos compared to observer assessed outcomes can be a result of various response biases [25]. Interestingly, expensive placebos and "double-strength" placebos work better than cheaper "regular-strength" placebos. Age and gender have been also seen to influence response to placebo in individual trials. Expensive placebos are more effective than cheaper ones [29], as also shown in a *JAMA* study that interestingly also won the 2008 Ig Nobel prize in Medicine [30]. However, opposite reviews exist, and another study concluded that more intense placebos do not consistently lead to a better response. Nevertheless, even if they did, ethical considerations do not justify the usage of a more invasive or more expensive placebo in clinical settings.

Right midfrontal gyrus connectivity has been identified as a biomarker that can predict placebo response in osteoarthritis patients [31]. Similarly, activity of other brain regions can predict intensity of the placebo analgesic response [32].

In summary, placebos work, although their effect size is highly variable and dependent on the setting, including the therapeutic ritual, expectations, and doctor–patient relationship. Intensive, invasive, expensive placebos work better, especially in subjective outcomes such as pain.

Hopefully, with progress in big data and artificial intelligence, we will be able to have complex scores [33] and prediction algorithms that will be able to predict an individual's tendency to respond to placebos, and development of clinical decision support tools for such precision medicine.

18.6 How Do Placebos Work?

The pathways of this mind–body connect, through which conditioning about an intervention leads to actual development of a physical response due to expectancy without actual intervention, are still not completely characterized. They are best characterized for the placebo analgesia response, Parkinson's disease, and depression, as neurotransmitters (endorphins, dopamine, and serotonin), pathways, and areas of brain are already defined for it. Researchers have argued that broadly placebo/nocebo effect involves the same biochemical pathways as the actual drugs they are said to be.

Expectations do not always hurt. They may frequently benefit! In a study, the analgesia by a heat stimulus doubled when participants were expectant about the opioid they were receiving. The blockade of the placebo analgesia by open or hidden naloxone initially showed that some of the effects of placebo analgesia could be through endogenous opioids [34, 35]. In later studies, significant activation of μ-opioid receptor-mediated neurotransmission was seen in parts associated with pain modulation (cingulate and insular cortex, thalamus, etc.) through PET scan in participants given placebo compared to controls [36]. Placebos have been shown to activate the same dopamine receptors as the actual anti-Parkinson dopaminergic drugs, and cause significant change in basal ganglia activity [37]. People warned about risk of headaches at high altitude indeed had more headaches, but also more prostaglandins than the control group. This increase was inhibited when they were given placebos [38]. A meta-analysis of functional MRI (fMRI) studies on placebo analgesia showed that placebos show a small but statistically significant widespread reduction of pain-related activity and neurological pain response compared to controls, especially in areas associated with pain modulation [39].

18.7 Uses and Advantages of Placebo in the Field of Dermatology

Placebos do not seriously harm the patients, in line with the Hippocratic oath, and can be beneficial for the patients. Their uses can be described in the following categories:

18.7.1 Research

18.7.1.1 Interventional Trials

As in other branches, the most commonly cited use of placebo in dermatology is their use in randomly controlled trials (RCTs). With the development of evidence-based medicine in the latter half of twentieth century, many interventional trials require comparison of newer interventions like new drugs and procedures with either preexisting interventions or placebos to demonstrate efficacy. Interestingly, use of a placebo control is still prevalent in trials with newer modalities like biologics for psoriasis despite the existence of proven conventional therapies and older biologics [40]. Active controls rather than placebo controls as the first evidence/trial of any new biologic in psoriasis should be considered more ethical; however they may not yield a difference that is sensational enough for pharmacological companies. A nuanced reading of trials is frequently lacking even in healthcare providers.

18.7.1.2 Placebo Studies

For researchers interested in studying the mechanisms and effects of placebo, placebos are the primary "interventions" used.

18.7.2 Clinical

18.7.2.1 Lack of an Effective Treatment

In difficult-to-treat diseases, an effective treatment may not exist. Placebos can make the patient feel better. The dictum states that "if the patient is helped by the placebo, discontinuing the placebo, in absence of a more effective treatment, would be unethical" [41]. They also maintain hope in the patients. It is also imperative to counsel the patients regarding the possibility of a better treatment in the future.

18.7.2.2 Prevention from Seeking Alternative Therapies and Treatment from Quacks

Dejected patients may resort to quacks or alternative therapy, and can incur significant cost and side effects of alternative medication. Vitiligo patients, especially skin of color patients, have significantly impaired quality of life and are willing to pay significant proportion of their salaries or household incomes for potential treatments [42]. Patients of acrofacial vitiligo have resorted to alternative medications leading to significant out-of-pocket and out-of-insurance-network expenditure, along with severe adverse effects like chronic arsenicosis [43]. Patients of lichen planus pigmentosus, a hyperpigmentary disorder, have significant distress and can spend a lot for treatment. But unfortunately, many options including depigmenting agents and pigmentary lasers yield an unsatisfactory response and can lead to worsening of pigmentation through ochronosis and post-inflammatory pigmentation. Often, patients with pigmentary disorders (like generalized or acrofacial vitiligo, recalcitrant melasma, and lichen planus pigmentosus) and genodermatoses (like ichthyosis and epidermolysis bullosa) may end up receiving topical or systemic corticosteroids from unregulated quacks and end up developing topical steroid-damaged face, steroid-induced atrophy and even cushingoid features. It is sometimes difficult to wean off topical steroids in stable vitiligo patients even if they have failed adequate duration of trial to induce repigmentation without switching with placebos. The perception of getting a treatment and expectation of treatment early in the course can prevent them from seeking alternate practitioners. Later, when a good rapport is established, patients can be slowly sensitized to make peace with their disease and adapt to a life with it. Approaching even qualified practitioners other than those covered in their insurance like non-government private practitioners can prove expensive to the patients without necessarily offering a new treatment approach for these difficult-to-treat diseases. In self-limiting diseases too, like pityriasis rosea and viral exanthems, a prescription of a placebo can frequently prevent anxious patients or their attendants to seek alternative therapies with quacks. It is argued that this practice is ethical [41].

18.7.2.3 Ensuring Follow-Up

Often, the diagnosis at presentation is uncertain. Patients often do not like the uncertainties associated with lack of diagnosis or multiple differentials and can change practitioners or treatment modalities. A placebo is a good way to allay their anxieties while a wait and watch approach can be followed to observe the evolution of the disease. Similarly, in chronic diseases like vitiligo or psoriasis, patients may have mild flares without the requirement of any additional treatment over and above their previous treatment. Increase of body surface area involvement from 1 to 2% in psoriasis and 1–2 new depigmented lesions 4 months ago in vitiligo may not warrant any addition of a systemic treatment. Often patients who complain more about their disease get stronger treatment or earlier systemic therapy, although this might not be in these patients' best interests. Systemic therapy may not alter the course of disease. Therapies like methotrexate require more frequent monitoring in patients with who have achieved a threshold total cumulative dose. Starting them earlier may lead to achievement of this threshold dose earlier in life in chronic diseases like psoriasis. An oral placebo can be prescribed in such mild flare situations, along with adequate counseling, to prevent the adverse effects of unwarranted systemic therapy.

18.7.2.4 Chronic Pruritus: Analogous to Chronic Pain

A problem unique to the domain of dermatologists is refractory itch, whether primary in form of prurigo, or secondary to an inflammatory disorder. In the group of prurigo disorders, often no cause of itching is identified. It is not uncommon to see cases refractory to or only partially responding to maximum doses of anti-histamines, topical steroids, thalidomide, etc. Such cases are analogous to chronic pain syndromes and fibromyalgia in terms of a chronic symptom with suboptimal/less than desirable response. Similar to the way the general practitioners use placebos for some relief in refractory pain, dermatologists use them for refractory itch. A normal saline injection placebo in dermatology in-patients of toxic epidermal necrolysis, psoriatic or reactive arthritis, etc. with severe pain on maximal permitted limit of opioids or with contraindication for opioids often provides pain relief. Such practice is commonplace [41]. Similar relief is obtained for in-patients of endogenous dermatitis, connective tissue disorders such as dermatomyositis, etc. with refractory itch. The action of placebos on itch pathways should be explored similar to the action on pain pathways.

18.7.2.5 Suspected Functional Symptoms

In patients of hypochondriasis, conversion disorders, or those with symptoms of pain and itch out of proportion to the signs, physicians often resort to placebo to alleviate the patient's complaints and to figure out any component of primary or secondary gain/malingering. Some clinicians may prescribe a topical moisturizer to a patient with minimal scars if their distress is perceived out of proportion to the noticeability of the scars.

18.7.2.6 Differing View of Illness

There are differing views about treatment of some disorders, especially those who can be considered "premalignant," or can have a low but unpredictable rate of transformation to malignancy. Parapsoriasis and early-stage mycosis fungoides spectrum of disorders is such a condition, where treatments such as topical steroids, methotrexate, or phototherapy may lead to resolution of symptoms and plaques, but do not alter the course of disease or transformation to malignancy. In such cases, the treatment and anxiety of a pre-malignant diagnosis, and burden of an aggressive treatment approach might be worse for the patient than the burden of the disease. Some clinicians may opt for a wait and watch observational approach rather than treating the asymptomatic existing plaques. Placebos help in allaying the anxiety of patients who might have googled mycosis fungoides and get worried to death if offered the strategy of "no-treatment" in a potentially malignant condition.

18.7.2.7 For Reducing Active Drug

Drug-extending placebos, as mentioned above, are used along with or in rotation with active drugs. They can be useful in patients with painful psoriatic or reactive arthritis, or even uncontrolled itch.

18.8 Criticisms

Do placebos actually do no harm? There are several controversies associated with the use of placebo.

18.8.1 Research

18.8.1.1 Not a Suitable Alternative to the No Treatment Group

As have been mentioned before, placebos may not be a superior alternative to the no-treatment group as a control while measuring the impact of an intervention in clinical trials. They may complicate the interpretation and analysis of the results.

18.8.1.2 Difficulty in Interpretation and Significance of Effect Size

For example, in a hypothetical scenario, if an intervention in such a disease and placebo both lead to a modest improvement in 30% patients in a trial, the results usually lead to clinicians continuing with counseling with no treatment option. In such cases, usage of placebo could have proven useful in 30% of the patients, which might have been more than the no-treatment group. A real life prospective or retrospective study of response rate or comparison with no-treatment group can better highlight its utility. Proportional contextual effects need to be emphasized while interpreting the results of placebo [26, 27]. The magnitudes of the effect sizes of placebo even for the same indication are also highly variable and dependent on the actual clinical setting.

18.8.1.3 Lack of Consensual Definitions

As highlighted above, the understanding on what constitutes placebo, placebo effect, placebo response, and nocebo varies widely. This makes comparisons between studies difficult. Many studies are difficult to generalize.

18.8.2 Clinical

18.8.2.1 Lack of Consensual Usage

For interventions of diseases where there's no treatment yet, a placebo if shown to improve patient reported parameters might be a good option. But there's no consensus to its usage. Although most clinicians do use placebos, the forms and indications of its usage are highly variable in doctors, and so are its justifications.

On changing practitioners, the new clinician might find the prescription of a multivitamin for acrofacial vitiligo or lichen planus pigmentosus by an old clinician bizarre. The usage of a drug as a placebo is usually not indicated on the records handed to the patient. The new doctor may not have access to internal records of the previous one, and may not even understand the role of the multivitamin tablet as a placebo. There might be even a doubt about the competency of the past clinician. Even pharmacists dispensing the medication or friends/relatives suffering from the same disease can point the patients towards the "weirdness" of their treatment. It is difficult to limit the information of usage of placebo to the desirable.

18.8.2.2 Lying to the Patient

Are placebos ethical? They involve inherent deception to the patient. In the current era of Google doctor and tech-savvy patients, they may very well come to discover that they have been prescribed placebos. The indication for placebos in them might not be apparent to them. The patients may feel hurt, and can think that their symptoms are not perceived to be "real" enough, or they have been perceived as attention-seeking or psychiatric patients. They may perceive to be experimented upon. There is a significant breach of trust in the doctor–patient relationship while prescribing a placebo. As per American Medical Association's Code of Medical Ethics opinion, "in the clinical setting, the use of a placebo without the patient's knowledge may undermine trust, compromise the patient–physician relationship, and result in medical harm to the patient [44]."

18.8.2.3 Informed Consent or Paternalism?

Informed consent approach in medical ethics implies that the patient is informed of all the options in details how to proceed next with management. The patient is enabled to make an educated choice and his/her wishes are respected. It can be argued that the statement "I am giving you this pill for your disease, it has shown to benefit some patients" is technically correct but withholds much information from the patient [41, 44]. Such an approach where the doctor chooses what is best for the patient without even giving him/her all the options constitutes paternalism. Open-label placebos can bypass this limitation of placebos and can be considered more ethical, while not being less effective than conventional placebos.

18.9 Conclusion—The Art of the Placebo

Perhaps what must be emphasized for today's clinician, apart from the relevance of placebo, is the art of the placebo. The placebo effect is not akin to doing nothing, but it's actually doing everything except giving the actual considered "intervention," and making the patient believe that he/she is getting that intervention or an intervention that works. How these fit into the transition of medical ethics from a paternalistic approach to complete-disclosure-with-options approach, is individualistic. We must recognize with better accuracy which patients are likely to respond to placebo, and optimize ethical placebo usage to maximize benefits.

References

1. de Craen AJ, Kaptchuk TJ, Tijssen JG, Kleijnen J. Placebos and placebo effects in medicine: historical overview. J R Soc Med. 1999;92(10):511–5.
2. Kienle GS, Kiene H. The powerful placebo effect: fact or fiction? J Clin Epidemiol. 1997;50(12):1311–8.
3. Shang A, Huwiler-Müntener K, Nartey L, Jüni P, Dörig S, Sterne JAC, et al. Are the clinical effects of homoeopathy placebo effects? Comparative study of placebo-controlled trials of homoeopathy and allopathy. Lancet. 2005;366(9487):726–32.
4. Tilburt JC, Emanuel EJ, Kaptchuk TJ, Curlin FA, Miller FG. Prescribing "placebo treatments": results of national survey of US internists and rheumatologists. BMJ. 2008;337:a1938.
5. Howick J, Bishop FL, Heneghan C, Wolstenholme J, Stevens S, Hobbs FDR, et al. Placebo use in the United Kingdom: results from a National Survey of primary care practitioners. PLoS One. 2013;8(3):e58247.

6. Linde K, Atmann O, Meissner K, Schneider A, Meister R, Kriston L, et al. How often do general practitioners use placebos and non-specific interventions? Systematic review and meta-analysis of surveys. PLoS One. 2018;13(8):e0202211.
7. Hull SC, Colloca L, Avins A, Gordon NP, Somkin CP, Kaptchuk TJ, et al. Patients' attitudes about the use of placebo treatments: telephone survey. BMJ. 2013;347:f3757.
8. Padgett DA, Sheridan JF, Dorne J, Berntson GG, Candelora J, Glaser R. Social stress and the reactivation of latent herpes simplex virus type 1. Proc Natl Acad Sci USA. 1998;95(12):7231–5.
9. Schmidt SAJ, Sørensen HT, Langan SM, Vestergaard M. Perceived psychological stress and risk of herpes zoster: a nationwide population-based cohort study. Br J Dermatol. 2021;185(1):130–8.
10. Cohen S, Tyrrell DA, Smith AP. Psychological stress and susceptibility to the common cold. N Engl J Med. 1991;325(9):606–12.
11. Gouin JP, Kiecolt-Glaser JK. The impact of psychological stress on wound healing: methods and mechanisms. Immunol Allergy Clin N Am. 2011;31(1):81–93.
12. Rousset L, Halioua B. Stress and psoriasis. Int J Dermatol. 2018;57(10):1165–72.
13. Arndt J, Smith N, Tausk F. Stress and atopic dermatitis. Curr Allergy Asthma Rep. 2008;8(4):312–7.
14. Ray O. How the mind hurts and heals the body. Am Psychol. 2004;59(1):29–40.
15. Vitetta L, Anton B, Cortizo F, Sali A. Mind-body medicine: stress and its impact on overall health and longevity. Ann N Y Acad Sci. 2005;1057:492–505.
16. Ikemi Y, Nakagawa S. A psychosomatic study of contagious dermatitis. Kyushu J Med Sci. 1962;13:335–52. https://www.semanticscholar.org/paper/A-psychosomatic-study-of-contagious-dermatitis-Ikemi-Nakagawa/65442ac9d4e7a800a55734c65601d591957a39a9.
17. Luparello TJ, Leist N, Lourie CH, Sweet P. The interaction of psychologic stimuli and pharmacologic agents on airway reactivity in asthmatic subjects. Psychosom Med. 1970;32(5):509–13.
18. Evers AWM, Colloca L, Blease C, Annoni M, Atlas LY, Benedetti F, et al. Implications of placebo and nocebo effects for clinical practice: expert consensus. Psychother Psychosom. 2018;87(4):204–10.
19. McCambridge J, Witton J, Elbourne DR. Systematic review of the Hawthorne effect: new concepts are needed to study research participation effects. J Clin Epidemiol. 2014;67(3):267–77.
20. McDonald CJ, Mazzuca SA, McCabe GP. How much of the placebo "effect" is really statistical regression? Stat Med. 1983;2(4):417–27.
21. Hróbjartsson A, Kaptchuk TJ, Miller FG. Placebo effect studies are susceptible to response bias and to other types of biases. J Clin Epidemiol. 2011;64(11):1223–9.
22. Fent R, Rosemann T, Fässler M, Senn O, Huber CA. The use of pure and impure placebo interventions in primary care—a qualitative approach. BMC Fam Pract. 2011;12:11.
23. Lembo A, Kelley JM, Nee J, Ballou S, Iturrino J, Cheng V, et al. Open-label placebo vs. double-blind placebo for irritable bowel syndrome: a randomized clinical trial. Pain. 2021;162(9):2428–35.
24. Colloca L, Enck P, DeGrazia D. Relieving pain using dose-extending placebos: a scoping review. Pain. 2016;157(8):1590–8.
25. Hróbjartsson A, Gøtzsche PC. Placebo interventions for all clinical conditions. Cochrane Database Syst Rev. 2010;2010(1):CD003974.
26. Hafliðadóttir SH, Juhl CB, Nielsen SM, Henriksen M, Harris IA, Bliddal H, et al. Placebo response and effect in randomized clinical trials: meta-research with focus on contextual effects. Trials. 2021;22(1):493.
27. Tsutsumi Y, Tsujimoto Y, Tajika A, Omae K, Fujii T, Onishi A, et al. Proportion attributable to contextual effects in general medicine: a meta-epidemiological study based on Cochrane reviews. BMJ Evid Based Med. 2023;28(1):40–7.
28. Horing B, Weimer K, Muth ER, Enck P. Prediction of placebo responses: a systematic review of the literature. Front Psychol. 2014;5:1079.
29. Espay AJ, Norris MM, Eliassen JC, Dwivedi A, Smith MS, Banks C, et al. Placebo effect of medication cost in Parkinson disease: a randomized double-blind study. Neurology. 2015;84(8):794–802.

30. Waber RL, Shiv B, Carmon Z, Ariely D. Commercial features of placebo and therapeutic efficacy. JAMA. 2008;299(9):1016–7.
31. Tétreault P, Mansour A, Vachon-Presseau E, Schnitzer TJ, Apkarian AV, Baliki MN. Brain connectivity predicts placebo response across chronic pain clinical trials. PLoS Biol. 2016;14(10):e1002570.
32. Benedetti F, Piedimonte A, Frisaldi E. How do placebos work? Eur J Psychotraumatol. 2018;9(Suppl 3):1533370.
33. Trivedi MH, South C, Jha MK, Rush AJ, Cao J, Kurian B, et al. A novel strategy to identify placebo responders: prediction index of clinical and biological markers in the EMBARC trial. Psychother Psychosom. 2018;87(5):285–95.
34. Levine JD, Gordon NC, Fields HL. The mechanism of placebo analgesia. Lancet. 1978;2(8091):654–7.
35. Gracely RH, Dubner R, Wolskee PJ, Deeter WR. Placebo and naloxone can alter post-surgical pain by separate mechanisms. Nature. 1983;306(5940):264–5.
36. Zubieta JK, Bueller JA, Jackson LR, Scott DJ, Xu Y, Koeppe RA, et al. Placebo effects mediated by endogenous opioid activity on μ-opioid receptors. J Neurosci. 2005;25(34):7754–62.
37. Benedetti F, Colloca L, Torre E, Lanotte M, Melcarne A, Pesare M, et al. Placebo-responsive Parkinson patients show decreased activity in single neurons of subthalamic nucleus. Nat Neurosci. 2004;7(6):587–8.
38. Benedetti F, Durando J, Vighetti S. Nocebo and placebo modulation of hypobaric hypoxia headache involves the cyclooxygenase-prostaglandins pathway. Pain. 2014;155(5):921–8.
39. Zunhammer M, Spisák T, Wager TD, Bingel U, Placebo Imaging Consortium. Meta-analysis of neural systems underlying placebo analgesia from individual participant fMRI data. Nat Commun. 2021;12(1):1391.
40. Afach S, Evrenoglou T, Oubaya N, Le Cleach L, Sbidian E. Most randomized controlled trials for psoriasis used placebo comparators despite the availability of effective treatments. J Clin Epidemiol. 2021;133:72–9.
41. Lichtenberg P, Heresco-Levy U, Nitzan U. The ethics of the placebo in clinical practice. J Med Ethics. 2004;30(6):551–4.
42. Mehta N, Gupta V. Psychosocial impact of vitiligo in patients with skin of color. Dermatol Rev. 2022;3(5):269–75.
43. Dev T, Mehta N, Goldust M, Khan E, Gupta S. Iatrogenic arsenicosis in a young female causing cosmetic distress. J Cosmet Dermatol. 2022;21(12):7235–6.
44. Use of Placebo in Clinical Practice | ama-coe [Internet]. https://code-medical-ethics.ama-assn.org/ethics-opinions/use-placebo-clinical-practice. Accessed 6 Mar 2023.

Procedural Dermatology: What Dermatologists Can Do and What They Cannot—A Resident Doctor's Perspective

19

Arunachalam Narayanan

Aging is inevitable. However, none of us like to have an aged appearance. While surgical procedures have been done since time immemorial, the rage towards obtaining the perfect supple young skin in the twenty-first century has led to a boom in procedural dermatology. In addition to consumer demand, the resultant attractive financial rewards have encouraged more and more dermatologists to take up procedural dermatology [1]. Professional needs also compel patients to undergo cosmetic procedures. In addition, economic growth, improved middle-class affordability, and increased social media influence have increased the demand for cosmetic procedures. These factors have created a unique scenario where more and more dermatologists are taking up procedures which were not routinely considered under the ambit of dermatology.

From the times of Sushruta to modern times, surgical treatments for aesthetic concerns have come a long way. Sushruta worked on rhinoplasty to repair disfigured noses of those who were punished with amputation of the nose for theft and other crimes as early as 600 BC. Modern dermatologic surgery evolved only in the last 150 years. Dermatologists started using peels in the late 1800s to smooth wrinkles and facial scarring [2]. Cryosurgery was first used by Campbell White in 1899 to remove skin lesions including naevi, warts, and epitheliomas [3]. Mackee started using phenol for treating facial scars in 1903. In 1905, Kromeyer introduced an early form of dermabrasion. Mackee also introduced electrosurgical fulguration to dermatology in 1909. Dermatologists like Noel were actively performing blepharoplasty and facelifts during the 1920s. Mohs' work during the 1930s in the treatment of cutaneous malignancies changed the way melanomas and non-melanoma skin cancers are treated even today [4]. In the latter part of the twentieth century, multiple procedures like soft tissue augmentation, liposuction, and laser surgeries were

A. Narayanan (✉)
Department of Dermatology (Skin and STD), Jawaharlal Institute of Postgraduate Medical Education and Research, Puducherry, India

S. Gupta et al. (eds.), *Critical Thinking in Contemporary Dermatology: Cognitive Essays*, https://doi.org/10.1007/978-981-97-0411-8_19

introduced. Professor Howard Green's pioneering work in culturing keratinocytes was initially in the field of burns treatment [5]. Green's method was later adopted to treat vitiligo and non-healing ulcers and wounds. Similarly, the concept of platelet-rich plasma was conceived initially by haematologists and platelet-rich fibrin was used a decade later in maxillofacial surgery. However, platelet-rich plasma has become the go-to treatment option in cosmetic dermatology in the current day. The work of Carruthers (dermatologist) and Carruthers (ophthalmologist), a husband-and-wife team, enabled the cosmetic use of botulinum toxin [6]. That widened the therapeutic uses of botulinum toxin, which was primarily used to treat strabismus and blepharospasm till then.

Over the last few years, dermatologists have had the opportunity to get trained in various aspects of procedural dermatology during or after completing their residency. The spectrum of procedures practised by dermatologists includes botulinum toxin, fillers, microneedling, subcision, vitiligo surgery, and sclerotherapy. There are also a number of procedures that have been introduced by other specialties only to be adopted by dermatologists later on. This raises a question: where is the line of distinction? Is it with respect to a procedure? Can a dermatologist do fat transfer or liposuction? If one dermatologist is trained to do fat transfer, does it mean every dermatologist can do it? Can a dermatologist do sclerotherapy of all veins? I will discuss in this chapter what kind of procedures dermatologists can do and what they cannot, or should ideally not do.

During my early training days, my seniors would ensure we did not handle trichloroacetic acid application or electrosurgical procedures over the face. Frustrated over this restriction, one of my friends decided to do a trichloroacetic acid application over the face of a patient on his own. It ended disastrously when a drop of the trichloroacetic acid sticking to his gloves touched the patient's forehead, and she winced with pain. Thankfully, the patient did not have any lasting pigmentation or scarring. In that scenario, the distinction on what procedures we could do and could not do was decided by our training or, more specifically, the lack of it at that point of time. Once we get trained under an expert's guidance and assist in a sufficient number of cases, we can practice the said procedure independently. In our case, we had the benefit of doing procedures while a senior observed and ensured that we did it the right way. Breaking this ladder and skipping a step backfires often. **Dermatologists can do procedures they are trained for and should refrain from doing procedures they are not trained for.**

Dermatologists should have a clear idea about the profile of their patients. This helps in addressing their concerns. A professional need-based client would want to 'look good'. A few other clients may want to 'feel good' by removing their seborrheic keratosis and skin tags. Yet another patient may come to us with an emotional need requiring only reassurance and counselling. Clients with special occasion-based needs would like to look good on a particular day. Children/adolescents with symptoms suggestive of body dysmorphic disorder might require a liaison with a psychiatrist or psychotherapist. Understanding the needs of a patient is essential before taking up a procedure. When a dermatologist does not spend adequate time to understand a patient's needs, it results in an incongruence of objectives between the dermatologist and the patient. A procedure with significant downtime might not be appropriate for a professional need-based client or bride. **Dermatologists should do procedures after understanding the needs of a patient.**

The first time we utilised the R20 technique in an Indian patient, we were not aware of the side effects due to repeated exposure of laser on Indian skin. We explained the chance of blistering and residual scarring to our patient before we started. One day after the procedure, the patient presented with blistering over the areas (Fig. 19.1) where the tattoo was band-like and had received repeated exposures. The patient was calm since we had explained the chance of that side effect. If not, he would have been under significant mental duress. **Dermatologists should do procedures only after explaining the risk and likelihood of side effects to the patient** [7].

In addition to side effects experienced post-procedure, dermatologists should also be aware of the changes patients experience post-procedure. In one of our leprosy patients, we undertook radial cutaneous nerve biopsy after explaining the risk of sensory loss post-biopsy to the patient. One week after the biopsy, he presented to us in a worried state with loss of sensation in a small patch on the hand. While he had heard what we had told before the procedure, he had not considered it seriously till then. Often, it requires more than one session to educate the patient regarding the procedure and the side effects which are likely to occur. Patients might not be able to grasp everything we say due to their anxious state of mind. In such a scenario, it is essential to discuss the issues properly with the patient and ensure they have time to digest the information and ask questions.

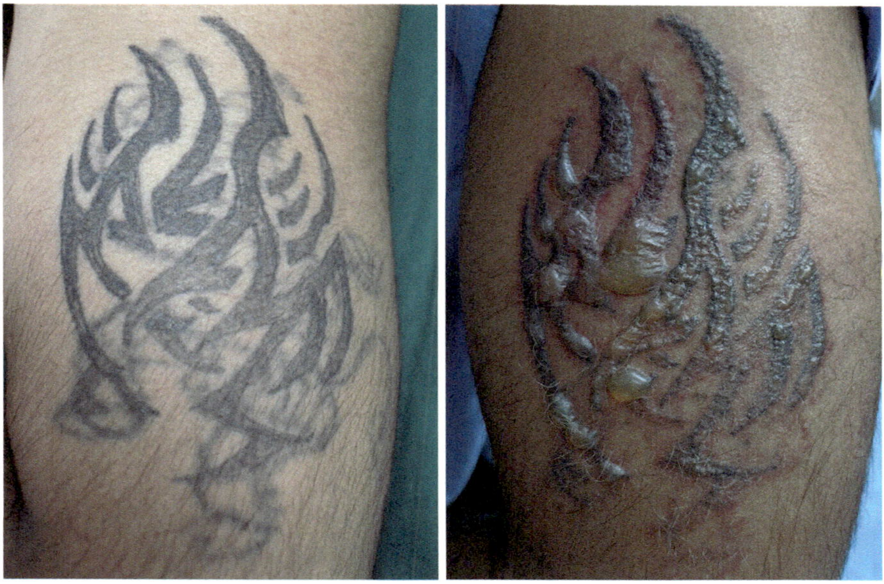

Fig. 19.1 Pre- and post-treatment photographs of a patient who underwent repeated exposures of QS Nd:YAG tattoo

In private practice, we are sometimes enticed to take up procedures by patients who keep requesting us to do more and more procedures one after another. While the financial incentive is enticing, such patients are often never satisfied [8]. Some of those patients have body dysmorphic disorder (BDD). They would keep coming back after every procedure with dissatisfaction with the outcome. "Beauty is in the eye of the beholder". This stands for how one perceives one's own body too. If one's perception of one's own body doesn't change, no procedure will satisfy one's desires. Incidence of body dysmorphic disorder among patients seeking cosmetic treatment is as high as 53.6% [9]. It is important to screen patients for BDD before performing aesthetic procedures [10]. These patients often end up being lawsuits-in-waiting for dermatologists. More importantly, as long as the patient isn't happy, the dermatologist will never get to savour the success or fruits of their efforts. **Dermatologists should not do procedures on patients with unrealistic expectations.**

I was once consulted by a patient with keloidal tendency for tattoo removal. He had undergone a laser session 2 years ago with keloids at that tattoo site (Fig. 19.2). He wanted to continue the procedure despite the high risk of keloidal tendency and was willing to sign a high-risk informed consent. In that scenario, what is the right thing to do? Can I take him up for laser sessions since he has given high-risk

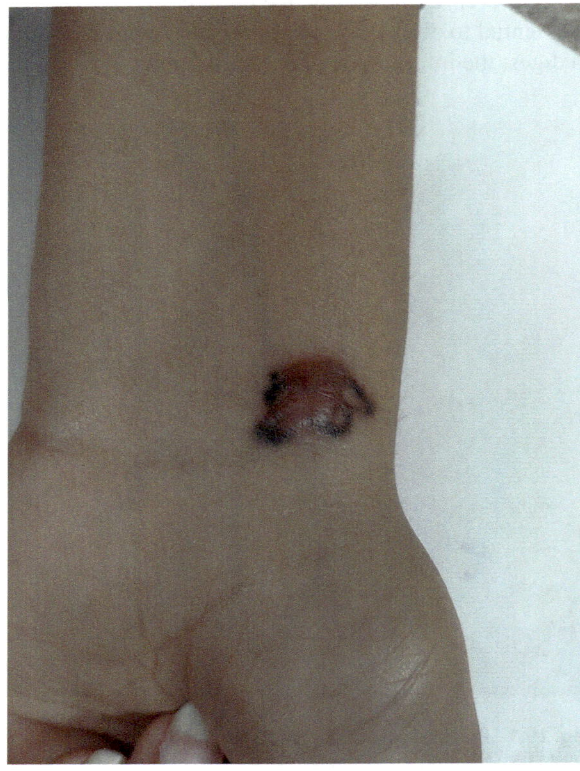

Fig. 19.2 Patient presenting with keloid over the tattoo site after a session of laser

consent, or should I refuse? While taking a call to treat the patient or not is a personal clinical decision depending on the treating physician, we should never forget the first rule of medicine—'primum non nocere'. As a physician, it is our solemn duty not to harm the patient.

With time and experience, we gain a sense of security with what we do. But adverse side effects or unexpected complications can strike anytime. Few years back, we performed a skin biopsy procedure in a leg swelling with a differential diagnosis of mycetoma. During the procedure, there was a spurt of bright-red blood from the biopsy site as soon as the skin sample was extracted. It was an arteriovenous malformation that we had misdiagnosed clinically as mycetoma. After multiple unsuccessful attempts to arrest the bleed, we asked our surgery colleagues to assist us in controlling the bleed. They were kind enough to come immediately, and the patient was eventually fine. This was an important lesson for me. **Dermatologists should take up elective procedures in procedure rooms equipped with adequate facilities to manage complications.** Taking up a procedure assuming it wouldn't meet any hurdles is a sure-shot way of setting oneself up for failure.

While dermatologists recognise that not all patients respond well to all treatments, expecting the same understanding from patients is unfair. Recently, I had prescribed glycolic acid peels to a patient of facial melanosis. We had repeated three sittings with no improvement following which the patient got frustrated and angry regarding the lack of improvement and the wastage of his time. This could have been avoided if proper communication had been established with the patient. Every dermatologist must explain the expected improvement to the patient and make sure she/he is willing to undergo the procedure. Educating the patient on the predicted response and chance of resistance to treatment is also an integral part of our clinical practice. **Dermatologists can do procedures after communicating the expected outcome to the patient and after confirming that the patient has realistic expectations.**

Recently we saw a woman with basal cell carcinoma over the post-auricular area overlapping the lobule (Fig. 19.3). There was a discussion regarding the possibility of taking up the case for excision or referring her to plastic surgery. After discussion, we decided to refer her to a plastic surgery colleague. While we had the training to do excision of basal cell carcinoma, we did not have the expertise to do pinna-reconstruction in an aesthetically appealing way. Our plastic surgery colleagues were trained to deal with challenging cases and would provide a cosmetically better result. Standard of care provided by us to a patient should be based on the best evidence available. **Dermatologists should be willing to refer patients to other experts if they are not sure of the results they can provide.** While it is never easy to accept one's limitations, taking ownership of aesthetically unappealing results is much more damaging.

The sanctity of informed consent can never be understated [11]. We should undertake procedures only after written informed consent. While all physicians get written consent religiously, most doctors worldwide fail to meet patients' expectations regarding the 'informed' part in the consent. **Dermatologists should do procedures only after written informed consent, and never without.**

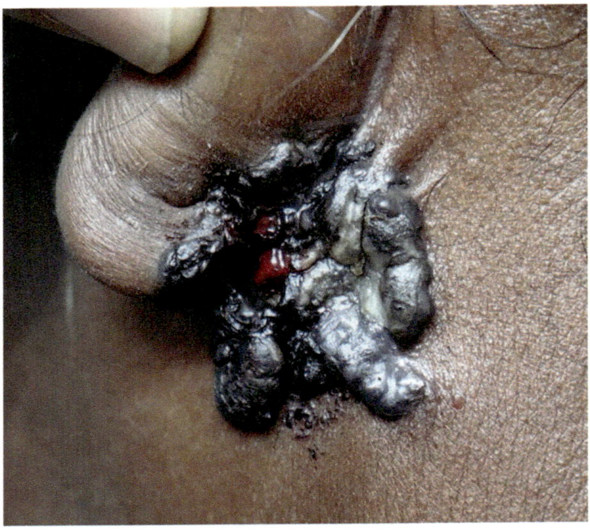

Fig. 19.3 Pigmented basal cell carcinoma over the post-auricular area with involvement of the lobule (Courtesy: Dr. Jayakrishna A)

Table 19.1 Examples of cosmetic surgical procedures that can be performed by dermatologists and procedures which are best avoided (number of procedures performed by ASPS member surgeons inside parentheses) [12]

Procedures that can be performed	Procedures that are best avoided
Rhytidectomy (234 thousand procedures) Liposuction (211 thousand procedures) Dermabrasion (139 thousand procedures) Malar augmentation (108 thousand procedures) Forehead lift (88 thousand procedures)	Rhinoplasty (352 thousand procedures) Blepharoplasty (325 thousand procedures) Augmentation mammoplasty (193 thousand procedures) Abdominoplasty (97 thousand procedures) Mastopexy (87 thousand procedures) Otoplasty (53 thousand procedures)

The American Society of Plastic Surgeons (ASPS) report showed that the most common minimally invasive cosmetic procedure performed by ASPS member surgeons in 2020 was botulinum toxin followed by soft tissue fillers [12]. The most common cosmetic surgical procedure in 2020 was rhinoplasty followed by blepharoplasty. While the minimally invasive procedures can be taken up by dermatologists, prudent dermatologists would stay away from surgical procedures like rhinoplasty and blepharoplasty, unless they are specifically trained (Tables 19.1 and 19.2).

While hair transplantation, botulinum toxin, soft tissue fillers, and radiofrequency ablation have always been practised by dermatologists, younger dermatologists have also started performing liposuction and fat transfer successfully. The need for Mohs surgery is rapidly raising with over 876,000 tumours excised using Mohs surgery in the United States in 2012 [13]. Dermatosurgeons have also started excision of xanthelasma with aesthetically appealing results. While dermatologists are

Table 19.2 Examples of minimally invasive cosmetic procedures that can be performed by dermatologists (number of procedures performed by ASPS member surgeons inside parentheses) [12]

Minimally invasive cosmetic procedures that can be performed by dermatologists
Botulinum toxin (4.4 million procedures)
Soft tissue fillers (3.4 million procedures)
Laser resurfacing (990 thousand procedures)
Chemical peels (930 thousand procedures)
Intense pulsed light treatment (827 thousand procedures)
Laser hair removal (757 thousand procedures)
Microdermabrasion (522 thousand procedures)
Non-invasive fat reduction (357 thousand procedures)
Sclerotherapy (295 thousand procedures)
Non-surgical skin tightening (188 thousand procedures)
Injection lipolysis (135 thousand procedures)

adequately trained to deal with these conditions, they are not well-trained to deal with tendon transfer surgeries or surgeries conducted under general anaesthesia. **Prudent dermatologists would stay away from such invasive surgeries unless they have received a special training in them.**

Lasers have conventionally been used by dermatologists for the treatment of ageing skin, tattoos, pigmentation, and unwanted hair. However, specialised lasers like endovenous lasers should be used only by trained physicians. Such specialised training may not be available to everyone and it is better to stay away from procedures in which one is not properly trained. When used by an untrained person, even pigmentary lasers might cause significant blistering and other complications.

In addition to aesthetic procedures, dermatologists sometimes take up procedures like circumcision. While a few training centres provide appropriate training during the undergraduate course, not all training centres provide that. Any dermatologist should take up such surgeries only if she/he is confident of their ability. Similarly, skin grafting for skin ulcers was earlier done by plastic surgeons. The uptake of the graft depends on the skill of the surgeon and due diligence must be taken to assess one's ability before taking up a patient for surgery.

Once we leave our parent institute and move out, often we find ourselves in situations where there is no senior to guide us. This raises the question: how does one learn new skills? While it is enticing to learn new dermatological procedures as we practice and improve ourselves without a break in clinical practice, one must develop the habit of looking at it from the patient's point of view. Would we be willing to put ourselves in the hands of a dermatologist who has not performed the procedure earlier? I find asking myself this question to often solve the question of whether I can do a particular procedure or not.

The decision on whether to do a procedure or not depends on the dermatologist and their patient. If a dermatologist decides they have the required skill and infrastructure to do the procedure and knowledge to anticipate and prevent complications, they are justified in doing it.

References

1. Hibler BP, Eliades PJ, Kagha KC, Avram MM. Litigation arising from minimally invasive cosmetic procedures: a review of the literature. Dermatol Surg. 2021;47:1606–13.
2. Coleman WP, Hanke CW, Orentreich N, Kurtin SB, Brody H, Bennett R. A history of dermatologic surgery in the United States. Dermatol Surg. 2000;26:5–11.
3. Zacarian SA. The art and science of cryosurgery. J Dermatol Surg Oncol. 1977;3:401–2.
4. Mohs FE. Chemosurgery: microscopically controlled surgery for skin cancer—past, present and future. J Dermatol Surg Oncol. 1978;4:41–54.
5. Green H. The birth of therapy with cultured cells. BioEssays. 2008;30:897–903.
6. Carruthers JD, Carruthers JA. Treatment of glabellar frown lines with *C. botulinum*-A exotoxin. J Dermatol Surg Oncol. 1992;18:17–21.
7. Hamasaki T, Takehara T, Hagihara A. Physicians' communication skills with patients and legal liability in decided medical malpractice litigation cases in Japan. BMC Fam Pract. 2008;9:43.
8. Situm M, Buljan M. How to protect medical professionals from unrealistic expectations of clients in corrective dermatology? Acta Clin Croat. 2010;49:509–13.
9. Ribeiro RVE. Prevalence of body dysmorphic disorder in plastic surgery and dermatology patients: a systematic review with meta-analysis. Aesthet Plast Surg. 2017;41:964–70.
10. Malick F, Howard J, Koo J. Understanding the psychology of the cosmetic patients. Dermatol Ther. 2008;21:47–53.
11. Rathor MY, Rani MFA, Shah AM, Akter SF. Informed consent: a socio-legal study. Med J Malays. 2011;66:423–8.
12. American Society of Plastic Surgeons. Plastic Surgery Statistics. https://www.plasticsurgery.org/news/plastic-surgery-statistics. Accessed 12 Jan 2022.
13. Asgari MM, Olson J, Alam M. Needs assessment for Mohs micrographic surgery. Dermatol Clin. 2012;30:167–75.

Core Concepts of Dermatologic Surgery 20

Nikhil Mehta, Narayanan Baskaran, and Somesh Gupta

Dermatologic surgery has become an integral and essential component of dermatological practice. The American Society for Dermatological Surgery refers to dermatologic surgery as a "specialty dealing with the diagnosis and treatment of medically necessary and cosmetic conditions of the skin, hair, nails, veins, mucous membranes and adjacent tissues by various surgical, reconstructive, cosmetic and nonsurgical methods" [1]. They propose that the purpose of dermatologic surgery is to repair and/or improve the function and cosmetic appearance of skin tissue. There are various dermatologic surgery procedures ranging from conventional dermatologic surgery techniques like cryotherapy, nail surgeries, and vitiligo surgeries; to more advanced cosmetic procedures like facial rejuvenation, lip augmentation, and fillers; to use of lasers, light sources, and energy-based devices. In addition to all the advances taking place in this field, one needs to be aware of the core concepts of dermatologic surgery which hold true for all these advancements. While the basics of dermatologic surgery like patient selection, Operation Theatre (OT) setup, and asepsis are covered in dermatologic surgery textbooks, the themes underlying the development and rationale of these procedures are not discussed. These fundamental concepts are learned through experience and do not translate well in textbooks. They can also guide goals and direct the development of further innovations.

N. Mehta · S. Gupta (✉)
Department of Dermatology and Venereology, All India Institute of Medical Sciences, New Delhi, India
e-mail: someshgupta@aiims.edu

N. Baskaran
Department of Dermatology and Venereology, Post Graduate Institute of Medical Education and Research, Chandigarh, India

S. Gupta et al. (eds.), *Critical Thinking in Contemporary Dermatology: Cognitive Essays*, https://doi.org/10.1007/978-981-97-0411-8_20

20.1 Surgical Frugality/Tissue Saving

One of the most important core concepts of dermatologic surgery is surgical frugality. It is based on the simple approach of "first do no harm." Surgical frugality is the hallmark of cosmetic dermatologic surgery. While others refer to "frugality in dermatologic surgery" as saving resources and operating with limited means, [2] we here refer to frugality as being frugal with the skin tissue rather than with resources. Frugality in surgery refers to the approach causing minimal collateral damage thereby maximizing the safety of the patient and thereby also achieving an optimal cosmetic outcome. The most dreaded complication for a dermatologic surgeon would be a worsening of the appearance of the patient as compared to pre-procedure, which is especially applicable for cosmetic procedures. The development of complications due to the overzealous and over-ambitious procedures could lead to a dissatisfied patient and also hamper the confidence of the operating dermatologic surgeon. Formation of dog-ears due to large elliptical excision on the face; development of complications like brow ptosis, spock eyebrows, and asymmetry of the face due to inexpert administration of botulinum toxin; excision of keloids at sites having high rates of recurrence (such as presternal skin) are examples of the above.

Lasers exemplify this approach as they are selective to their chromophores and cause minimum damage to surrounding tissue [3]. Newer lasers and methods like pinhole techniques lead to even lesser collateral tissue damage than the previous ones.

Subungual tumors like glomus tumors are difficult to remove owing to their location underlying the nail plate and/or the proximal nail fold. Conventional methods like removal of partial/entire nail plate to access the area would lead to a larger raw area, and subsequently delayed healing and pain and discomfort. To overcome these hurdles and reduce patients' suffering, Bhatia et al. developed a simple, radiofrequency-assisted "*onychostomy*" for minimally invasive extraction of subungual tumors. In this technique, radiofrequency is used to create a small hole in the nail plate to gain access to the tumor in the subungual region, which is then dissected and the excised plate of the nail plate is put back in its place as a biological dressing (Fig. 20.1) [4].

Melanocytic nevi are common benign proliferations of melanocytes that can be a cosmetic concern over the face. Punch excision is a preferred modality of elimination of these nevi, but this technique is associated with the formation of tissue protrusions or dog-ear formation. To evade this complication, Gupta et al. proposed the use of a punch graft taken from the postauricular area of the patient to fill the defect caused by the punch excision [5]. This saves some loss of normal skin associated with elliptical excision. Also, they propose the use of serial excision at spaced out intervals as the best approach for larger nevi, as it would expand the tissue during each excision and help to carry out subsequent closure without tension. It also reduces the loss of normal tissue and prevent the formation of a dog-ear during excision of a round nevus (Fig. 20.2) [6].

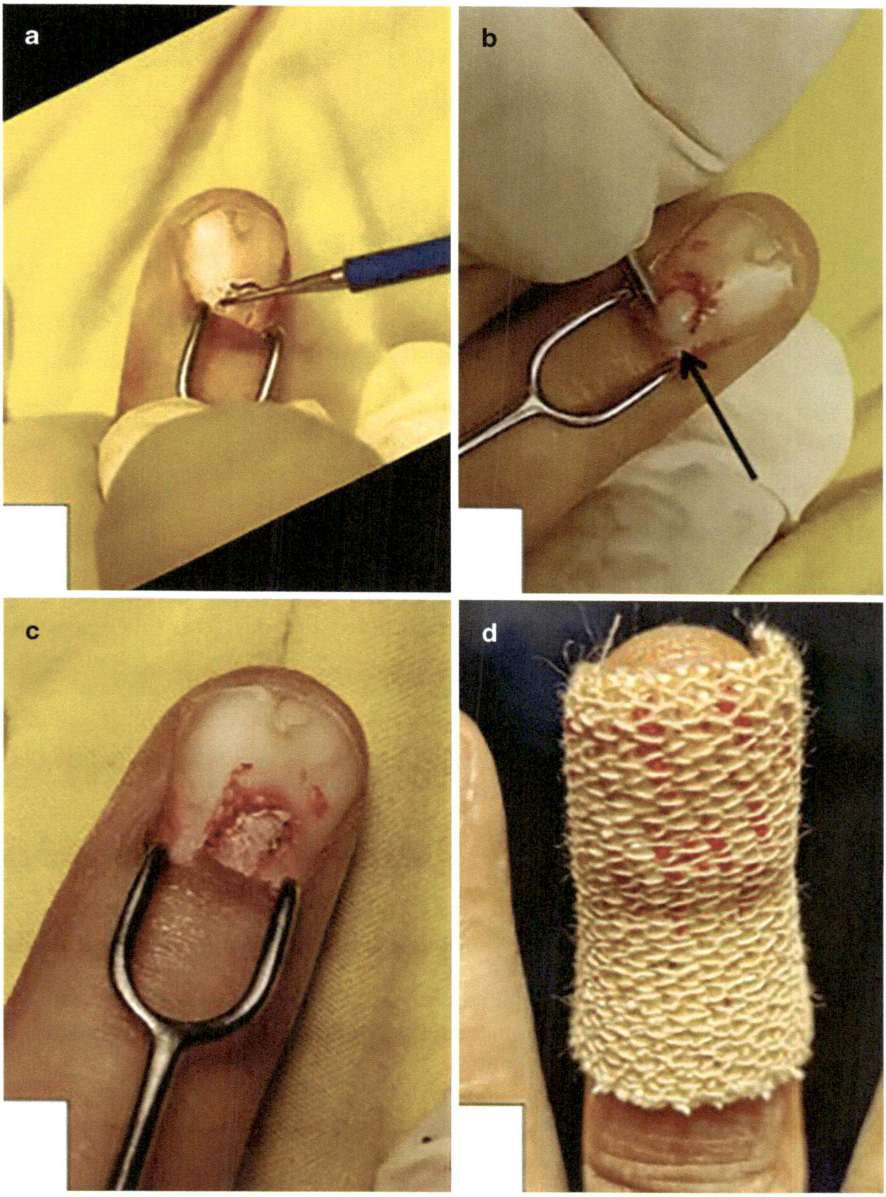

Fig. 20.1 Radiofrequency assisted onychotomy. (**a**) Retraction of proximal nail fold and creation of a window at the proximal nail plate above a glomus tumor using radio-frequency probe; (**b**) extraction of glomus tumor using blunt dissection [arrow], (**c**) placing the nail plate fragment back into the defect, (**d**) dressing with adhesive bandage. [Reproduced with permission from authors from- Bhatia S, Chauhan J, Grover C, Gupta S. Radiofrequency-assisted onychostomy for minimally invasive extraction of subungual tumors. J Am Acad Dermatol. 2022 Jan;86(1):e5–6]

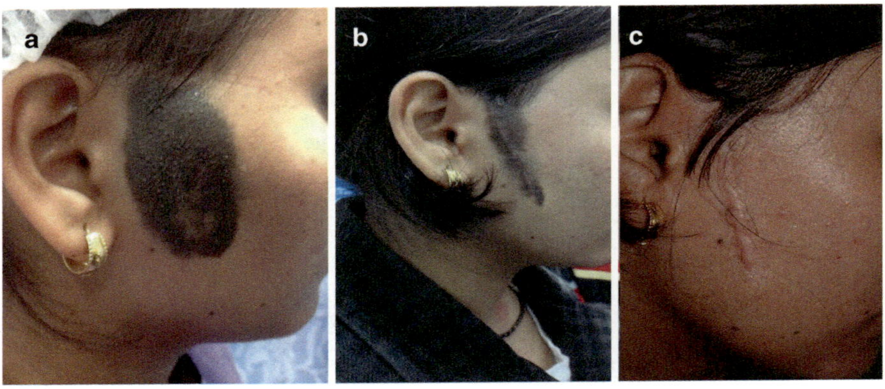

Fig. 20.2 Serial excision of compound melanocytic nevus (**a**) baseline. (**b**) Two months after first surgical excision of a part of the nevus. (**c**) After all sessions

20.2 Minimalistic Approach

Dermatologic surgeons are not native to surgery, but immigrants. They are more hesitant and less adventurous as opposed to other surgeons. This inherent nature can be utilized to our advantage. Since we deal with surgeries that primarily have a cosmetic outcome, our goal of surgery must be optimal desirable outcomes while maximizing safety. The minimalistic approach in dermatologic surgery refers to surgeries and procedures that are minimally invasive, with minimal healing time and minimal downtime for the patients, being minimally painful, with minimal risk of complications, yet delivering the maximum outcome. Minimally invasive surgery not only improves cosmetic outcomes but also has the potential to restrict the magnitude of the surgical injury, which in turn can attenuate the inflammatory and neuroendocrine response resulting in less postoperative pain and quicker recovery. The invasiveness of the surgical procedure and the patients' tolerance to pain and complications are least for a cosmetic procedure when compared to a non-cosmetic procedure; thereby emphasizing the importance of a minimalistic approach in dermatologic surgery. The advent of chemical peels, fillers, and the use of botulinum toxin in facial rejuvenation are examples of the minimalistic approach [7].

A sub-concept of the minimalistic approach is the use of minimal essential tissue for transplants. The aesthetic outcome is always inversely proportional to the amount of tissue that has been transplanted; the smaller the unit of transplantation, the better would be the aesthetic outcome in the majority of the cases. Minimum essential tissue harvesting would also lead to minimal damage at the donor site. The concept of minimal tissue transplant has been maximally utilized in the field of vitiligo surgeries. Vitiligo surgeries have advanced from the basic old tissue transplant procedures like suction blister grafting, and split-thickness skin grafting which would lead to a donor—recipient ratio of 1:1 to the newer advanced cellular grafting techniques like the noncultured epidermal cell suspension (NCES) and cultured melanocyte grafts which have donor–recipient ratio ranging from 1:10 to 1:100. When we obtain the tissue sample from the donor site in NCES, it should be ultrathin to avoid donor site scarring. Dermal component in the graft is not only unnecessary but also disadvantageous. It leads to delayed healing at the donor site and scarring. And, a graft with a lot of dermis attached to it is difficult to digest with trypsin to prepare a single cell suspension. Thus minimizing the thickness of the harvested tissue prevents complications and adds to the success [8, 9]. Similarly, in mini-punch grafting for vitiligo, initially 2–2.5 mm punch grafts were used which would cause a lot of cobblestoning, subsequently the graft size was reduced to 1.5 mm and now micropunch grafts of 0.5–0.8 mm diameter as proposed by Bae et al. [10].

Another example of a minimalistic approach is the "manhole cover technique" for nail matrix biopsy, which involves using a deep 2 mm punch through the proximal nail fold blindly till the bone, without needing to retract it, horizontal separation of nail fold and nail matrix tissue from the biopsy specimen, and placement of the tissue of the nail fold back, saving tissue and time [11].

Another sub-concept of the minimalistic approach is the targeted pathological tissue ablation and preservation of normal surrounding tissue to achieve a good surgical outcome. Metaphorically, this can be compared with a "surgical strike" and a "terror strike." The former is done in a precise manner to destroy the target without much collateral damage. The latter is done to cause a lot of indiscriminate damage to generate fear in people's minds. Targeted pathological tissue ablation is like surgical strike, aimed to destroy the pathological tissue while sparing the normal tissue.

Cryotherapy is a method aimed at targeted destruction of pathological tissue. Although the method has many advantages in terms of being easy to perform, noninvasive, and inexpensive, it is associated with its fair share of complications like blistering, hypopigmentation, ulceration, and necrosis. To reduce its complications and expand its utility in rejuvenation and aesthetics, Gupta et al. proposed the use of thin plywood or transparent plastic plates with multiple uniform holes to deliver fractionated cryotherapy. Such plates can be custom-made and used to deliver targeted cryotherapy for indications like keloids, post-herpes zoster hypertrophic scars, cold slush peels, and facial rejuvenation (Fig. 20.3) [12]. This allows controlled minimal fractional freezing while sparing some tissue in between frozen area, which allows rapid regeneration of affected tissue resulting in less complications, such as depigmentation, which are inevitable sequelae of the conventional freezing.

Radiofrequency is an indispensable tool for a dermatologist for the treatment of various benign conditions. The use of intralesional electrosurgery has gained

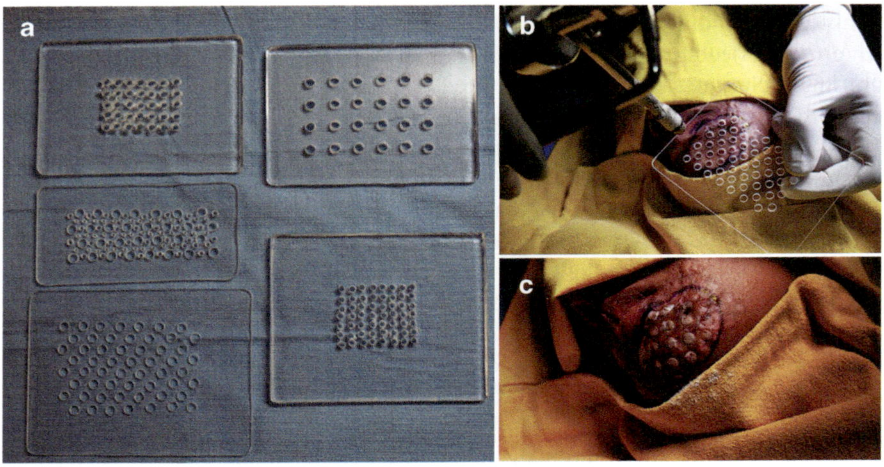

Fig. 20.3 Fractionated cryotherapy. (**a**) Multiple transparent plastic plates with holes of different sizes and arrangements to be used for different indications. (**b**) Liquid nitrogen sprayed over the transparent plastic plate with multiple holes placed over the chin of the patient with post-herpes zoster hypertrophic scars. (**c**) Skin with frozen areas in a grid pattern with spared normal skin in between the frozen areas. [Reproduced with permission from authors from- Gupta S, Yadav S, Patra S, Gupta S. Fractionated cryotherapy. J Am Acad Dermatol. 2017;77(3):e69–e71]

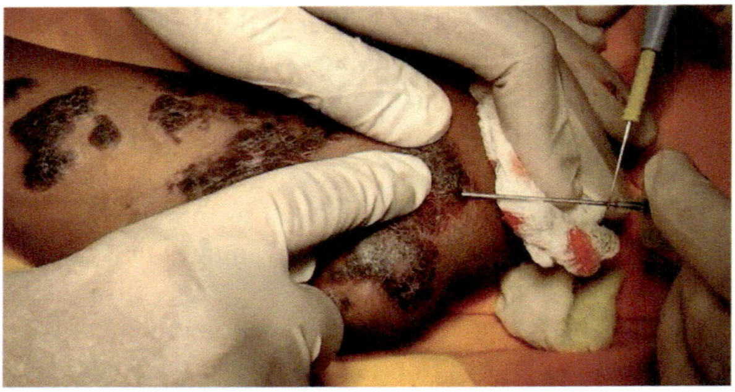

Fig. 20.4 Intralesional radiofrequency for a verrucous venous malformation. An intravenous cannula is taken and a small window in its plastic sheath near the proximal end of the cannula near the hub is made. Intralesional radiofrequency using RF probe is delivered by touching the metallic needle through the window

popularity in the treatment of a variety of benign and vascular conditions of the skin as it allows us to deliver maximum energy of the radiofrequency to the pathological part of the deep-seated lesion while sparing the normal, uninvolved epithelial tissue. By minimizing the surface complications like pigmentation, ulceration, scarring, and collateral damage, it serves as an excellent example of surgical frugality too.

The application of this novel method of insulated intralesional radiofrequency ablation was found to be safe and effective in vascular lesions including pyogenic granuloma, lymphangioma circumscriptum, venous and capillary venous malformations, and various deep dermal and subcutaneous lesions including hypertrophic scar, hidradenitis suppurativa, ganglion, acne cysts and sebaceous cysts in addition to angiolymphoid hyperplasia (Fig. 20.4) [13–17]. The technique can be combined with the intralesional deposition of steroids in the treatment of hypertrophic scars and keloids.

Pangti and colleagues also proposed the use of bipolar forceps of a high-power electrosurgical unit for the precise removal of small benign skin lesions. The authors propose that the use of bipolar forceps results in targeted destruction of pathological tissue and minimal collateral damage to surrounding skin as the flow of energy is restricted between the tips of the active and the return electrode. This method can be effectively used for the ablation of any benign lesion with a diameter of 1–2 cm like genital warts (Fig. 20.5) [18].

Electromechanical resection refers to the simultaneous use of electrocoagulation energy with mechanical resection. The technique of electromechanical resection for small, benign growths like acrochordons, filiform warts, and neurofibromas was

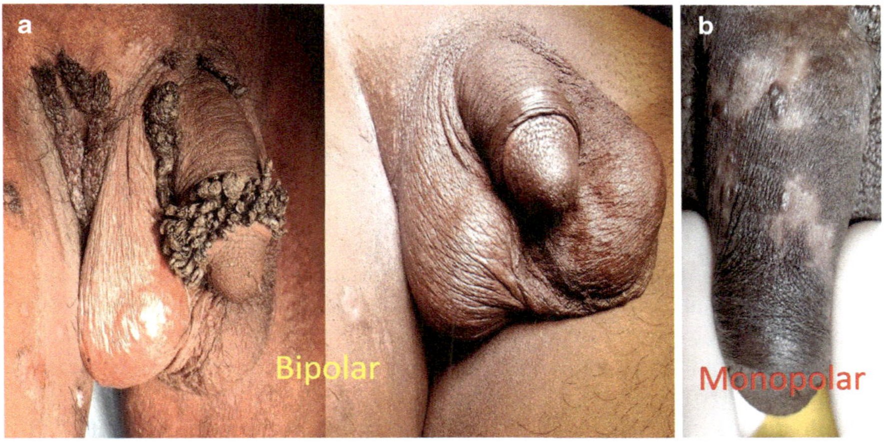

Fig. 20.5 (**a**) A patient with multiple genital warts, and six months after removal of warts with bipolar forceps without scarring. (**b**) In comparison, persistence of warts and presence of depigmentation is seen in a case where monopolar electrode was used for radiofrequency ablation. [Reproduced with permission from authors from- Pangti R, Dixit A, Gupta S. Bipolar forceps of a high-power electrosurgical unit for precise removal of small benign skin lesions. J Am Acad Dermatol. 2020 May;82(5):e155–6]

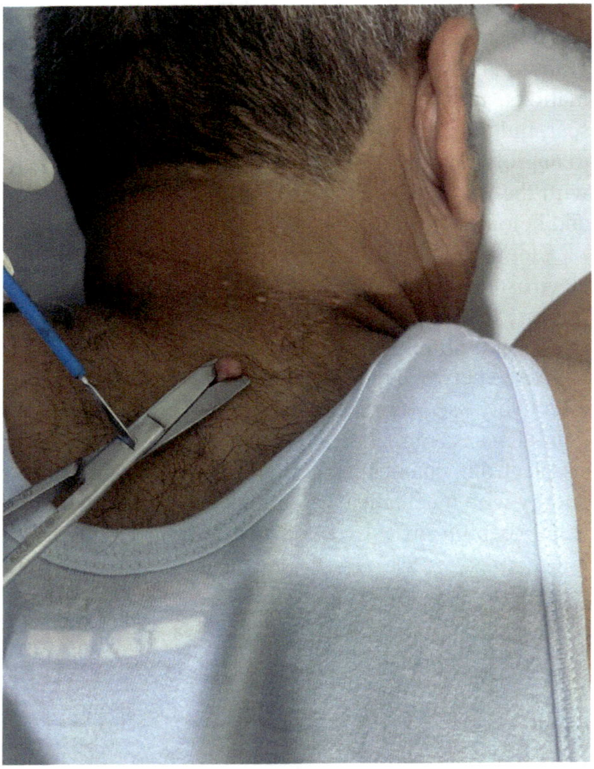

Fig. 20.6 Resection of skin tag using the electromechanical resection technique

proposed by Pangti et al. In this technique, the lesion is grasped with a toothed forceps, and its base is cut with a scissor while simultaneously touching the hinge of the scissor with monopolar electrode tip in coagulation mode. This would ensure faster excision, obviate the need for anesthesia, eliminate bleeding, reduce the total amount and duration of radiofrequency energy delivery, and achieve faster scar-free healing (Fig. 20.6) [19].

Hidradenitis suppurativa is difficult to manage. Appropriate surgery is the only potentially "curative" modality, at least for the site where it is done, but it entails significant morbidity and prolonged healing times, and in some cases, practically not feasible. Permanent hair removal through lasers or radiofrequency epilation is a minimally invasive intervention targeting the likely site of origin of pathology in it. It does not cure, but reduces the severity and morbidity (Fig. 20.7) [20].

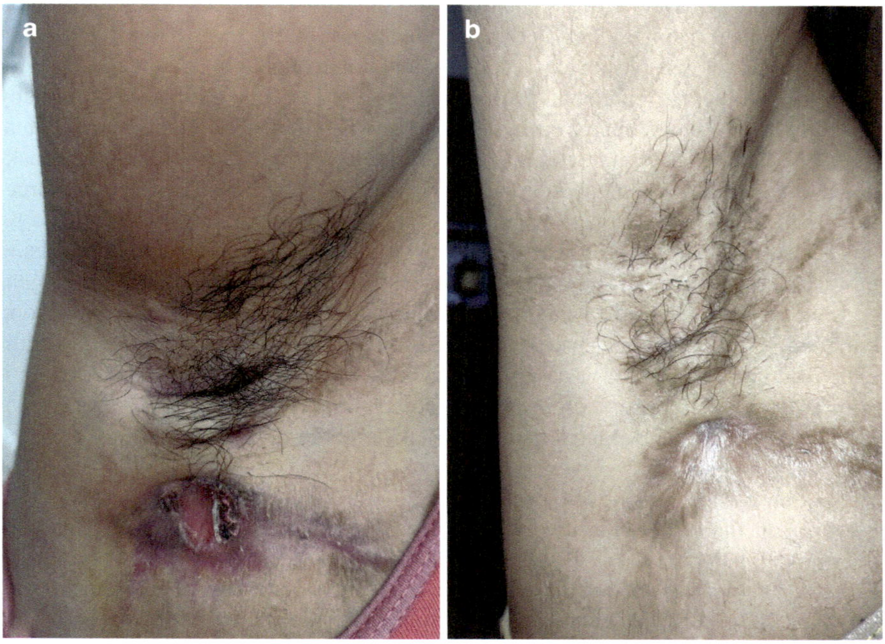

Fig. 20.7 Result of radiofrequency epilation using acupuncture needles in hidradenitis suppurativa. (**a**) Before treatment. (**b**) Four months after a single session. All lesions have healed, and no recurrence without any requirement of antibiotics. [Reproduced with permission from authors from- Mehta N, Khan E, Gupta S. Radiofrequency Epilation Using Acupuncture Needles to Decrease the Disease Burden in Hidradenitis Suppurativa. Dermatol Surg Off Publ Am Soc Dermatol Surg Al. 2022 Jul 1;48(7):788–9]

20.3 Anti-fragility/Adaptability in the Procedure Room

The next important core concept of dermatologic surgery is anti-fragility in the operating room. Anti-fragility is a desirable trait of a dermatologic surgeon, which makes one adaptable and innovative while facing adversities and constraints. Antifragile would embrace the adversity and use it to their advantage. One who is anti-fragile would learn from their previous mistakes and others' mistakes and would get better. They would also learn to be innovative and resourceful while faced with limitations. Although such innovations, when done to bypass resource constraints, have been cited as examples of "frugality," [2] we believe that they better represent the mettle of surgeons to adapt to change. Innovation technically means something new; a new idea, method, or device. It also refers to a new way of approaching and doing things or improving existing ones to give a better outcome. It also helps in overcoming problems associated with existing techniques or instruments like cost and feasibility, and providing effective and cheaper alternatives to them. As the old saying goes, necessity is the mother of invention.

For cellular grafts in vitiligo, the extracted shave biopsy needs to be incubated at 37 °C with the trypsin-EDTA solution in an incubator for the trypsin to act. However, incubators are expensive, space-occupying and not available in all centers. To overcome this problem, Gupta et al. proposed the use of patients' axillary vault thereby the body heat as an incubator during the period when they undergo dermabrasion at the recipient sites [21]. Interestingly, this technique was invented due to the breakdown of the door of the incubator on that particular day, demonstrating the resourcefulness of innovative dermatologists .

Dermabrasion of the recipient sites during vitiligo surgeries is usually done using motorized or manual dermabraders. However, they are associated with aerosol generation, which may lead to inadvertent injury and require an expensive diamond burr. This problem can be overcome by the use of collodion paint containing salicylic acid and lactic acid for de-epithelialization of the recipient site and rubbing it with a dry woven gauze to remove the already loosened epidermis [22]. Similar procedures can be invented on days when dermabraders get suddenly missing from OT!

Suction-blister grafting is a useful surgical modality in the treatment of vitiligo; however, in the initial stages it was limited by the requirement of expensive and heavy suction apparatus. Gupta et al. made a revolutionary change in this technique by using an apparatus consisting of a cylindrical funnel/cup connected with a three-way tap. One end of the cannula was connected to a vacuum gauge and the other end to a 50 mL syringe for suction [23]. The technique was further simplified by the use of disposable syringes used upside down on the patient's skin replacing the funnels/cups [24].

Patients with lipomas on cosmetic sites like the face desire excision; however, the limiting factor was the resultant linear scar of standard excision that may fail to improve the cosmetic outcome of the patient. The use of a "pot-lid" technique in which a 5 mm skin punch is inserted deep into the lesion, the punched-out skin is preserved in saline, the lipoma is extruded with a hemostat and squeezing pressure, following which the excised skin is repositioned to cover the defect like a pot-lid was shown to improve the aesthetic outcome [25].

There are several occasions when conventional dermatologic surgery equipment might not be available for use. This has led to the advent of easily available and cheaper alternatives that can practically be utilized for various procedures. The examples include the use of a hypodermic needle as a disposable skin hook, using the rim of the tip of a ballpoint pen without refill instead of a comedone extractor, utilizing kitchen chimney as a smoke evacuator in procedure rooms, and the use of sterile acupuncture needles as disposable electrosurgical electrodes [20, 26–28].

Subcision is a commonly used technique for the treatment of depressed scars including post-acne scars. To circumvent the risk of injury to deeper structures with the conventional technique, Khunger et al. proposed a modification where the procedure is done with a hypodermic needle bent at right angles at the end. This makes the procedure safer, easier, and ensures better orientation to the surgeon [29].

All these innovations display anti-fragility in the OT. Many of them were spur-of-the-moment thoughts necessitated by some sudden problem or deficiency, or came after deep contemplation for recurrent problems in OT.

20.4 Appropriate Procedure for Appropriate Indication

Not all procedures are appropriate for all patients. A basic screening of patients should be done to determine suitability. Expectations should be managed. Patients with unrealistic expectations despite counselling should not be taken up for surgery. Patients suspected to have body dysmorphic disorders should be referred for counselling.

The surgery should be done as per patient's need rather than patient's desires. For example, the general consensus is to have lesional and disease stability for at least 6 months before the surgical management of vitiligo, and patients should be counselled regarding the same rather than hurrying the procedure on patients' requests [30]. A patient coming to you for the first time with a self-reported history of lesional stability for 6 months but with ill-defined borders, trichrome pattern, and other signs of activity is definitely not suitable for immediate procedures. When in doubt, it is better to err on the side of caution.

Similarly, it can be argued whether a small superficial basal cell carcinoma in a debilitated 90-year-old warrants the gold standard surgical removal, or radiofrequency ablation, or if no intervention at all. Multiple sessions of a less-effective procedure might be more suitable rather than less sessions of a more-effective procedure. For example, a patient of post-acne scars might opt for microneedling rather than CO_2 laser ablation if the former is more affordable to her. Similarly, another might opt for just chemical peeling if she has blood phobia and does not want microneedling and fractional CO_2. A patient with a previous perceived adverse effect (example post-inflammatory pigmentation after CO_2 laser) with one procedure will prefer another procedure, even though that adverse effect might be transient and may not recur on decreasing fluence or using safe parameters.

Patients' inclinations do not always favor minimally invasive surgeries. Some patients and circumstances warrant a more aggressive procedure despite having more adverse effects. Patients may choose a complicated procedure with more adverse effects if that does not require multiple sessions. In a leprosy patient with large nonhealing ulcers who is not able to follow-up regularly for multiple sessions of platelet-rich fibrin therapy, a split-thickness skin graft might be preferable. Some patients of hidradenitis suppurativa or acne keloidalis nuchae may opt for a morbid surgery of wide local excision with healing by secondary intention, rather than primary closure or grafting, thinking about better results or to prevent scar at donor areas.

Being frugal is not always the way to go, and occasional spendthriftness might be required! The procedure most appropriate for a patient must be chosen after detailed consultation with him/her, after giving informed choices with pros and cons of the procedures, and addressing his/her concerns.

20.5 Under-Promise and Over-Deliver

An important core concept of procedural dermatology is to downplay the expected results to the patient. An important contraindication to any aesthetic procedure would be a patient with unrealistic expectations. It is important to always under-promise on the level of improvement that would be expected out of a procedure to the patient, thereafter choose appropriate patients and then try and over-deliver the results. This especially holds for aesthetic procedures like treatment of post-acne scars, facial scars, facial rejuvenation, chemical peels, dermabrasion, thread lifts, fillers, chemical peels, and lasers.

20.6 Combination for Synergism

Change is the only constant in life. Paraphrasing Darwin, it is not the strongest that survives, nor the most intelligent, it is the one that is most adaptable to change. Like many things, change is unpredictable. Things may remain static for a long time, followed by a sudden upheaval, fit to be termed revolutionary. The evolution of Dermatology from a medical branch to one that accommodates numerous procedures and surgeries demonstrates a renaissance, and in some cases a full-blown revolution. A century ago, humanity did not have so many medical options for diseases. The treatment for lupus vulgaris was primarily surgical excision. Similarly, excision was considered as the only option for various dermatological diseases including many granulomatous diseases. Since the discovery of topical glucocorticoid analogues, dermatology evolved primarily as a medical branch for some decades, before the evolution of many procedures. These procedures were minimally invasive, compared to the crude procedures before. It is not as if dermatology has turned full circle back to procedures, but a plethora of both medical and surgical options have evolved simultaneously in the last half century. Getting medical options for a variety of diseases and procedural options for others in the last 50 years has truly made dermatology a hybrid branch where both types of modalities are complementary to each other. No longer are procedures considered last in hierarchy. Instead of referring patients to surgeons for procedures after all medical interventions fail, procedures are incorporated by dermatologists themselves in their practice early in their management protocols [7]. Some centers also evaluate procedural dermatology as a part of final residency examination [31].

Excess of everything is bad. These numerous options have created a paradox of choices. Many procedures are available for any given indication. There are over 120 different three-procedure combinations possible from just 10 treatment modalities for post-acne scars [32]. Individually, the efficacy of these procedures might not constitute much, but their combination may yield better results and lesser number of sessions than those with either alone. They may target different components by different mechanisms and could be synergistic, for example, combining subcision, trichloroacetic acid CROSS and microneedling, with or without platelet-rich plasma in the same sitting, for post acne scars. Chemical peeling can also be added to the mix. Evidence-wise, we have barely scratched the surface of the potential of these combinations [32]. Interestingly, such combinations are much more common in private practice than in academia. Now academia is catching up, and trying to separate wheat from the chaff. There is skepticism about these procedures in a section of general public and the academia that many of these procedures and their combinations might be gimmicky and profit-oriented rather than evidence-based. More trials on these combinations are needed.

20.7 Aesthetic Socialism and Dishonest Signaling

As defined by the World Health Organization, "*health is a state of physical, mental and social well-being and not merely an absence of disease or infirmity*" [33]. Treatment of dermatological disorders and cosmetic enhancement procedures are in a continuous spectrum. Dermatological disorders mostly lead to a social disadvantage and a drop in the quality of life below baseline, and treatment of these disorders is aimed at restoring the normal quality of life. On the other hand, cosmetic procedures are aimed at aesthetic enhancement, gaining a social advantage and increasing the quality of life above the baseline. While the transfer of knowledge occurs usually from academic dermatology to practising dermatology during the treatment of dermatological disorders, there is a transfer of knowledge regarding cosmetic dermatology from practising dermatologists to academic dermatology. This is because of academic dermatology's reluctance to accept the significance of improved cosmesis in social well-being. This resulted in ignoring the research and training of aesthetic procedures in academic institutions. Cosmetic dermatologic surgery should be a field driven by science and ethics, and not by commerce.

Beauty is a part of evolutionary fitness of an individual. There are considerable obvious and hidden advantages of being beautiful. Likewise, considerable disadvantages of being perceived as "ugly" or not beautiful. Cosmetic surgery to counter the effects of skin aging creates a "dishonest signaling," where we increase the evolutionary fitness of an individual through artificial means. Should any reproductive advantage through this means be termed "artificial selection?" The development of such procedures by our species represent the ways, including more natural methods and camouflage by make-up, in which individuals unconsciously try to enhance their reproductive fitness. As usual, the resources to avail these procedures are limited to the select few. But similar points were applicable to all such historical ways to enhance beauty. Perhaps our society as a whole should not deride cosmetic procedures as "dishonest signaling."

20.8 What Procedures Should One Do

Dermatologic surgical techniques can be divided into conventional dermatologic surgery, cosmetic dermatologic surgery, and lasers, light sources, and energy-based devices. Several procedures fall under the above headings. Each of these procedures varies in the level of skill required, the monetary investment involved and the return of investment. Knowledge of the same is required to determine the area where a dermatologic surgeon initially chooses to expertise in initially and thereafter broaden the horizon once he/she attains a firm footing in the field. Broadly speaking, conventional dermatosurgical techniques require a high skill level and have a steeper learning curve, low to moderate monetary investment, and a moderate return on investment. Cosmetic dermatologic surgery requires a moderate skill level, low to moderate investment, and a moderate to high return on investment. On the other hand, lasers and energy-based devices usually require the highest monetary investment. Low-to-moderate skill level because of automation, and have a low return on investment for the initial periods, which increases as more patients get treated [7].

Also, some procedures have a low monetary investment and start providing a high return of investment from the word go. These include procedures like hair restoration surgeries, acne scar surgeries, injectable fillers, botulinum toxin, and facial rejuvenation. On the other hand, device-based procedures like lasers and microneedling radiofrequency require a large initial monetary investment, and a longer latent period to get back the money invested and thereafter gain profits [7].

Conventional dermatosurgical techniques are exciting and require active thinking and decision making on a case-to-case basis and thus do not cause boredom and monotony. On the contrary, machine-based procedures are automated, safer and less prone to human errors, and are easy to deliver by minimally trained professionals as they are easy to learn. They also generate more money after an initial phase. However, they are more mechanized and thereby are less exciting. One needs to maintain a balance between both skill-intensive and technology-intensive procedures in practice [7]. Nevertheless, machines have revolutionized the therapeutic scenario in dermatology by providing therapeutic tools associated with minimal risk of complications.

20.9 Conclusion

Dermatologic surgery is a rapidly expanding field with many advancements. The above core concepts of dermatologic surgery apply to all advancements in this field. The fundamentals mentioned above can make a big difference in clinical practice. It is important to bear in mind these concepts while embarking on a career in procedural dermatology.

References

1. Skin Experts [Internet]. https://asds.net. Accessed 18 Aug 2023.
2. Bhatti Y, Basu R, Barron D, Ventresca M. Frugal innovation: models, means, methods. Cambridge: Cambridge University Press; 2018.
3. Bogdan Allemann I, Kaufman J. Laser principles. Curr Probl Dermatol. 2011;42:7–23.
4. Bhatia S, Chauhan J, Grover C, Gupta S. Radiofrequency-assisted onychostomy for minimally invasive extraction of subungual tumors. J Am Acad Dermatol. 2022;86(1):e5–6.

5. Gupta S, Handa S, Kumar B, Rai R. Surgical pearl: punch excision and grafting for removal of mole. J Am Acad Dermatol. 1999;41(4):635–7.
6. Pangti R, Gupta S. Surgical removal of moles. Cosmoderma. 2021. https://cosmoderma.org/surgical-removal-of-moles/. Accessed 18 Aug 2023.
7. Mehta N, Sharma A, Sindhuja T, Dudani P, Sahni K, Khanna N, et al. Procedural dermatology and its unmet need. Indian J Dermatol Venereol Leprol. 2022;89:807–18.
8. Taneja N, Sahni K, Gupta S. Autologous noncultured epidermal cell suspension for treatment of iatrogenic variegate repigmentation, textural changes, and color mismatch in vitiligo. Dermatol Ther. 2020;33(6):e14399.
9. Mehta N, Taneja N, Gupta S. Non-cultured epidermal cell suspension and laser resurfacing to improve the appearance of thick post-burn skin graft. Indian J Dermatol Venereol Leprol. 2023;1–3.
10. Bae JM, Lee JH, Kwon HS, Kim J, Kim DS. Motorized 0.8-mm micropunch grafting for refractory vitiligo: a retrospective study of 230 cases. J Am Acad Dermatol. 2018;79(4):720–727.e1.
11. Bhatia S, Mehta N, Gupta S. Manhole cover technique: a novel modification for nail matrix biopsy. Dermatology. 2020;237:291–2.
12. Gupta S, Yadav S, Patra S, Gupta S. Fractionated cryotherapy. J Am Acad Dermatol. 2017;77(3):e69–71.
13. Fruth K, Gouveris H, Kuelkens C, Mann WJ. Radiofrequency tissue volume reduction for treatment of auricle keloids. Laryngoscope. 2011;121(6):1233–6.
14. Poonia K, Kumar A, Thami GP. Intralesional radiofrequency treatment for venous lake. Int J Dermatol. 2019;58(7):854–5.
15. Singh S, Dayal M, Walia R, Arava S, Sharma R, Gupta S. Intralesional radiofrequency ablation for nodular angiolymphoid hyperplasia on forehead: a minimally invasive approach. Indian J Dermatol Venereol Leprol. 2014;80(5):419–21.
16. Huang LP, Zhang L, Wang XL, Liu XC, Jiang TY, Lin BW. A technique for periorbital syringomas: intralesional radiofrequency ablation. Int J Ophthalmol. 2012;5(2):181–5.
17. Singh S, Passi S. A 4-year multicentric experience of intravenous cannula-based intralesional radiofrequency ablation as an effective and safe office procedure for common cutaneous nodules. Indian J Dermatol Venereol Leprol. 2021;87(3):433–5.
18. Pangti R, Dixit A, Gupta S. Bipolar forceps of a high-power electrosurgical unit for precise removal of small benign skin lesions. J Am Acad Dermatol. 2020;82(5):e155–6.
19. Pangti R, Gupta S. Electromechanical resection: a novel method for quick, bloodless removal of multiple benign lesions. Indian J Dermatol Venereol Leprol. 2022;88(3):435–6.
20. Mehta N, Khan E, Gupta S. Radiofrequency epilation using acupuncture needles to decrease the disease burden in hidradenitis suppurativa. Dermatol Surg. 2022;48(7):788–9.
21. Bhatia S, Rajput L, Gupta S. Axillary incubator for cell-based therapies in vitiligo. J Am Acad Dermatol. 2021;85(5):e279–80.
22. Rajput L, Kharghoria G, Patel U, Gupta S. Chemically assisted gauze abrasion: an economical and convenient alternative to mechanical dermabrasion in vitiligo surgery. J Am Acad Dermatol. 2021;89(4):e141–2.
23. Gupta S, Shroff S, Gupta S. Modified technique of suction blistering for epidermal grafting in vitiligo. Int J Dermatol. 1999;38(4):306–9.
24. Gupta S, Ajith C, Kanwar AJ, Kumar B. Surgical pearl: standardized suction syringe for epidermal grafting. J Am Acad Dermatol. 2005;52(2):348–50.
25. Gupta S, Pandhi R, Kumar B. "Pot-lid" technique for aesthetic removal of small lipoma on the face. Int J Dermatol. 2001;40(6):420–4.
26. Gupta S, Kumar Jain V, Aggarwal K, Jindal S, Khanna M. Disposable skin hook. Int J Dermatol. 2005;44(12):1063–4.
27. Ashique KT, Srinivas CR. Pen punching: an innovative technique for comedone extraction from the well of the concha. J Am Acad Dermatol. 2015;73(5):e177.
28. Gupta S, Jangra RS, Gupta S, Mahendra A. An economical alternative to disposable electrodes for electrosurgical devices. J Am Acad Dermatol. 2016;75(6):e225–7.

29. Khunger N, Khunger M. Subcision for depressed facial scars made easy using a simple modification. Dermatol Surg. 2011;37(4):514–7.
30. Lahiri K, Malakar S. The concept of stability of vitiligo: a reappraisal. Indian J Dermatol. 2012;57(2):83.
31. Mehta N, Dudani P, Sahni K, Gupta S. Procedural dermatology evaluation for residents: a system in progress. Indian J Dermatol Venereol Leprol. 2023;89(4):640–2.
32. Gupta A, Kaur M, Patra S, Khunger N, Gupta S. Evidence-based surgical management of post-acne scarring in skin of color. J Cutan Aesthet Surg. 2020;13(2):124–41.
33. Constitution of the World Health Organization [Internet]. https://www.who.int/about/governance/constitution. Accessed 18 Aug 2023.

Breaking the Scar 21

Narayanan Baskaran, Pankhuri Dudani,
and Somesh Gupta

We are imperfect beings; our bodies aren't truly symmetrical, our brains definitely aren't, and our perception is always biased. Beauty is a matter of perception, and that which is geometrically perfectly symmetric (as well as grossly asymmetric) is quite often *not* beautiful to us [1]. The most beautiful thing one has seen is almost always a natural phenomenon such as a sunset, aurora lights, a stunning bird, or their child growing. It's never the perfectly symmetrical building, or the perfectly square piece of stationery. Imperfection is natural, and hence, beautiful. From the perfect single-celled ovum, our bodies form to become a human child; with left just a bit different from right, with fingers that aren't equal in length, hair that aren't the same all over the body, curved limbs, and a crooked smile. And as we grow, the differences grow more pronounced; our hands don't match exactly, we favor one hand or one foot over the other, our gait isn't the same from both sides.

Beautiful faces, when seen closely, often have clear asymmetry [1]. Symmetry is odd to our eyes; just superimpose someone's left face on their right and you get an "unnatural" looking face (Fig. 21.1).

In this sea of beautiful irregular lines of the face and body, anything regular, straight or geometric in shape attracts the attention as an oddity (paradox). Most traumatic scars tend to be straight or defined as per the trauma-causing object, and the ones following infection tend to be jagged, irregular, and depressed.

Principles of "breaking" a scar
We cannot make scars disappear, but we *can* create an illusion of their absence. By breaking them, hiding them in skin creases and natural lines, shifting them in areas less visible, and by irregularizing them to mimic natural lines
Elongate a broad scar, so the same amount of tension is redistributed along a thin longer line

N. Baskaran · P. Dudani · S. Gupta (✉)
Department of Dermatology and Venereology, AIIMS, New Delhi, New Delhi, India
e-mail: someshgupta@aiims.edu

S. Gupta et al. (eds.), *Critical Thinking in Contemporary Dermatology: Cognitive Essays*, https://doi.org/10.1007/978-981-97-0411-8_21

Principles of "breaking" a scar
Distort a geometrically defined scar to make it irregular, as no natural lines on the face are geometrically defined. More irregular the scar, the more invisible it is
Hide the revised scar in natural lines of face. Create an illusion of scar being a natural line
Reorient a scar to align it along the skin tension lines. It remains thin as the natural pull is shifted to the longitudinal axis of the scar
Human face is a highly disordered structure, not conforming to any geometrically defined shape. Any geometrically defined scar attracts undue attention. Irregularity of a scar is more forgiving
A scar crossing aesthetic subunits of the face is best divided into two scars, one each for each aesthetic subunit with the scarline connecting the two lines at the junction of two subunits

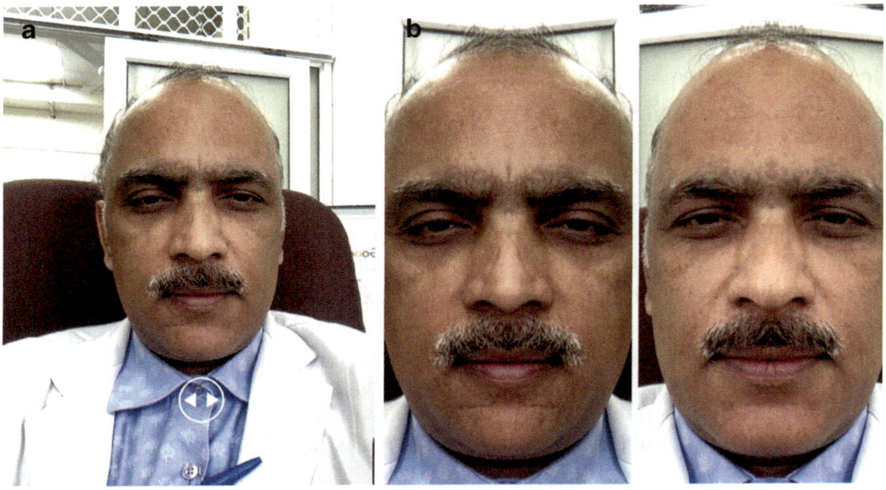

Fig. 21.1 (**a**) Photograph of a face (Courtesy Dr. Somesh Gupta). (**b**) Constructed facial image for perfect symmetry, where the two halves are identical

21.1 Illusion of Non-existence

Scar formation is an inevitable outcome of wound healing that occurs due to a traumatic or an iatrogenic injury. The most important criteria to judge the aesthetic outcome of any procedure is the appearance of the resultant scar. Any abnormality like a scar cannot be made to disappear; however, it can be revised in a way to create an optical illusion of its non-existence. A good example of optical illusion is the Muller-Lyer illusion, wherein two lines of similar length appear to be of different lengths. Any scar that is symmetrical or regular on the face is more likely to catch the attention of the observer. The key principle of scar revision surgery is to distort and break the scar and introduce asymmetry and disorder which would make it less visible and create an optical illusion of its non-existence. The visibility of an irregular scar is less because it is more similar to natural lines and thereby is less easy for the eyes to follow when compared to a straight linear scar. The location of skin tension lines on the face is not consistent and may vary from patient to patient. A good scar surgeon should respect the skin tension lines (STL), as any excision done along the lines would result in a far better surgical and aesthetic outcome as opposed to an excision done against them. Also, it is prudent to utilize the normal anatomical skin folds like the eyelid and infraorbital fold, ala of the nose, nasolabial fold, fold beneath the lip, submental fold, and the neck folds to merge and position the revised scar there, thereby blending the surgical scars in them.Certain factors improving the outcome of the scar are, incisions parallel to the RSTL, atraumatic handling of the tissues, judicious undermining for mobilization of surrounding skin and tension-free wound repair, layered wound closure, everted wound edges, choosing appropriate suture material, size, and technique, and ensuring good hemostasis. According to Gupta et al. the fundamental principle of scar revision is to minimize the scar regularity and deformation, as much as possible [2]. There are various techniques used for scar excision. Fusiform elliptical excision is used for revising a mature scar along the skin tension lines. W-plasty is a technique aimed at irregularizing a linear scar, thereby making it less noticeable. Z-plasty helps lengthen a contracted scar, restricting the movement across a joint and aligning them along the RSTL (Fig. 21.2).

W-plasty is indicated for linear scars that are more than 2 cm in size and are at an angle greater than 35° to the STL, short scars on prominent areas like the forehead and cheek, and for closures in pre-trichial areas and curved surfaces like the jaw. In W-plasty, the dots of the apex of the triangles are placed 5–6-mm apart from each other and at a distance of 3–5 mm from the scar. The limbs of each triangle should be 3–5-mm long and the angle of the triangular apex is usually angled between 60°–90°. The angle at the ends of the W-plasty should be less than 30° to avoid dog-ear or standing cone deformity formation. After excising the scars along these lines and undermining, re-approximation is done by interdigitating the triangles to form a single zigzag line (Fig. 21.3) [3].

Geometric broken line closure is the most sophisticated technique aimed at creating maximum scar irregularization and camouflage. The outline of the revision is made using a series of random irregular geometric designs like semicircles, squares, rectangles, and triangles, and a mirror image of this pattern is made on the other side. Each segment should have a length between 3 and 7 mm and the angles at the end should be less than 30° [3].

The use of autologous fat transfer has also been done to improve the aesthetic appearance of scars. Adipose stem cells have regenerative potential and can improve scars and the quality of the overlying tissue [4].

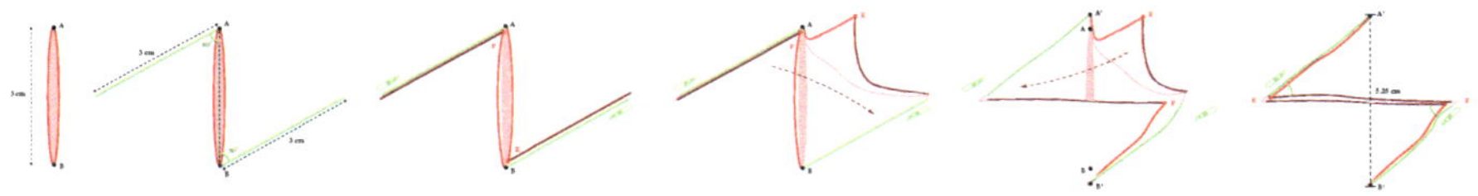

Fig. 21.2 Z-plasty. Please note the lengthening achieved

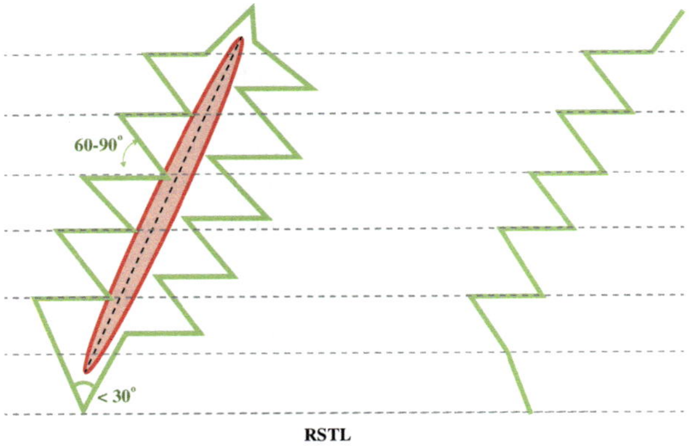

Fig. 21.3 W-plasty for a long oblique scar

In summary, scars bring regular or well-defined shapes on otherwise naturally irregular and disordered human bodies. The irregularity in the human body is acquired during the fetal growth, the rate of which varies in different parts of the body, thus creating an irregular structure, the human baby. This disproportionate growth makes all natural lines irregular. Therefore, any regular scar needs to be broken, distorted, and made irregular. Other correction principles involve chemical and energy-based ablation of elevated scars, refilling the depressed scars with natural or synthetic substances, correcting the contour abnormalities, matching the color with the surrounding skin, and resurfacing methods to deal with uneven surfaces.

References

1. Zaidel DW, Cohen JA. The face, beauty, and symmetry: perceiving asymmetry in beautiful faces. Int J Neurosci. 2005;115(8):1165–73. https://doi.org/10.1080/00207450590914464.
2. Garg S, Dahiya N, Gupta S. Surgical scar revision: an overview. J Cutan Aesthet Surg. 2014;7(1):3–13.
3. Rodgers BJ, Williams EF, Hove CR. W-plasty and geometric broken line closure. Facial Plast Surg. 2001;17(4):239–44.
4. Klinger M, Marazzi M, Vigo D, Torre M. Fat injection for cases of severe burn outcomes: a new perspective of scar remodeling and reduction. Aesthet Plast Surg. 2008;32(3):465–9.

Why Do We Need Teledermatology?

22

Paola Pasquali

22.1 Introduction

Telemedicine is the use of telecommunication technology to address medical services. From the perspective of the World Health Organization, information and communication technologies (ICTs) would be the answer to address some of the challenges in providing accessible health care services [1]. What was envisioned as a necessity for developing countries has now become—with the COVID pandemic—a worldwide requisite.

Telemedicine was originally envisioned to overcome geographical barriers and increase access to specialized medicine. The concept of exchanging medical information for the purpose of patient management is probably as old as medicine, and its development is intrinsic to the advancements, increasing availability and democratization of ICTs by both health providers and patients. Exchange of medical information has had many purposes: helping to diagnose, giving therapeutic suggestions, following-up on a patient's condition, giving psychological support and reassurance, teaching, triaging, and prioritizing conditions that deserve to be seen in person. Our concept of telemedicine has changed with time. Probably a physician's phone call at the beginning of twentieth century using the recent Bell's invention should be considered as such; another example can be taken from 100 years ago, when Willem Einthoven (1860–1927), a Dutch physician and physiologist, founder of modern electrocardiography, and winner of the Nobel Prize in Physiology or Medicine 1924, transmitted an electrocardiogram via telephone wire [2].

Mobile phones have probably been revolutionary in this sense as 83.96% of the world's population now owns a smartphone [3]. Indeed, the general population has

P. Pasquali (✉)
Pius Hospital de Valls, Tarragona, Spain

Universidad de Alcalá, Madrid, Spain

S. Gupta et al. (eds.), *Critical Thinking in Contemporary Dermatology: Cognitive Essays*, https://doi.org/10.1007/978-981-97-0411-8_22

been the biggest driver of telemedicine over the past decade, rapidly creating new possibilities for health care service and delivery [1].

If telemedicine seems to address relevant medical issues such as accessibility, cost-effectiveness, and democratization of medicine, why do we still find resistance to it?

22.2 Why Teledermatology?

The world's health care force is unevenly distributed. Regarding medical doctors, the highest density is found in Europe (around 43 per 10,000 population); the lowest in Africa (around 2 per 10,000 population) [4].

There are two conditions that collide to generate the perfect storm: on the one hand, a relatively fixed number of dermatologists trained worldwide per year, a significant number of which go exclusively into private practice and many dedicate most of their time to cosmetic procedures; on the other hand, a growing world population where skin and subcutaneous diseases represent the fourth leading cause of disability worldwide [5].

The burden of skin disease together with the maldistribution of dermatologists task force has brought an increase in nonphysicians taking care of skin diseases [6]. We need "more eyes." But access has to come by the hand of quality. The responsibility to guarantee the quality of care lies on the trained dermatologists, who, by taking an active role in training those "extra eyes," can make sure that the future Artificial Intelligence (AI) algorithms are properly trained.

22.3 Types of Teledermatology

To speak about teledermatology (TD) before the COVID pandemic may be a futile exercise, as few were interested; many insisted it was an unnecessary practice that needed to be reserved to reach patients in the Antipodes, where second class medicine was better than none. Dr. Anne Burdick's famous title *"The teledermatology train is coming: get on board, get out of the way, or get run over"* [7] has been frequently cited in TD conferences as a subtle warning to skeptics that TD was here to stay and would soon become part of our daily practice.

TD received a push in those countries with socialized medical systems that needed to attend to a large population and did not have enough specialists to attend the flood of face-to-face patients. Large waiting lists (some around a year-long) motivated the inclusion of TD as part of the workflow to facilitate access to those patients that needed to have their appointments prioritized. In countries with a large incidence of skin cancer, the possibility to refer patients with suspicious skin lesions by store-and-forward (SAF) TD proved to be superior to conventional referral as patients were seen sooner. For a melanoma patient, this could be a lifesaving decision, as patients with melanoma seen through TD had on an average a thinner Breslow at diagnosis and therefore, better prognosis [8].

TD can be delivered through several modalities [9]. The main and most-often used one is the *"Asynchronous", also known as "Store-and-Forward"* workflow. Clinical, dermoscopic, and other specialized images are sent as a bundle for consultation. The provider responds at a later time spending as much time as required; in addition, the image remains for future reference and monitoring. The face-to-face examination gives a short moment of time and no second opportunity to evaluate a condition. An additional advantage of this method is that connectivity is required only during downloading the consultation and when sending the answer.

Another modality is *Real-Time (RT) Video Consultation (Live Interactive)* which employs live video conferencing. The advantage is that it gives the opportunity to ask pertinent questions that might have been missed by the consultant who sends only images and text. There is additional information that could be referred to by the patient themselves regarding pain, other symptoms, and texture. It has the disadvantage that it is more time-consuming, video images are still not as good as photographs, and for patients in different areas of the world, difference in time zones imposes additional logistics to consider. Furthermore it requires high-quality connectivity during the entire consultation.

Hybrid TD combines the first two modalities. One possibility is a SAF and phone call to get information directly from the patient or video call and high-quality images (clinical and/or dermoscopy) of the lesions sent as a complement.

Phone calls are a good option particularly for monitoring medication or healing. During the 2020 COVID pandemic and subsequent lockdown [10–12] they became probably the sole means to reach patients, as most of the population—both patients and physicians—had to stay at home. The impact of a simple phone call was very relevant as it helped solving medical issues and, more importantly, it allowed patients to feel accompanied and cared for. Compassion played a role during this period where there was a lot of uncertainty and fear of death. This word, compassion, encompasses many aspects: generosity, altruism, solidarity, hospitality, accompaniment and solace, among others [13]. It is not to be confused with pity, condescension, or paternalism [14]. It involves a relationship of equals who share an understanding of suffering: it is "the sensitivity shown in order to understand another person's suffering, combined with a willingness to help and to promote the well-being of that person, in order to find a solution to their situation" [15]. Phone calls can be formally incorporated as part of the dermatologists' workflow and play a role in monitoring diseases, medications, or postsurgical concerns. Some departments have included them as part of the routine work (personal reference) after the first COVID lockdown.

Direct-to-consumer TD allows direct access of patients to specialist's care. The required platforms can be in the form of non-for-profit mobile phone app like https://www.mdipsoriasis.com/ which is meant to help dermatologists individualize therapeutic decisions of their psoriasis patients and bases its recommendations on technical sheets and on the clinical guidelines and consensus of scientific societies [16]. Others are commercial companies that streamline care—diagnosis, prescription, and the sale of medications—on a single platform. Their offer is to be more affordable and accessible [17]. To protect the patient, it is pivotal to understand the nature of the relationships with physicians and the company that provides the platform.

22.4 Learning Through Images

Photography has been a *disruptive innovation* right from the beginning. For authors Molella and Beidi [18] photography reframed how we look at the world and ourselves. One of the big impacts of the incursion of photography into the medical world, besides the possibility to take images of patients to register a condition, was the possibility to reproduce that image by the thousands without introducing any changes. These images were not contaminated by interpretation. Dermatological photographs were among the first medical images to be reproduced in series for atlases which were used to spread medical knowledge. Just as Gutenberg's printing press caused a dramatic social and cultural revolution by making printed work available to everyone [19] (before it, books were handwritten, very rare, and accessible only to a few, mostly the Catholic Church), photography revolutionized medical education, particularly dermatology. In this sense, photography can be considered an instrumental part of the emergence of dermatology as a discipline. Soon after photography was invented (1826), the first atlases appeared which were published between 1865 and 1900 [20]. Since then, dermatologists' main source of learning has been through images, from textbooks, conferences, and patients' photographs. Many rare conditions have been seen only through photographs. We are specialists that have been trained through images before seeing patients; therefore, diagnosing, monitoring, and teaching using images, which is what TD is all about, should be as natural and intuitive as examining a patient face-to-face.

There is an additional advantage to TD—we can evaluate an image for long periods of time. By doing so, we might be able to point out important findings that we had missed at first glance. A face-to-face consultation does not give a second chance.

22.5 Pattern Recognition

> *The best thing we have going for us is our intelligence, especially pattern recognition, sharpened over eons of evolution* [21]
>
> *Neil de Grasse*

Pattern recognition, according to IQ test designers, is a crucial determinant of a person's potential to think logically, verbally, numerically, and spatially [22].

Compared to other all mental abilities, pattern recognition is best correlated with the so-called general intelligence factor [23].

We hear about pattern recognition and machine learning, but it is humans that have an unsurpassed ability to spot patterns; which improves with time as more "data" is filled in; supported by intuition. It is indeed a crucial skill for decision-making [24]. Pattern-formation represents one of the most fundamental principles that nature enlists for system organization, the quintessential skill of a dermatologist [25].

Dermatologic diagnosis relies primarily on vision and an accurate diagnosis is predicated first on seeing and then comparing the visual data with one's working mental database of dermatologic diagnoses [26]. That vision can be of a person or of a picture.

Furthermore, we can teach others—those "extra-eyes"—to recognize lesions [27, 28]. In the study by Rimoin et al. [29] clinical images were shown to a group of medical students and an answer was selected; the learner was given immediate feedback on the correct answer. These Perceptual and Adaptive Learning Modules were effective and efficient in teaching pattern recognition. By giving an immediate answer, the student had the opportunity to match the image with the correct diagnosis. This is the same teaching effect of TD over consulting family physicians: sending an image and receiving a diagnosis during the next few hours/days has a learning effect [30].

22.6 The World of Images

We live in a world surrounded by images. In 2020 alone humanity took 1.4 trillion photos. This is more than all the photographs taken since photography was invented. We see icons everywhere. Images have become a communicative necessity. Medical sciences and visual arts tend toward an intensive use of iconic codes. People are communicating more and more using emoticons. In the words of Samsung: *"8 out of 10 users communicate daily through images…image is a new language where the main channel is the smartphone as a universal device that has modified the communication habits of people"* [31].

Arnheim's concept says that all visual perception is already in itself a cognitive activity, even before receiving the endorsement of reason [32] and medicine has not escaped this universal tendency. We cannot imagine a medical conference if not with a powerpoint presentation full of images. We are becoming experts at diagnosing by looking at images.

22.7 Image Quality

Once the correct patient with a medical condition suitable for TD has been selected, the next step is to take a picture that meets the standards. Although it seems a simple task, there are some simple but necessary rules that need to be considered for warranty quality. This includes:

- *Focus and Depth of Field.* Images need to have a deep depth of field. This means, every element in the picture needs to be in focus. If it is a face, the nose and ears have to be in focus as well.

- *Color Calibration/White Balance.* Whatever is white needs to appear white in the photograph. Depending on the hour of the day or the type of bulb, there will be a different light temperature and as such, different colors that will "dye" the picture in reddish, bluish, or greenish hue.
- *Light (Illumination).* Flash light is commonly recommended for medical photography as it has a temperature similar to the ambient light. It needs to appear from the sides and not the center (builtin flash) to avoid central whitening of the image.
- *Resolution.* Pictures should be taken at the highest possible resolution.
- *Backdrop.* It is mandatory to have a neutral solid-colored backdrop to eliminate background distractions and help focus the image.
- *"Distractions" on patients.* All jewelry, make-up, amulets, glasses, and masks should be removed before the picture is taken. Proper exposure must be ensured and clothes must not be included in the photographs as far as possible. If holding of the part being clicked is necessary; the hand coming into the frame should also be without jewelry/makeup and should be gloved if possible.
- *Field of view.* It is important to send an adequate number of pictures. If it is a skin tumor, a close-up and a mid-view are required to understand the size of the tumor in regards to the area where it is located. A scale can also help in objectivizing the size. All this information is useful to properly refer a patient for further evaluation and management.
- *Position.* Patients should be placed in standardized anatomical positions.
- *Scale.* It can be helpful to understand how large a tumor is.

It is important that image "senders" learn these basic rules, regardless of whether they are medical professionals or patients themselves. Good quality images are necessary to make a proper diagnosis, and also help to build a library of images which can later feed algorithms intended to help physicians in triaging dermatology patients [33].

22.8 Diagnostic Error in Dermatology

The term 'gold standard' is used to describe a diagnostic test that is regarded as definitive for a particular disease, and thereby becomes the ultimate measure for comparison. A 'perfect' gold standard may only exist in theory [34].

TD studies are constantly asked to demonstrate how they stand in regard to the gold standard face-to-face consultation. Curiously, very little has been written on the diagnostic error in dermatology. In general, 10% and 15% of all diagnoses are inaccurate with cognitive errors contributing to 74% of these diagnostic errors [35]. It would seem that visual specialties have a somewhat lower diagnostic error rate, close to around 5% [36]. To support the search for this information, studies should be done among specialists with similar years of experience and similar educational background to reduce variability in the studied sample. In a study by Lozzi et al. [37] a group of patients were seen face-to-face and also via TD. Although the study group was very small, there were instances where the diagnoses was incorrect by both (F-to-F and TD), and also a few with incorrect diagnosis in the F-to-F but correct by the TD physician. This goes to show that before judging the modality, the participating physicians must be adjudged to be of similar competence.

22.9 The Incidental Lesion

A TD consultation puts the focus on a medical condition; sometimes, other lesions are commented on as well. In any case, it is not the result of a total body skin examination (TBSE). Indeed, TBSE is the ideal exam given the fact that the skin is an exposed organ and dermatologists have a unique opportunity to examine it completely (or almost completely) in search of all possible lesions. This is particularly true in skin cancer patients. A study by Omara et al. [38] showed that up to 21.7% of malignancies in patients who had been sent to the clinic for treatment of a malignancy had another lesion detected incidentally through TBSE. However, TBSE is not performed routinely by all dermatologists. Some studies report that over 80% of dermatologists routinely do TBSE [39] while in other studies this was as low as 30% [40].

While TBSE is not possible in a TD consult, TD is not meant to replace face-to-face consult; but rather, be a mode of consultation where the latter is not possible due to logistic regions.

When a patient uses a direct-to-consumer app to reach a specialist or a family physician sends a TD consultation, there is always a selection of the skin. It is not the dermatologist who decides where the focus is placed. When a patient is referred by the conventional route, there is also a previous selection. Ideally, the patient that is seen face-to-face should be undressed and the entire skin surface examined. This would reduce the possibility of missing those incidental lesions. For high-risk cancer patients, the solution will probably be given by the generation of total body scanners (there are already prototypes) which can photograph the entire body surface, with polarized light and generate an *avatar* that can be sent to dermatologists to check-up. These scanners should eventually be available in family physicians' offices but also in pharmacies and other locations, to facilitate access.

For most consultations, the incidental lesion is not an issue. Over 70% of TD consultations are solved and the patient does not need to come to see the doctor face to face.

22.10 COVID-19 Pandemic: The Inflection Point

With the lockdown, we were all obligated to rethink our profession. Attending to our patients from a distance, keeping our medical knowledge updated, or communicating with colleagues were some of the issues we were confronted with overnight. All this, in addition to our concern for our families, friends, and ourselves.

With regard to TD, many government regulations and policies suddenly faded. We were given the green signal to use any system to make TD possible: Google, WhatsApp, Telegram, etc. Protocols were created and adapted [41]. We were faced with the issue of older people facing difficulty with technology; taking a picture of a lesion and sending it is intuitive for the younger generation but is not so for most seniors. Reimbursement was made possible. Some insurance companies paid for the specialist online consultation the same as face-to-face. This favored a further increase in acceptance.

The most important aspect of this was a reduction in resistance by many professionals regarding TD. On the other hand, policymakers have understood the importance of favoring TD and hopefully understood the need to reduce unnecessary regulations.

22.11 Conclusions

With the COVID pandemic, there was an impressive increase in the interest for consultation through TD [42, 43]. Many dermatologists experienced TD for the first time because of the need for social distancing and found it effective. Many have expressed their intention to continue using it.

There are still issues that raise concern regarding security, patient's privacy, license regulations (some countries have different state regulations regarding telemedicine), reimbursement, dependence on effective connectivity, age-related impediments to use technology, and fast changes caused by technological innovation. There is a need to generate simple but effective workflows to select the best conditions to be consulted through TD. Image quality is pivotal and we need to explain how we want those images to be taken.

TD needs to be incorporated in the medical programs as it will become increasingly more important with time. Physicians need to be involved in the development of new technologies, not just as passive donors of information but in the design of applications, algorithms, and platforms that can improve their daily work and, most importantly the life of their patients.

There is a need to reduce the dependence on face-to-face consultations because the patient demand is expected to rise and the number of specialists is insufficient to handle that number. It is important to train nurses, medical students, pharmacists, and the general population to increase the number of "trained eyes" that can help us reach a larger number of patients, and lessen the number that truly need a specialist's consultation. Not everyone has to come to the hospital. We need to spend more effective face-to-face time with those patients with critical and complex conditions. For the majority of patients, visiting a hospital poses unnecessary cost, discomfort, and risk.

The future will provide algorithms that will pre-screen patients. TD on a one patient-to-one doctor will soon be part of the past.

By rethinking dermatological care, we will benefit our patients, improve our workflow, and help the environment.

References

1. Telemedicine. Opportunities and developments in Member States. WHO. 2010. https://www.who.int/goe/publications/goe_telemedicine_2010.pdf. Accessed 7 Jan 2022.
2. Einthoven W. The telecardiogram. Am Heart J. 1957;53(4):605–12. https://doi.org/10.1016/0002-8703(57)90367-8.
3. Bankmycell. How many smartphones are in the world? https://www.bankmycell.com/blog/how-many-phones-are-in-the-world. Accessed 7 Jan 2022.
4. WHO. Global Health Workforce statistics database. https://www.who.int/data/gho/data/themes/topics/health-workforce. Accessed 7 Jan 2022.
5. Karimkhani C, Dellavalle RP, Coffeng LE, Flohr C, Hay RJ, Langan SM, et al. Global skin disease morbidity and mortality: an update from the global burden of disease study 2013. JAMA Dermatol. 2017;153(5):406–12. https://doi.org/10.1001/jamadermatol.2016.5538.
6. Bystryn JC. Dermatology manpower needs. Dermatol Clin. 2000;18(2):303–12. https://doi.org/10.1016/s0733-8635(05)70176-5.
7. Burdick AE, Simmons SC. The teledermatology train is coming: get on board, get out of the way, or get run over. Cutis. 2011;88(5):213–4.
8. Ferrándiz L, Ruiz-de-Casas A, Martin-Gutierrez FJ, Peral-Rubio F, Mendez-Abad C, Rios-Martin JJ, Moreno-Ramirez D. Effect of teledermatology on the prognosis of patients with cutaneous melanoma. Arch Dermatol. 2012;148(9):1025–8. https://doi.org/10.1001/archdermatol.2012.778.
9. Pasquali P, Sonthalia S, Moreno-Ramirez D, Sharma P, Agrawal M, Gupta S, Kumar D, Arora D. Teledermatology and its current perspective. Indian Dermatol Online J. 2020;11:12–20. https://doi.org/10.4103/idoj.IDOJ_241_19.
10. Fritz C, Claude LA, Hamada S, Trosdorf M, de la Barre H, Yavchitz A, Clausse D, Lemogne C, Godier A, Flahault C. Daily telephone call during the COVID-19 pandemic: perceptions of families and providers. Am J Crit Care. 2022;31(1):77–81. https://doi.org/10.4037/ajcc2022797.
11. Johri M, Agarwal S, Khullar A, Chandra D, Pratap VS, Seth A, Gram Vaani Team. The first 100 days: how has COVID-19 affected poor and vulnerable groups in India? Health Promot Int. 2021;36(6):1716–26. https://doi.org/10.1093/heapro/daab050.
12. García-Sierra R, Moreno-Gabriel E, Badia Perich E, Sabaté Cintas V, Bonet Simó JM, Violán CF, Gil NP, Rodríguez MP, Torán-Monserrat P. Evaluation of a support system for health professionals confined by COVID-19. Rev Saude Publica. 2021;55:108. https://doi.org/10.11606/s1518-8787.2021055003735.
13. Jiménez A, Triana M, Washburn J. Compasión y salud. Revista De Filosofía Moral Y Política. 2002;27:211–23.
14. Pellegrino ED. Humanism and the physician. Knoxville: University of Tennessee Press; 1979.
15. Perez-Bret E, Altisent R, Rocafort J. Definition of compassion in healthcare: a systematic literature review. Int J Palliat Nurs. 2016;22:599–606. https://doi.org/10.12968/ijpn.2016.22.12.599.
16. MDPsoriasis. https://www.mdipsoriasis.com/. Accessed 7 Jan 2022.
17. Ranpariya VK, Lipoff JB. Direct-to-consumer teledermatology platforms may have inherent conflicts of interest. J Am Acad Dermatol. 2021;85(4):e259–60. https://doi.org/10.1016/j.jaad.2021.04.102. Epub 2021 Jun 5.
18. Gillespie SK. The early American daguerreotype: cross-currents in art and technology. In: Bedi J, Daemmrich A, editors. . Cambridge: MIT Press; 2016. p. 232.
19. Littlejohn A. Social and cultural impact. Johannes Gutenberg and the Printing Press; 2022. https://owlcation.com/humanities/Johannes-Gutenberg-and-the-Printing-Press-Revolution.
20. te Hennepe M. Depicting skin: visual culture in nineteenth-century medicine. Maastricht: Maastricht University; 2007. p. 192. https://doi.org/10.26481/dis.20070920mh.
21. Tyson de NG. Cosmos: A Spacetime Odyssey-transcripts (Episode 3), When Knowledge Conquered Fear. 2015.
22. Robert CB. Why the human brain is so good at detecting patterns. https://www.psychologytoday.com/us/blog/singularperspective/202105/why-the-human-brain-is-so-good-detecting-patterns. Accessed 7 Jan 2022.

23. Kurzweil R. How to create a mind- the secret of human thought revealed. New York: Penguin Books; 2012.
24. Miemis Venessa. Pattern recognition. https://www.disruptorleague.com/blog/2010/08/18/essential-skills-for-21st-century-survival-part-1/. Accessed 7 Jan 2022.
25. Chuong CM, Dhouailly D, Gilmore S, Forest L, Shelley WB, Stenn KS, et al. What is the biological basis of pattern formation of skin lesions? Exp Dermatol. 2016;15:547–64. https://doi.org/10.1111/j.1600-0625.2006.00448_1.x.
26. Ko CJ, Braverman I, Sidlow R, Lowenstein EJ. Visual perception, cognition, and error in dermatologic diagnosis: key cognitive principles. J Am Acad Dermatol. 2019;81(6):1227–34. https://doi.org/10.1016/j.jaad.2018.10.082. Epub 2019 Feb 21.
27. Simonetta C, Eric AE. Patient identification of benign and malignant skin lesions: can a simple pictorial intervention make a difference? J Am Acad Dermatol. 2017;76(6):AB189.
28. Lacy FA, Coman GC, Holliday AC, Kolodney MS. Teaching intuitive visual diagnosis of melanoma: a randomized controlled study. J Am Acad Dermatol. 2018;79(3):AB279.
29. Rimoin L, Altieri L, Craft N, Krasne S, Kellman PJ. Training pattern recognition of skin lesion morphology, configuration, and distribution. J Am Acad Dermatol. 2015;72(3):489–95. https://doi.org/10.1016/j.jaad.2014.11.016. Epub 2015 Jan 13.
30. van Sinderen F, Tensen E, van der Heijden JP, Witkamp L, Jaspers MWM, Peute LWP. Is teledermoscopy improving general practitioner skin cancer care? Stud Health Technol Inform. 2019;264:1795–6. https://doi.org/10.3233/SHTI190652.
31. Pasquali A. Epilogue: the future of imaging. In: Pasquali P, editor. Photography in clinical medicine. 1st ed. Springer; 2020. p. 727–31.
32. Arnheim R. Art and visual perception: a psychology of the creative eye. University of California Press; 1974.
33. EADV. How to take a good picture. Patient's corner. https://eadv.org/patient-corner. Accessed 7 Jan 2022.
34. Gold R, Reichman M, Greenberg E, Ivanidze J, Elias E, Tsiouris AJ, et al. Developing a new reference standard: is validation necessary? Acad Radiol. 2010;17(9):1079–82. https://doi.org/10.1016/j.acra.2010.05.021.
35. Dunbar M, Helms SE, Brodell RT. Reducing cognitive errors in dermatology: can anything be done? J Am Acad Dermatol. 2013;69(5):810–3. https://doi.org/10.1016/j.jaad.2013.07.008.
36. Norman GR, Eva KW. Diagnostic error and clinical reasoning. Med Educ. 2010;44:94–100. https://doi.org/10.1111/j.1365-2923.2009.03507.x.
37. Lozzi GP, Soyer HP, Massone C, Micantonio T, Kraenke B, Fargnoli MC, et al. The additive value of second opinion teleconsulting in the management of patients with challenging inflammatory, neoplastic skin diseases: a best practice model in dermatology? J Eur Acad Dermatol Venereol. 2007;21(1):30–4. https://doi.org/10.1111/j.1468-3083.2006.01846.x.
38. Omara S, Wen D, Ng B, Anand R, Matin RN, Taghipour K, Esdaile B. Identification of incidental skin cancers among adults referred to dermatologists for suspicious skin lesions. JAMA Netw Open. 2020;3(12):e2030107. https://doi.org/10.1001/jamanetworkopen.2020.30107.
39. Oliveria SA, Heneghan MK, Cushman LF, Ughetta EA, Halpern AC. Skin cancer screening by dermatologists, family practitioners, and internists: barriers and facilitating factors. Arch Dermatol. 2011;147(1):39–44. https://doi.org/10.1001/archdermatol.2010.414.
40. Federman DG, Kravetz JD, Kirsner RS. Skin cancer screening by dermatologists: prevalence and barriers. J Am Acad Dermatol. 2002;46(5):710–4. https://doi.org/10.1067/mjd.2002.120531.
41. Yeboah CB, Harvey N, Krishnan R, Lipoff JB. The impact of COVID-19 on teledermatology: a review. Dermatol Clin. 2021;39(4):599–608. https://doi.org/10.1016/j.det.2021.05.007.
42. Moscarella E, Pasquali P, Cinotti E, Tognetti L, Argenziano G, Rubegni P. A survey on teledermatology use and doctors' perception in times of COVID-19. J Eur Acad Dermatol Venereol. 2020;34(12):e772–3. https://doi.org/10.1111/jdv.16843.
43. Kennedy J, Arey S, Hopkins Z, et al. Dermatologist perceptions of teledermatology implementation and future use after COVID-19:demographics, barriers, and insights. JAMA Dermatol. 2021;157(5):595–7. https://doi.org/10.1001/jamadermatol.2021.0195.

Patient-Reported Outcome Measures (PROMs) in Dermatology: An Idea Whose Time Has Come

23

Nikhil Mehta and Somesh Gupta

23.1 Introduction

The second half of the twentieth century saw the development of evidence-based medicine. Gradually, objective measures were introduced to characterize and measure the outcomes. The ways in which outcomes were expressed were quantified and tried to be standardized for uniform application. Simultaneously, there was an evolution of medical ethics too. It involved shifting of focus from paternalism to an informed consent-based approach. This empowered patients and provided them with greater agency. The treatment approach became more patient-centric. *"The surgery was successful; the patient is dead"* grew less acceptable.

Patient-reported outcome measures (PROMs) are the result of the application of evidence-based medicine to a patient-centric approach. They represent the belief that for patients of a particular disease, the best intervention is the one that maximally improves their quality of life. Hence to gauge the effectiveness of interventions, it became necessary to develop tools that can measure the impact on the quality of life, as reported by the patients themselves. The use of PROMs started in the 1970s and 1980s, and gradually increased as more evidence poured in, and now they are used in research trials, routine clinical use, policy formulation, resource allocation, and provider assessment [1].

N. Mehta · S. Gupta (✉)
All India Institute of Medical Sciences, New Delhi, India
e-mail: someshgupta@aiims.edu

S. Gupta et al. (eds.), *Critical Thinking in Contemporary Dermatology: Cognitive Essays*, https://doi.org/10.1007/978-981-97-0411-8_23

23.2 Definition

As per the United States, Food and Drug Administration's (USFDA) guidance for industry documents regarding PROMs, a patient-reported outcome (PRO) is any report of the status of a patient's health condition and its therapy that comes directly from the patient, without interpretation of the patient's response by a clinician or anyone else [2]. The outcome can be static, measured in absolute terms (e.g., the severity of a symptom, sign, or state of disease) at a point in time or a specific period preceding the reporting of the outcome; or dynamic, measured as a change from a previous measure. Use of a PRO instrument in a clinical trial is advised when measuring a concept best known by the patient or best measured from the patient perspective, for example, pain as a symptom [2]. PRO measures often represent the effect of disease on health and functioning from the patient perspective, for example, difficulty in sleeping due to itch of an inflammatory skin disease.

The level of evidence required to demonstrate improvement in a PRO measure is the same as required for any other objective parameter [2]. For example, to label that a particular biologic is useful in moderate-to-severe psoriasis, an objective way is to demonstrate achievement of PASI75 (a reduction by 75% in the psoriasis area severity index) in a significantly more proportion of trial participants who were on that biologic, compared to those who were on placebo or a comparator drug. To say that biological therapy improves the quality of life of those patients, a similar demonstration must be done for a reduction in an impairment of quality-of-life measures, such as DLQI (Dermatology Life Quality Index) [3]. PROMs are now an integral component of patient assessment (Fig. 23.1).

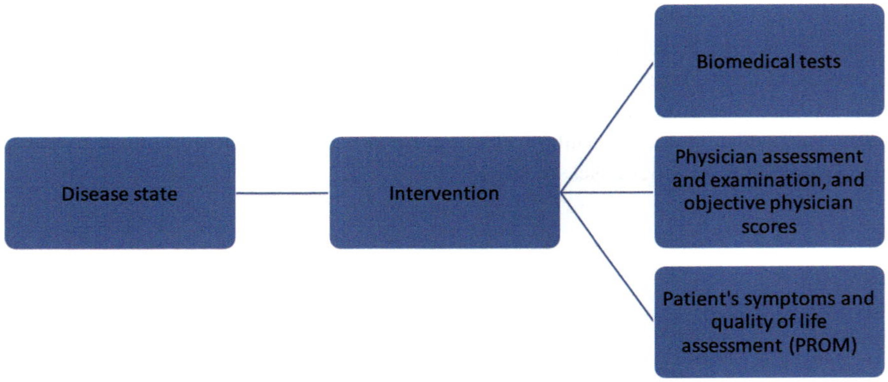

Fig. 23.1 Assessments of response to a specific treatment. PROM is now becoming an integral part of this model

23.3 Classification

PROMs are classified on a variety of basis—as general health-related, specialty-related (or 'dermatology-related' for dermatologists), and the most precise disease-specific. They range from simple measures of intensity of a single symptom (example numerical rating score for pain or itch) or complex multidimensional measures. Multidimensional PROMs have various sections/domains like physical, mental (including cognitive and emotional), and social, each measuring a different concept/aspect of the impact of the disease on the patient's well-being. Depending on use case, they may be divided into those simple enough for clinical practice, or comprehensive questionnaires for usage in clinical trials.

23.4 Development Process of a PROM

What makes the so-called objective biomarkers, laboratory parameters, and clinicians' ratings better than PROMs? The fact that they were used first in evidence-based medicine while PROMs are relatively newer? The normative values of biomarkers are defined from a reference range from an apparent population, and healthy outliers may be normal but will be considered diseased, or some diseased people have biomarker values within the normal range. The 95% reference range will be different for different populations and labs; hence these parameters require standardization for different population groups for their use. For example, erythrocyte sedimentation rate (ESR) is higher and platelet count is lower in Indians compared to commonly provided values [4]. The development and validation of PROMs also follow the same rigorous and robust methods as used for clinicians' scoring systems and laboratory parameters, and their usage in different populations require standardization and validation for those populations. PROMs do not seem to be inferior to biomarkers.

While developing a PROM, the first step is setting a clear goal for the use of that PROM—the patient population and setting for which the PROM will be used. The next step involves qualitative research, that might use semi-structured interviews, to find out various aspects or domains by which it impacts people. The next step entails formulating various questions and their responses in a language compatible with target people. The questions might be worded responses or scores on an ordinal/Likert scale, with an increase point scoring denoting a greater impact of disease on the quality of life. They may measure the impact at a particular time or in a recent duration. Questions from other quality of life instruments can be used as an example. The questions are divided into various domains, and redundant and irrelevant questions are removed through multiple iterations of interviews and expert discussions. The draft questionnaire is pretested on some participants and is further revised. After finalizing the questionnaire, it is tested on a sample population against a gold standard, like a single global health question or physician/patient's global assessment, for sensitivity, accuracy, and reliability. Various cut-offs/ranges of total scores are decided grouping the impact on quality of life from mild to severe. It can also be used in healthy populations as a control, although many questions might be meaningless when applied to control population. Further studies are done in other populations to validate the PROM or to validate it in different languages and populations. A minimally effective/least amount of change in the value of PROM that translates to a clinically meaningful change is calculated.

23.5 Characteristics

The characteristics of an ideal PROM are the following:

23.5.1 Internal Consistency

If each item correlates well with the total score.

23.5.2 Validity

Validity means *if* the PROM indeed accurately measures the outcome of what it intends to measure. Criterion validity is tested by measuring correlation with the gold standard like a single global health question or physician/patient's global assessment. Construct validity implies *how well* the PROM measures what it intends to measure. Few ways of assessing it include using convergent validity (correlation with previous validated questionnaires for the same concept/condition/disease), divergent validity (low correlation with previous validated questionnaires measuring different concept/condition/disease), and known-groups validity (if the score is higher in the subgroups which are expected/known to have a higher impact of disease). Content validity refers to the extent by which *all facets* of the construct are measured.

23.5.3 Reliability

A test is considered reliable if its score does not vary significantly on repeating it after a short time during which the disease extent has not changed and its impact on quality of life is not expected to change.

23.5.4 Responsiveness

A test is considered responsive if the score change correlates with the change in the impact on quality of life with change in the activity and extent of the disease. Cross-sectional sensitivity is the ability to detect differences between two subgroups (which are expected to have some differences) at a point in time, while longitudinal sensitivity is the ability to detect change in a subgroup with time.

23.6 Some Examples of PROMs in Dermatology

As many as 36 dermatology-specific PROMs exist, and this number is ever increasing [5]. The number rises exponentially for dermatological disease-specific PROMs. Sixteen specific PROMs for psoriasis were identified in a recent review [6]. Similarly, many PROMs exist for dermatitis, including those for atopic dermatitis and chronic hand eczema. They include Patient-Oriented SCOring Atopic Dermatitis (SCORAD) index, Patient-Oriented Eczema Measure (POEM), Self-Administered Eczema Area and Severity Index (EASI), Atopic Dermatitis Quickscore, and the Nottingham Eczema Severity Score. As per the various Harmonising Outcome Measures for Eczema (HOME) meetings, although SCORAD has been the most commonly used PROM for AD, they have preferred EASI and POEM, and DLQI to measure impact on overall quality of life. Recap of Atopic Dermatitis (RECAP) is another tool to measure long-term control [7–9]. Itching and its various dimensions are measured using different scales, and recently HOME preferred Numerical Rating Scale-11 over past 24 hrs for itch in atopic dermatitis. Itching in dermatology is analogous to pain and fatigue in other specialties, having several multidimensional PROMs [10]. There has been a burgeoning collection of scoring systems and PROMs for hidradenitis suppurativa, used in a variety of trials [11]. Vitiligo, being an asymptomatic disease, is thought to have less impact on quality of life compared to a symptomatic disease with itching and flaking like psoriasis. But its psychosocial burden may match psoriasis, especially in skin of color. Vitiligo also has a plethora of PROMs developed in the last decade. One of the PROMs for vitiligo has a separate version for skin of color patients [12]. Acne and melasma also have specific PROMs [13, 14]. Recently, a PROM for vascular malformations has also been developed [15]. A detailed updated list can also be accessed through the Dermatology PRO Consortium website [16].

23.7 Advantages

PROMs offer some advantages over the more objective disease-centric parameters.

23.7.1 Holistic

Multidomain PROMs represent a holistic broader psychosocial view rather than a narrow medical view of conventional "objective" parameters. Few small acral lesions of vitiligo at visible sites are more bothersome to the patient than large patches at covered areas. The former, though lesser in extent and difficult to treat, might warrant a trial of surgical treatment as they are more bothersome to the patient [12, 17]. Similarly, palmoplantar psoriasis causes more disability to patients compared to rest of the body involvement with higher BSA involvement and higher Psoriasis Area Severity Index (PASI) [18]. PROMs, rather than BSA or PASI, correspond better with quality of life.

23.7.2 Combine Metrics of Advantages and Disadvantages of an Intervention

Pre- and post-intervention global PROMs combine the measure of efficacy with safety to assess the risk–benefit ratio. For example, a new chemotherapy regime might significantly improve survival time in a trial, but PROMs can identify that patients are not compliant due to side effects, complexity of the regime, or due to an overall poor quality of life [19]. A similar scenario might exist for different interventions of pemphigus. In surgeries too, outcome should also be gauged by PROMs. With cell-based therapies for vitiligo, postsurgery dyschromia may offset any improvement in the appearance and quality of life as per patient, even if the repigmentation area might be greater than 75%. A physician might assess repigmentation following a cellular grafting procedure as 90% hence an excellent response, while the patient might not be satisfied because his disease might be still very noticeable to others. A slightly more effective intervention might have many more side effects and inconvenience. The latter two are often not studied or quantified in detail in trials. With multiple measures on effectiveness, side effects, and convenience of any intervention, it might be difficult to combine these measures and gauge if that intervention is "worth-it" in the majority of patients. But a PROM combines these multiple matrices into a single statistic. The Patient Benefit Index (PBI) is one such example [20].

23.7.3 Sensitivity

They are more sensitive to change and impact of therapy, and can measure small changes which won't show up on other quantitative measures [21].

23.7.4 Use in Chronic Diseases

The good sensitivity of PROMs makes them very useful for chronic diseases which can't be cured but can be managed, and useful to evaluate potential safer but less-effective drugs. PROMs are better for chronic noncommunicable diseases, compared to outcome measures like morbidity and mortality, which are more suited for acute infective conditions. It's no coincidence that rheumatology was one of the first medical fields to design and adopt PROMs [22]. In this light, it must be recognized that psoriasis, eczema, vitiligo, and many other dermatological diseases behave similarly. They too are chronic noncommunicable diseases that can be managed but not always cured, have a relapsing and remitting course, and unpredictable flares followed by uncertain periods of remission. Justifying a prolonged period of medications with many side effects requires data with PROMs.

23.7.5 Irreplaceable Use

Many diseases can be monitored best through patient-reported symptoms, for example, pain in rheumatoid or osteoarthritis (or for that matter, arthritis in systemic sclerosis or psoriasis) is a much more sensitive marker compared to joint swelling. For a trial with any new analgesic, a pain score is the primary outcome measure rather than any inflammatory biomarker and X-rays of joints. Similarly, to evaluate an antacid or a prokinetic in systemic sclerosis, questions such as "how frequently do you get reflux episodes while on treatment" can be answered only by patients. It is neither practical nor desired to use 24-hour esophageal pH monitoring rather than symptoms as the preferred marker. Similarly, reduction in scores measuring intensity of itching will be the primary outcome measures in a clinical trial of a new anti-histamine or a new anti-pruritic agent, compared to reduction in tissue biomarkers which are more useful in preliminary proof-of-concept studies.

23.7.6 Cost- and Time-Effectiveness

Although PROMs can be obtained through an interview too, and not just through patients' self-administered questionnaires, usually the latter dominates. The interviews can be conducted by medical personnel other than the clinician. The PROM data can be prefilled and available to the clinician before interaction with the patient during follow-up visits. Monitoring patients using PROMs instead of biomarkers also saves cost to the system and patient. A PROM in a patient with mild-to-moderate psoriasis with psoriatic arthritis, DLQI is much more convenient to both patient and clinician for monitoring, compared to PASI, C-reactive protein, and X-rays of joints.

23.7.7 Telemedicine and Electronic Records

Another advantage of PROMs is their unique adaptability for telemedicine and integration with electronic medical records (EMR). The COVID-19 pandemic led to increased adaptation of telemedicine services throughout the various branches of medicine. Dermatology is thought to be quite amenable to telemedicine practice. Skin is an externally visible organ, and the inspection part of the clinical dermatological exam can be done with the help of photos sent by the patient, or through video consultations. There's a lack of standardization in photos sent by the patients. The two-dimensional nature of the photos makes evaluation of the elevation of lesions difficult. Many conditions require palpation of lesions. Thus, there are many difficulties in teledermatology. Usage of PROMs for follow-up patients can alleviate some of them. A PASI scoring might be difficult to perform using the photographs, due to difficulty in rating of elevation or induration from the photos, but DLQI or a psoriasis-specific score is easy to evaluate.

23.7.8 Policy-Making

PROMs are especially useful to evaluate a clinician or a healthcare service, audits and assessment of cost–benefit ratio, for quality improvement projects, and to dictate policy.

23.7.9 Provider Assessment

PROMs are useful in provider assessment. United Kingdom's National Health Service (NHS) routinely employs PROMs to assess healthcare provider's quality and decide bonuses, and to dictate policy, especially for elective surgeries like hip and knee replacement, hernia repair, and varicose vein surgery [1].

23.7.10 Clinical Practice

PROMs are useful not only as research tools but also are increasingly used in routine clinical practice. Their use in routine clinical practice has shown to improve doctor–patient communication and better identification and addressal of the commonly overlooked problems. Use of PROMs in routine clinical use to improve healthcare delivery has, to some extent, shown to improve patients' overall satisfaction and health-related quality of life.

23.7.11 Patient-Centric Guidance to Interventions

They embody the movement to give more agency to the patient in the decision-making process. Each person has a different tolerance to stressful conditions. A patient of psoriasis vulgaris may have minimal distress with body surface area (BSA) involvement of 15%, while another can be quite distressed with BSA involvement of 5%. Many stakeholders advocate that the degree of psychosocial distress and impact a disease has on a particular patient must be included as severity indicators. Multidomain PROMs which capture the impact of diseases on the multiple aspects of quality of life are best suited to quantify this distress. The extent of the disease which is not "severe" in the physicians' eyes is "severe" for that particular patient, and this might entail an aggressive therapy tailored to that patient. Although a patient-centric approach is tailored to a specific patient rather than population or policy decisions, demonstration of impairment of quality of life in a number of patients can very well lead to incorporation of a patient-centric indication of treatment in the guidelines or policy document itself. The recommendation to use isotretinoin in moderately severe acne patients significantly distressed by their disease, compared to limiting its use for severe nodulocystic acne, reflects the patient-centric approach.

23.8 Limitations of PROMs

The usage of PROMs has its limitations.

23.8.1 Lack of an Ideal PROM

Various reviews for various dermatology-specific and disease-specific PROMs argue that no PROM is good enough [5, 6]. It has been argued that the gold standard Consensus-based Standards for the selection of health Measurement Instruments (COSMIN) criteria for PROMs might be too strict [5]. However, many PROMs continue to be in use despite not fulfilling all the strict requirements and expected validations.

23.8.2 Separate Validation for Different Populations

Multi-domain PROMs developed using patients from a localized population group will have a specific language, words, and phrases, and specific culturally relevant questions. Their use in different populations with different translated versions requires revalidation in that language, and tailoring of some questions to suit a different culture. In a review of dermatology-specific PROMs, it was seen that many translated versions in use lack measurement invariance, a measure of cross-cultural validity. Hence, there is lack of evidence for many translated versions, if they actually measure the same construct as measured by the original version [5].

Developing these PROMs with patient populations from multiple centers, including both developed and developing countries, developing and validating versions in different languages simultaneously, and keeping the questions as culturally neutral as possible are the ways to minimize revalidation each time and to ensure widespread adaptability of a PROM. The questions must be such that patients from both the developing and developed world can relate to.

23.8.3 Patient Requirement

Self-administrated questionnaires require educated patients who can comprehend the questions. This excludes their use in a significant proportion of patients in underdeveloped countries where literacy rates remain unsatisfactory, and can significantly skew the data. Interviews can help, but they may have to explain some words and questions using unapproved nonstandardized language and phrases.

23.8.4 Trust

Despite increasing use, PROMs are not inherently trusted by clinicians and are treated as whimsical and inferior to the "more consistent and reliable" objective physician scores, although the latter too can show much intra-observer variation, and bias in open studies. It is thought that unrelated personal circumstances or misfortune of the patient can significantly affect his perception of the effect on the quality of life due to the disease, although this might not be the case.

23.8.5 Internal Controls and Partial Treatment

PROMs assess the impact of the whole disease on a patient. If a split-face or split-body trial is planned, or some lesions are treated with one intervention and the remaining with another, two sets of a PROM cannot be obtained to gauge both these interventions independently from a single patient.

23.8.6 Excessively Patient-Centric in Guiding Interventions and Defects in Routine Clinical Use

Although PROMs are good for policy decisions and assessing outcomes of interventions, their use for personalized medication is questioned by some. Advocates argue that if an otherwise "mild" or limited-extent disease is much bothersome for a particular patient and causing significant impairment in the quality of life, then the treatment must include counselling sessions to enable that patient to cope with the disease, instead of providing aggressive treatment for the disease. It has also been suggested that patients may report higher morbidity through PROM if they perceive that it will lead to an aggressive line of treatment for them, for example, a higher dosage of opioids for pain. Deciding incentives to clinicians based on PROMs reported by their patients can also lead to unnecessary and aggressive therapy. This argument, alas, has been frequently used by insurance companies and payers in denying such treatments or providing lesser reimbursements, although patient-centered advocacy groups like National Psoriasis Foundation frequently recommend PROMs as a trial outcome and target. They advocate for insurance companies to reimburse therapies which show better response in terms of better improvement in PROMs.

23.8.7 Too Sensitive

A spate of new PROMs have been proposed, many for usage in clinical trials of newer biologics, claiming them to be more sensitive in detecting a small change in otherwise difficult-to-treat and manage conditions. They aren't revalidated in different studies, and it is difficult to ascertain if the change in these PROM measures is truly clinically meaningful.

23.8.8 Variability in Assessment for Chronic Diseases

PROMs that are done only post-intervention can interpret the impact of intervention differently in comparison to those done serially pre- and post-intervention. A time-period-based PROM that asks the patient to assess symptoms over a short duration in the recent past differs from PROM which asks for responses with reference to the day on which that PROM was recorded. A PROM score in a patient who just developed a chronic disease might be significantly different from his score done a few years after living with the disease, although the extent of lesions at the two points might be the same.

23.8.9 Too Cumbersome

Some older PROMs are too lengthy and detailed, have redundant questions, and frustrating for patients to fill. They are also difficult to adapt to electronic systems. Researchers frequently shorten and simplify their PROMs in successive iterations to ease widespread adaptability and routine clinical use.

23.9 Patient-Centric Care and Patient-Reported Experience Measures (PREM)

For most patients, the better doctor is not necessarily the better clinician or diagnostician, or one who has an aggressive therapeutic approach, but one who's more patient-centric. What constitutes patient-centric care? Isn't all care patient-centric? Well, it's supposed to be. But frequently it isn't. In essence, patient-centric care implies appropriating a greater weightage of patients' agency in medical decision-making.

Almost all of us, in our formative years, would have witnessed wise experienced clinicians who could gauge appropriate treatment for a patient in an instant. They would have been efficient clinicians, loved by their patients, inspiring figures and role models. An important component in their art of patient-centric care is to presume what a patient might need, and then present that choice to the patient. With experience, we learn to identify particular needs of patients of different profiles without their verbalization or explicit stating. A daily wage laborer with palmoplantar psoriasis, who faces difficulty in manual work due to cuts in his hands, might warrant a more aggressive treatment than a retired person. A small stable focal vitiligo patch on the face can be treated with surgery or left alone, depending upon if the patient is a young television anchor or a middle-aged freelance software designer working from home. Patient-centric care comes from experience and empathy, and is not just desirable, but a necessary trait in medicine.

We may also discuss patient-reported experience measures (PREM) in brief. A patient may describe a high level of satisfaction with treatment outcome, they may find the experience of services suboptimal. Unlike PROM, PREM is administered to evaluate and enhance the patient experience of healthcare delivery and specific aspects of organization. In some comparative studies, PREMs are found to be a better assessment tool for discriminating practices and organizations than measures of satisfaction [23]. PREMs can guide about small interventions that can improve overall patient experience, and can help in monitoring and comparing services; however, in developing countries and resource-limited settings, PROMs are usually prioritized.

23.10 Conclusion

PROMs are very useful outcome measures of a clinical trial of any intervention. They reflect the shift from paternalism to a patient-centric approach through evidence-based medicine. Apart from clinical trials and policy-making, their use in routine clinical practice is also increasing, which reflects increased agency to patients and precision medicine. They have a distinct advantage in teledermatology, over scoring systems that rely on clinicians' examination. While developing PROMs, researchers must make efforts to encompass multiple domains, use a heterogeneous population from multiple centers, validate them simultaneously in multiple languages, keep universal questions relevant to patients from different cultures, and keep them short, simple, and easily adaptable for online/electronic platforms. The PROMs developed with the aid of public funding should be available for free unfettered use to ensure widespread adaptability.

References

1. Black N. Patient reported outcome measures could help transform healthcare. BMJ. 2013;346:f167.
2. U.S. Department of Health and Human Services FDA Center for Drug Evaluation and Research, U.S. Department of Health and Human Services FDA Center for biologics evaluation and research, U.S. Department of Health and Human Services FDA Center for devices and radiological health. Guidance for industry: patient-reported outcome measures: use in medical product development to support labeling claims: draft guidance. Health Qual Life Outcomes. 2006;4:79.
3. Jungo P, Maul JT, Djamei V, von Felten S, Kolios AGA, Czernielewsk J, et al. Superiority in quality of life improvement of biologics over conventional systemic drugs in a Swiss real-life psoriasis registry. Dermatol Basel Switz. 2016;232(6):655–63.
4. Sairam S, Domalapalli S, Muthu S, Swaminathan J, Ramesh VA, Sekhar L, et al. Hematological and biochemical parameters in apparently healthy Indian population: defining reference intervals. Indian J Clin Biochem. 2014;29(3):290–7.
5. Pattinson RL, Trialonis-Suthakharan N, Gupta S, Henry AL, Lavallée JF, Otten M, et al. Patient-reported outcome measures in dermatology: a systematic review. Acta Derm Venereol. 2021;101(9):adv00559.

6. Kitchen H, Cordingley L, Young H, Griffiths CEM, Bundy C. Patient-reported outcome measures in psoriasis: the good, the bad and the missing! Br J Dermatol. 2015;172(5):1210–21.
7. Murrell DF, Paul CF. What instruments should we add to our toolbox for measuring the severity and control of eczema? Br J Dermatol. 2021;185(1):13–4.
8. Thomas KS, Apfelbacher CA, Chalmers JR, Simpson E, Spuls PI, Gerbens LAA, et al. Recommended core outcome instruments for health-related quality of life, long-term control and itch intensity in atopic eczema trials: results of the HOME VII consensus meeting. Br J Dermatol. 2021;185(1):139–46.
9. Leshem YA, Chalmers JR, Apfelbacher C, Katoh N, Gerbens LAA, Schmitt J, et al. Measuring atopic eczema control and itch intensity in clinical practice: a consensus statement from the Harmonising outcome measures for eczema in clinical practice (HOME-CP) initiative. JAMA Dermatol. 2022;158(12):1429–35.
10. Schoch D, Sommer R, Augustin M, Ständer S, Blome C. Patient-reported outcome measures in pruritus: a systematic review of measurement properties. J Invest Dermatol. 2017;137(10):2069–77.
11. Mac Mahon J, Kirthi S, Byrne N, O'Grady C, Tobin A. An update on health-related quality of life and patient-reported outcomes in hidradenitis Suppurativa. Patient Relat Outcome Meas. 2020;11:21–6.
12. Mehta N, Gupta V. Psychosocial impact of vitiligo in patients with skin of color. Dermatol Rev. 2022;3(5):269–75.
13. Hopkins ZH, Thiboutot D, Homsi HA, Perez-Chada LM, Barbieri JS. Patient-reported outcome measures for health-related quality of life in patients with acne vulgaris: a systematic review of measure development and measurement properties. JAMA Dermatol. 2022;158(8):900–11.
14. Zhu Y, Zeng X, Ying J, Cai Y, Qiu Y, Xiang W. Evaluating the quality of life among melasma patients using the MELASQoL scale: a systematic review and meta-analysis. PLoS One. 2022;17(1):e0262833.
15. Ring NY, England RW, Motaghi M, Garg T, Gong AJ, Gullotti DM, et al. Responsiveness of the patient-reported outcome measure for vascular malformation questionnaire in patients with low-flow vascular malformations. J Vasc Interv Radiol. 2023;34(5):840–848.e5.
16. Derm PRO Consortium. Main PROs for dermatology. 2023. https://www.dermproconsortium.org/pro-list.
17. Ezzedine K, Eleftheriadou V, Jones H, Bibeau K, Kuo FI, Sturm D, et al. Psychosocial effects of vitiligo: a systematic literature review. Am J Clin Dermatol. 2021;22(6):757–74.
18. Chung J, Callis Duffin K, Takeshita J, Shin DB, Krueger GG, Robertson AD, et al. Palmoplantar psoriasis is associated with greater impairment of health-related quality of life compared with moderate to severe plaque psoriasis. J Am Acad Dermatol. 2014;71(4):623–32.
19. Gondek K, Sagnier PP, Gilchrist K, Woolley JM. Current status of patient-reported outcomes in industry-sponsored oncology clinical trials and product labels. J Clin Oncol. 2007;25(32):5087–93.
20. Augustin M, Radtke MA, Zschocke I, Blome C, Behechtnejad J, Schäfer I, et al. The patient benefit index: a novel approach in patient-defined outcomes measurement for skin diseases. Arch Dermatol Res. 2009;301(8):561–71.
21. Patrick DL, Burke LB, Powers JH, Scott JA, Rock EP, Dawisha S, et al. Patient-reported outcomes to support medical product labeling claims: FDA perspective. Value Health. 2007;10(Suppl 2):S125–37.
22. Callahan LF. The history of patient-reported outcomes in rheumatology. Rheum Dis Clin N Am. 2016;42(2):205–17.
23. Salisbury C, Wallace M, Montgomery AA. Patients' experience and satisfaction in primary care: secondary analysis using multilevel modelling. BMJ. 2010;341:c5004.

Personalized Medicine: Can We Really Achieve This in Dermatology?

24

Robert Norman

In the field of dermatology, there are promising opportunities for expansion beyond our valuable capabilities in pattern recognition, diagnosis, and treatment. To tailor a therapeutic regimen after due consultation with the patient, keeping in mind his/her specific wants and needs rather than running through an algorithm, is not Personalized Medicine, rather is just good Medicine! Giving more agency to the patients in a shared decision-making process is informed consent. The term "Personalized Medicine (PM)," as used in this essay, refers to the specific customization of healthcare using molecular analysis to influence medical decisions, practices, and therapies for the individual patient.

The concept of personalized medicine has ancient origins. In the 1190s, Maimonides advocated for tailoring medical treatment to each individual patient, emphasizing the need for personalized consideration. Instead of categorizing a patient's illness as similar to another case, a doctor should approach each patient independently, taking into account their natural constitution, individual psychology, and specific circumstances. Maimonides highlighted Galen's advice that, in determining a course of treatment, a physician should consider seven factors: the nature of the sickness, the nature of the patient, their age, habits, the nature of the town, the season of the year, and the constitution of the surrounding air [1–3]. Now, in addition, we are able to add occupation, genomics, and other tests to the diagnostic and treatment mix.

Fresh research findings will leverage evolutionary medicine and genomics to underscore the enhanced ability to identify suitable antibiotics, therapies, and optimal dosages tailored to specific diseases or pathogens. This approach aims to establish a competitive advantage through prevention and risk management against invasive viruses, bacteria, or incorrectly administered drugs. In various domains

R. Norman (✉)
Center for Geriatric Dermatology, Integrative Dermatology and Neuro-Dermatology, Nova Southeastern University, Davis, FL, USA

S. Gupta et al. (eds.), *Critical Thinking in Contemporary Dermatology: Cognitive Essays*, https://doi.org/10.1007/978-981-97-0411-8_24

such as oncology and reproductive medicine, genetic testing has been employed for an extended period. The ongoing efficacy of newly developed diagnostic tests in dermatology must be assessed to ascertain whether there is a necessity for the creation of additional and enhanced tests [4, 5]. If we could combine all individual variables that can influence the best therapy for a particular patient, including conventional factors like history, current symptoms, allergies, all testing results, and personalized genetic profile, we could have powerful and perhaps more immediate and cost-effective treatments.

Strictly speaking, precision medicine does not deal with individual patients per se but stratifies subpopulations of patients with different characteristics. The subpopulations differ in their susceptibility to particular diseases, how severely they manifest diseases, and in response to specific treatments. To treat a particular patient, instead of a "one-size-fits-all" approach and "average effect" algorithm yielded by evidence-based medicine analysis of trials, the precision medicine approach involves classifying them into appropriate subclassification and choosing the best treatment for them. This subclassification requires genetic, environmental, and lifestyle data of that particular patient, and the availability of large data to enable stratification into subpopulations of that disease. This big data is yielded not just by looking into subgroups in trials which did not respond or responded less but also by large-scale population studies. When comparing personalized medicine with evidence-based medicine, it becomes clear that the "individual treatment" effect is emphasized in the former compared to the "average treatment" effect in the latter [6].

Like in other areas of medicine, PM in Dermatology has found its primary and predominant role in Oncology. Skin cancers, particularly melanoma, are an area where the role of PM in Dermatology is not in the future, rather it is being used now. The multi-hit model of carcinogenesis is well accepted for many cancers, and patients with similar cancer phenotypes can have very different genetic mutation signatures. Similar to the treatment of various hematological cancers, the mutational analysis of malignant melanomas of individual patients dictates their targeted therapy. Vemurafenib is FDA-approved for unresectable or metastatic melanomas with the BRAF(V600E) mutation [7].

What factors contribute to the acceptance or opposition to genetic testing? Central considerations involve the trust in data accuracy, the actions required based on the results, the significance of clear guidelines for enhancing treatment, the decision-making process and timing for identifying the most effective vaccines for specific populations, and apprehensions about government intervention, unwarranted scrutiny, and improper utilization of obtained genetic information. For example, a test that determines what percentage of topical minoxidil is the most suitable for a person with androgenetic alopecia might not be useful in itself, but a panel of tests which yield a comprehensive score that predicts a poor prognosis in androgenetic alopecia and leads to a decision of more aggressive treatment from the beginning might be worthwhile.

Examining personalized medicine through a biocultural lens is crucial for strategically planning our future in healthcare. The fundamental question revolves around optimizing healthcare outcomes with limited resources. It is imperative to establish the significance and effectiveness of personalized medicine in dermatology, emphasizing that it is not merely an inevitable consequence of the genetic revolution. The prevailing economic climate in most Health Maintenance Organizations (HMOs) is geared towards minimizing expenses to maximize profits for shareholders. The political and economic context significantly influences the acceptance and implementation of any novel approach. A substantial paradigm shift is necessary to redefine the insurance concept of "shared risk" by incorporating the newer notion of "individual risk factors" in personalized medicine within dermatology. While this transformation is challenging, utilizing genetic testing holds the potential to enhance the likelihood of biological and evolutionary success.

To achieve the fundamental objectives of personalized dermatology medicine (PDM), it is imperative that we increasingly consider the genetic implications of skin disorders as we advance in our field. In our 2016 publication on Personalized, Evolutionary, and Ecological Dermatology (Springer), we explored strategies to augment the dermatology profession's critical abilities in pattern recognition, diagnosis, and treatment through the evolution of contemporary medical methodologies. This evolution encompasses the integration of personalized medicine and genomics. Some of these tools are now readily available, facilitating the customization of healthcare through molecular analysis, influencing medical decisions, practices, and therapies tailored to individual patients [8].

The progression of our understanding of skin evolution and the description and treatment of dermatological conditions underscores the necessity to take numerous personal factors into account. Furthermore, with increasing knowledge about the skin's biology and the impact of new antibiotics, biologics, and other therapies on its ecological balance, there is an elevated awareness of the significance and contributions of ecological dermatology.

The combination of PM with social medicine, along with an evolutionary and ecological perspective, can assist dermatologists and other physicians in becoming better treatment providers, if used ethically and carefully. Now that we have about 18 "biologic" therapies for psoriasis and eczema, would it not be much more efficient for everyone to have a genetic ID that would allow the dermatologist to state, "Medication X should work the best of all." And what about being able to readily detect the most effective antibiotic, anti-inflammatory, anti-pruritic, anti-depressant, or anti-cancer drug for each person? And the best plan to follow for prevention and immune stimulation?

Let's further explore the provocative and amazingly diversified field of personalized dermatology.

24.1 Big Data and Artificial Intelligence

What can we expect from Big Data and artificial intelligence? We now have data generated from vast numbers of longitudinal, observational multicenter clinical trials and registries across the world to teach us about disease features, treatment selection, and practice patterns. The information from real-world management of various disease cohorts is fed into robust computer analysis programs to help detect risk factors, clinical features, morbidity and mortality, genetic mutations, treatment choice, the timing of therapy, and outcomes. We can drill down to pinpoint individual variations.

In the current era of highly advanced computers and rapid communication, the challenge is to effectively process the vast amount of information available, discerning what is crucial for our future and shaping the direction of our healthcare. The rate at which we accumulate information is unprecedented. From the inception of civilization until 2003, we had amassed five exabytes, each equivalent to 1 billion gigabytes or roughly the capacity of 5.1 million computer hard drives. By 2010, we were generating information at a pace five times greater than the total accumulated by all of civilization before 2003—five exabytes every 2 days. In 2013, the speed further accelerated to an astonishing five exabytes every 5 minutes.

Over 2.5 quintillion bytes of data are created every single day. By 2020, it was estimated that 1.7 MB of data would be created per second per person. Every day in 2021, 2.5 quintillion bytes of data are produced by humans and there are 18 zeros in a quintillion, so that's 2,500,000,000,000,000,000 bytes daily (I mostly worry about backing up my computer!). By 2025, there will be an expected 175 zettabytes of data in the global datasphere. Just because you are reading my essay, I will save you the task of looking this up. A zettabyte is a unit of measurement used by technology professionals and, infrequently by the general public to describe a computer or other device's storage capacity. The number of bytes is equal to 2 to the 70th power, also expressed as 1 sextillion bytes. One zettabyte is approximately equal to one thousand exabytes or one billion terabytes. Wow.

Some 90% of the world's data has been created in the last 2 years.

In a perfect world, I would like to have at least a quarter of an exabyte running on a computer sitting right next to me, to help during each one of my examinations, with the hope that my new computer buddy would help me and my patient to instantly find the best possible solution for every one of my patient's problems right down to the molecular level. But life does not always play out as we want. Personalized medicine, however, when fueled by the most robust artificial intelligence, certainly does offer a way to create wonderful advances in our diagnostic and treatment skills.

If you possess a smartphone, you carry AI in your pocket, and encountering AI online is inevitable. Its impact has already transformed various aspects, ranging from how medical professionals diagnose diseases to influencing your interactions with friends and altering the way you consume news.

24.2 Our Microbiome

We must devote much more time analyzing the microbiome in comprehensive detail in order to help create a healthy human and a healthy society. As Paul Nurse writes, "When scientists look at our own bodies, they see that for each and every one of our 30 trillion or more human cells, we have at least one microbial cell. You – and every other human being – are not an isolated, individual entity, but a huge and constantly changing colony made up of human and nonhuman cells. These cells of microscopic bacteria and fungi live *on* us and *in* us, affecting how we digest food and fight illnesses." [9]

The surface of our skin harbors approximately as many bacteria and yeasts as there are individuals on Earth. The presence of this life not only provides a perspective on our existence but also offers a glimpse into a miniature world within the layers of our skin, a perspective that is both fascinating and perplexing. As humans, we are just one among more than two million species of animals and plants. Similar to our fellow inhabitants in the realm of mortality, we are susceptible to the influence of minuscule entities such as viruses, bacteria, and yeasts. At no time in recent history has this become clearer than with the devastation caused by COVID-19 [10].

24.3 Genomic Skin Testing

For the last year we have been participating in the Dermtech clinical testing and research project at our office for a variety of skin diseases by using "smart stickers." In the case of melanoma, we know that early detection saves lives, and the Dermtech device facilitates in this goal. The status quo has been, for many, to biopsy any mole that looks remotely suspicious; this process often results in excess biopsies. The result had been a very limited accuracy, with 96% of biopsies taken testing negative for melanoma and 17% of the time missing early-stage melanoma. Dermtech added a step before the scalpel and today the DermTech Melanoma Test is extremely accurate, with a 99% negative predictive value (a 99% probability that a negative test means you really don't have the disease). All of this is happening at the genomic level with molecules more than 10,000 times smaller than cells [11].

Although it looks like a simple sticker tape, the proprietary adhesive is strong enough to pull 1.5 milligrams of tissue from the epidermis of a lesion to assess its genomic information but is without enough pull to cause pain or damage. For our research we do several adhesive tests per lesion and a non-lesional test for comparison and then follow with a biopsy of the lesion to test in our pathology lab. The adhesive collects and stores the genomic material so it can be sent via FedEx to DermTech's Gene Lab for examination. Unlike a biopsy, which evaluates only 1–2% of the mole, DermTech's smart sticker captures cells from 100% of the mole's surface. We send Dermtech the results of our biopsies but we are unaware of the sticker results for comparison.

Upon arrival at Dermtech, the sticker samples go through an automated process that amplifies RNA molecules. For melanoma detection, a subsequent analysis is conducted to ascertain the presence of one or both genes, PRAME and LINC00518, which are highly indicative of melanoma. This is accomplished through a proprietary gene expression test utilizing an amplification process known as RT-PCR (reverse transcription-polymerase chain reaction), generating billions of copies of these genes for detailed examination by Dermtech scientists. Elevated levels of the PRAME and/or LINC00518 gene revealed in this analysis are indicative of the presence of melanoma [11].

The DermTech Melanoma Test™ is a laboratory-developed test (LDT) ordered by physicians, and its regulation falls under the Clinical Laboratory Improvement Amendments (CLIA). Dermtech is currently working on LuminateSM, a product designed to identify UV damage on a genomic level. Additionally, the Carcinome test, which is in the developmental phase, aims to detect the presence of non-melanoma skin cancers at the genomic level [11].

If the Dermtech and other genomic tests prove effective, we may have a marked decrease in the number of biopsies and surgeries needed. The computer algorithms for testing and diagnosis biopsy specimens are rapidly improving and helping to eliminate the need for expensive and time-consuming special staining, immunohistochemistry, and further examinations. When utilizing all the factors in a person's health investigation and history, as mentioned earlier, AI suggestions will alert us to disease and prevention patterns and provide improvements in personalized dermatology.

24.4 Polymerase Chain Reaction Testing

Polymerase chain reaction (PCR) testing involves a chemical process that replicates billions of copies of a specific DNA or RNA, facilitating their amplification and detailed examination. PCR has been fine-tuned for the diagnosis and analysis of various disease-causing agents, including viruses and bacteria. This test is currently employed in diagnosing a wide range of medical conditions, serving as a potent diagnostic and research tool known for generating highly accurate and reproducible results. PCR provides clinicians with a diagnostic advantage, enabling earlier identification and treatment initiation, ultimately improving outcomes. As highlighted in a Journal of Investigative Dermatology article, the discovery of polymerase chain reaction (PCR) marked a radical transformation in biological science. PCR allows for the specific detection and generation of large amounts of DNA, playing a pivotal role in significant scientific endeavors such as the Human Genome Project. Widely utilized by clinicians and researchers, PCR facilitates disease diagnosis, gene cloning and sequencing, and sophisticated quantitative and genomic studies, offering rapid and highly sensitive results. Notably, one of the key medical applications of the classic PCR method is the detection of pathogens [12].

24.5 The Future

We now have highly effective genetic testing and disease therapies, a plethora of information about health on the internet, and the tools and hopefully the motivation to move ourselves in the right direction including more prevention modalities than ever before. With the rise in personalized medicine, we will be able to enhance our health right down to the cellular and genetic levels.

Novel devices are in development for the detection of skin cancer and other skin conditions, utilizing image analysis and computer-assisted diagnosis. These devices examine skin lesions for abnormal features and track changes over time, enabling more informed assessments of potentially problematic lesions that may warrant testing or removal. This pattern-recognition technology proves particularly beneficial for individuals with extensive lesions or a family history of melanoma, where the risk of melanoma is heightened. Ongoing research and refinement are expected to lead to advancements in detection and treatment.

Teledermatology, involving the computer-assisted transmission of dermatological data over long distances, is set to extend detection and therapeutic suggestions to regions where hands-on dermatology is limited. According to Joe Kvedar from Harvard Medical School, the internet's capabilities provide an opportunity for care delivery anytime, anywhere, allowing dermatologists to offer services independently of location and potentially disrupting existing referral networks.

Looking ahead, there is curiosity about upcoming drugs, currently considered experimental, that may soon be used for both acute and chronic illnesses. Additionally, questions arise about the potential emergence of boutique medicine, offering genetic treatments within the next decade. The ethical considerations of illness and genetic manipulation are also a topic of discussion. If genetic testing reveals a child's susceptibility to systemic lupus or severe arthritis, some may contemplate genetic manipulation for future protection. Evaluating the benefits of eliminating an illness through detection and genetic manipulation depends on the severity of the corresponding symptoms. The broader ethical implications encompass religious, philosophical, and moral imperatives associated with illness. As society moves forward, decisions will need to be made regarding what to prevent, repair, and prioritize in an ever-changing world.

One way to decide these is to read *The Code Breaker: Jennifer Doudna, Gene Editing, and the Future of the Human Race* by Walter Isaacson [13]. The must-read book recently moved onto my list of top books. The 2020 Nobel winner Jennifer Doudna, who helped develop the gene-editing technology CRISPR (clustered regularly interspaced short palindromic repeats) is highlighted in the book that states, "CRISPR could open some of the greatest opportunities, and most troubling quandaries, of this century." As it reveals new secrets about human life, it creates moral questions that must be addressed. The announcement of the 2020 Nobel Prize in Chemistry read- "This year's prize is about rewriting the code of life. These genetic scissors have taken the life sciences into a new epoch." I loved the inspiration, the rivalries, the ambitions and enormous hard work, and the thrill of discovery that opens the door to fundamental understanding of how life works.

In the book *Rule of the Robots* [14], Martin Ford argues that the true revolution is yet to come. "With unsupervised learning we are asking the computer to find its own patterns based on the data," states engineer Martin Kleiner. "Let's say I am looking for a spot on an X-ray of the lungs and I want to know if it is cancer. I can program the computer to do a Raster scan and specifically look for the spot and help define what it may be. With AI-supervised learning, humans are telling the computer what to look for. We understand the patterns and the expected outcomes and we are asking the computer to sort through tons of data to come up with the answer. Or I can also just feed a million X-rays into the computer and not tell it what I am looking for at all. I can just say 'look at all these X-rays and find your own way to cluster them and tell me what you come up with.' Both, of course are different aspects of artificial intelligence but the more exciting one is the unsupervised learning. It will find things you don't even know exist or how to even ask the computer to look for."

In this sequel to his prescient New York Times best seller *Rise of the Robots* [15], Ford presents us with a striking vision of the very near future. He argues that "AI is a uniquely powerful technology that is altering every dimension of human life, often for the better. For example, advanced science is being done by machines, solving devilish problems in molecular biology that humans could not, and AI can help us fight climate change or the next pandemic. It also has a capacity for profound harm. Deep fakes - AI-generated audio or video of events that never happened - are poised to cause havoc throughout society. AI empowers authoritarian regimes like China with unprecedented mechanisms for social control. And AI can be deeply biased, learning bigoted attitudes from us and perpetuating them." [14]

Is this speculation or science fiction or are we channeling "I, Robot," Asimov's fascinating, cautionary tale, and opening up Pandora's Box?

"In short, this is not a technology to simply embrace or let others worry about," Ford writes. "The machines are coming, and they won't stop, and each of us needs to know what that means if we are to thrive in the 21st century."

DeepMind Technologies is a British artificial intelligence subsidiary of Alphabet Inc. and research laboratory founded in September 2010 and based in London, with research centers in Canada, France, and the United States. In 2015, it became a subsidiary of Alphabet Inc., Google's parent company.

In one example of its power and efficacy, DeepMind Health had access to diverse medical data from hospitals, including admissions, discharge, transfer information, accident and emergency records, pathology and radiology data, and critical care data. This encompassed personal details like HIV diagnosis, depression history, and abortion records. The purpose of accessing this information was for research aimed at improving outcomes for various health conditions. In February 2018, DeepMind announced a collaboration with the U.S. Department of Veterans Affairs to utilize machine learning for predicting the onset of acute kidney injury and more broadly, the general deterioration of patients during a hospital stay. The objective was to enable faster treatment by doctors and nurses for patients in need.

Benjamin Franklin's belief that "All diseases may by sure means be prevented or cured, not excepting that of old age, and our lives lengthened at pleasure even beyond the antediluvian standard," reflects an optimistic outlook on the potential of medicine. Similarly, Dr. Alfred Gilman, a 1996 Nobel Laureate, envisioned a new era of medicine, predicting that in about 50 years, every molecule in the human body would be known, enabling the design of drugs specific to targeted molecules.

Considering the roughly one million genetic variants present in each person, the increasing capacity for genetic manipulation raises profound questions about the future of human health and longevity. The central question becomes, "What defines our humanity?" Amidst these advancements, it is crucial to address global challenges, such as climate change, to ensure the preservation of our planet.

While embracing new technologies, caution is necessary to avoid unintended consequences, as expressed in the proverb, "The camel came to receive horns and they cut off its ears." Future developments include the incorporation of full-immersion virtual reality to enhance experiences through augmented reality, engaging all our senses. Additionally, advancements in nanotechnology are poised to extend human intelligence, longevity, and disease prevention capabilities by interfacing biologic systems with human-created technology, as envisioned by Kurzweil and Grossman [16].

We should be optimistic; however, multiple challenges remain. The association with various alleles in various polygenic inflammatory dermatological diseases and their treatments lack the specificity and effect size for current clinical relevance. Although various strides have been made in atopic dermatitis and psoriasis, we are yet to identify strong associations that can predict the response to a particular biologic agent. Despite huge money being poured in machine learning and Big Data to crunch the numbers, we are yet to get to a model which can accurately predict the risk of development of atopic dermatitis and identify strongly associated variables that can predict its persistence into adulthood. The existence of such models in field of cardiology to very accurately identify, categorize, and predict the risk of heart disease in an individual shows that it is possible to have such models. We have limited resources and brainpower and are not able to prioritize research in precision medicine for noncancerous diseases. Despite predictions of a technologically advanced future in the past, we have not met the many of the expectations in healthcare with time. Mankind should not rest on its laurels but should come together and strive to actually achieve the technological prowess often predicted or hoped for in science fiction.

24.6 Summary

We now live in exciting and interesting times and have made wonderful advancements in the key areas of medical diagnosis and therapy. Although we live in the long shadow of Maimonides and other great past leaders, we now have our own unique battles and dreams. With the enormous power of Personalized Medicine to help influence our decisions, we can harness molecular analysis to influence medical decisions, practices, and therapies for the individual patient. Our goal remains—to utilize every means necessary to help our fellow mortals. But we are mortal, and we must carefully choose which is the best path to take.

References

1. Leibowitz JO. Maimonides on medical practice. Bull Hist Med. 1957;31(4):309–17.
2. Kottek SS. Maimonides (1138-1204): rabbi, physician and philosopher. IMAJ. 2005;7:547–53.
3. Barzel US, editor. Maimonides, art of cure: extracts from Galen (ed and trans). p. 108. cited in On Asthma, ed. and trans. G. Bos, p. 123.

4. Hamburg MA, Collins FS. The path to personalized medicine. N Engl J Med. 2010;363(4):301–4.
5. Mancinelli L, Cronin M, Sadée W. Pharmacogenomics. The promise of personalized medicine. AAPS PharmSci. 2000;2(1):E4.
6. Blackstone EH. Precision medicine versus evidence-based medicine. Circulation. 2019;140:1236–8.
7. Wang JY, Sarin KY. Dermatology advances into an era of precision medicine. JAMA Dermatol. 2021;157(7):770–2.
8. Norman RA, editor. Personalized, evolutionary, and ecological dermatology. Springer; 2016.
9. Nurse P. What is life?: five great ideas in biology. W. W. Norton & Company; 2021. p. 8.
10. Norman RA. The blue man and other stories of the skin the hidden life on the skin. University of California Press; 2014. p. 32.
11. DermTech. www.dermtech.com.
12. Garibyan L, Avashia N. Polymerase chain reaction. J Invest Dermatol. 2013;133(3):1–4.
13. Isaacson W. The code breaker: Jennifer Doudna, gene editing, and the future of the human race. Simon & Schuster; 2021.
14. Ford M. Rule of the robots. Basic Books; 2021.
15. Ford M. Rise of the robots. Basic Books; 2015.
16. Kurzweil R, Grossman T. Fantastic voyage. The Science Behind Radical Life Extension: Penguin; 2005.

Treating the Patient, Not the Disease: Holistic Dermatology Can Benefit

25

S. R. Narahari, S. N. Sourabha, and R. Yotsu

25.1 Treating the Patient, Not the Disease: Holistic Dermatology Can Benefit

When religion was strong and science weak, men mistook magic for medicine; now, when science is strong and religion weak, men mistake medicine for magic [1]. How can a physician turn into a health magician when the treatment and cure are received from the assembly of many sources? The knowledge available in biomedicine and complementary and alternative systems of medicine (CAM) shows that such a perceived magical response to treatment depends on the disease conditions, body constitutions (not entirely understood by genetics and epigenetics), and therapeutic forms. Therapies may react in different ways; suitable and active, repulsive, inactive, practical, and more effective. While some patients may get relieved by just a few biomedicine drugs, others look for better relief from their illness by combining medicines and procedures from traditional systems of medicine. Holistic or integrative medicine bases its evaluation on the understanding that individuals have exclusive receptivity and vulnerability to expedite cures or augment disease. Integrative medicine assesses the response to treatment based on the impact of care on patients. Holistic dermatology, as practised now, mainly focuses on chronic care

S. R. Narahari (✉)
Institute of Applied Dermatology, Kasaragod, Kerala, India

S. N. Sourabha
Sri Jayadeva Institute of Cardiovascular Science and Research, Bangalore, India

R. Yotsu
Department of Dermatology, National Center for Global Health and Medicine, Tokyo, Japan

School of Tropical Medicine and Global Health, Nagasaki University, Nagasaki, Japan

Department of Tropical Medicine, Tulane School of Public Health and Tropical Medicine, New Orleans, LA, USA

S. Gupta et al. (eds.), *Critical Thinking in Contemporary Dermatology: Cognitive Essays*, https://doi.org/10.1007/978-981-97-0411-8_25

and those patients who develop chronic conditions after very satisfying acute care provided by mainstream biomedicine.

25.2 Why Is the Paradigm Shift Happening in Patients' Perception of Deliverables by a HealthCare Facility?

The private sector dominates health care in the USA and many nations worldwide. In developing nations, it increased the number of corporate and tertiary hospitals without a required focus on primary care. The fee for service in the dominant private healthcare sector contributed to this belief and expectation of patients that biomedical health care services could answer all ailments. The commercialisation of the healthcare industry persuaded the change in the health-seeking behaviour of patients to seek speciality care ignoring primary care or a doctor in their locality. Often, patients seeking quicker relief tend to doctor-shopping in specialised private clinics, if cost allows. The pharmaceutical industry's promotions also contribute to the frequent use of high-technology products and devices in health care. Such patronage for specialities, coupled with research and newer treatment options, led to the compartmentalisation of biomedicine, and doctors trained in sub-specialities developed more knowledge on disease management. It proved excellent for acute care, but patients who developed chronic comorbidities are referred to multiple specialists because these comorbidities almost always involve multiple systems, and no single medical discipline takes ownership of the problem. Although it works well for acute care, such a disease-specific approach leaves patients suffering from chronic ailments dissatisfied despite the advances made by biomedicine. Those unhappy patients with chronic conditions explore other treatment options, especially CAM. Social media trumpets holistic medicine, whether self-medication or as patient-centric.

The patient-centricity of holistic medicine has a vital element in listening to the patient. However, listening to patients and counselling requires time that biomedical doctors do not have because of the demanding nature of medical science. Moreover, being a dominant system of health care, e.g. 97% of the Indian Government's budget is for the biomedical sector compared to 3% for CAM, leading to overcrowding in clinics, and biomedical doctors cannot spare the time needed for chronic patients. So, most patients feel confident with the CAM doctors, who do not have the crowd seeking quicker relief from illness and stress demanded by the acute care, and their capability to build rapport with them and their family members. Such is the rapport that patients reveal that they wish to continue the biomedical treatment simultaneously, while their biomedical physicians may or may not be aware of the holistic treatment regimens. The bond is initiated by the time allocated to the patient, which brings up patient-related issues along with symptoms of the disease: the first step in holistic medicine. Holistic medicine opens the door to understanding the patient and the context of their illness, problems, social situations, and beliefs, not just their disease. Sir William Osler said, '*The good physician treats the disease; the great physician treats the patient who has the disease.*' In practice, where most health delivery facilities are overstretched with the increasing workload, it is often the doctor's discretion to decide which elements of the patient's story are relevant. The current medical training focuses on what is relevant or fits the patterned thinking of disease management, especially after evidence-based medicine took a central position in the protocol- and guidelines-driven treatment approaches. Biomedical doctors must enhance their skills to treat patients and their diseases together, balancing technology-driven, pharmaceuticals-directed, evidence-based health care with patient-centric protocols.

25.3 How Could One Assess the Patient and Not Just the Disease?

Dermatology and cardiology, like other disciplines, have primarily chronic conditions and acute events over often unrecognised chronic diseases and some diseases with an acute presentation. Managing a chronic condition requires different skills than treating an acute condition. As the disease gets established, treatment options get limited; the doctor's role becomes more of an advisor. Diagnosis of a disease is only a starting point in patients' journey with chronic conditions. Once patients get a diagnosis, they have to manage their finances for treatment, treatment adherence, adverse effects of drugs, nutrition, self-care of the disease, and coping with their routine, including dealing with their job. In addition, a severe illness causes disability, and patients become dependent on their family members. Often, personal life can be compromised, such as sexual dysfunction, change in social status, and divorces due to psychosocial stress in visible skin diseases, such as vitiligo, especially in the skin of colour. Due to the chronicity of the disease, such developments in patients' lives may cause severe constraints on the family's income and achievement goals. Finally, the compartmentalisation of morbidities based on organ systems through referrals to other disciplines becomes more complex for patients as the disease gradually affects other organ systems. Such situations are demanding to patients, and they try to seek solace in holistic and patient-centric care services.

Oslerian wisdom advocates that a patient-centric approach to disease management could be developed through more intense bedside teaching in medical schools. Three decades ago, in Indian medical schools, there used to be intense bedside teaching during the ward's grand rounds (attended by the entire unit, i.e., faculty, residents, interns, undergraduate students, and nurses) and clinical case studies in outpatient departments (OPD). Grand rounds used to be conducted by the senior faculty in the unit, while the OPD discussions used to be conducted by different levels of faculty. During the busy OPD hours, the postgraduate students would pick up cases they could not diagnose and show them to the supervising faculty. If the faculty felt the presenting condition was worth discussing, they would either assign the patient to the same or a different resident and the discussion used to happen at a corner of the OPD in the seminar room. These bedside discussions used to start from the presenting history of the illness and move to the clinical signs, investigations, and the differential diagnosis; further investigations to confirm the diagnosis such as biopsy (those days, many imaging modalities were not available). Discussion would revolve around the disease and comorbidities. Many aspects of logistics also would get cited for lapses in care and hardships experienced by the care team and patients. There would be advocates for the 'gold standard' treatment as described in textbooks and experiences that such treatments may not work as well. The affordability of patients, potentially causing low treatment adherence was always part of the discussion, emphasising the tailoring of treatment for poor or affording patients. There are many incidents where patients discharged from the ward would get donations from doctors to buy medicines for a few days or even to travel home.

Bedside teaching rounds and seminar presentations mostly revolved around 'standard textbooks' except on journal club days. The senior faculty member would frequently refer patients to other departments, such as internal medicine or surgery. A resident or an intern had to accompany the patient and present the case to the expert to whom the patient was referred. During that time, PubMed, mobile phones, and the internet were unavailable, and literature could only be found by manually searching the departmental library, which used to be the source for reference during clinical hours. Post-clinic hours, resident doctors would rush to the college library that had a collection of bound volumes of foreign journals. The journal citations were obtained through the big books of Index Medicus. The library had racks of books, but they were limited compared to today's millions of books and articles on the web pages. One had to search for books in the classified racks manually. It allowed stumbling on a new or exciting book, intensely engaging clinicians who never intended to search for them, such as Shelly and Shelly's Dermatology; a highly patient-centric narration by Walter B. Shelley. Sir William Osler's Aequanimitas writes, 'full knowledge cannot be reached without drawing on supplies from other lands' and 'a student should be a citizen of the world'. These books inspired clinicians not to give up on a patient but encouraged them to look up all possible treatments available and offer them to patients. As the flow of information was not easy, all these gave scope for discussions across the disciplines.

When acquired immunodeficiency syndrome (AIDS) began to appear in the 1990s, the disease involved all organ systems and challenged the scompartmentalised care of biomedicine. Since antiretrovirals were not in the market, international policy-making bodies briefly focussed on CAMs as a possible treatment option for symptomatic AIDS patients. Academicians in Ayurveda medical colleges began discussing the parallel descriptions of AIDS. Ayurveda is the leading traditional medicine of India, governed by the Ministry of AYUSH, the acronym for Ayurveda, Yoga, Unani, Siddha, and Homoeopathy. AYUSH junior doctors in many provincial states of India undergo short training courses in biomedical hospitals. As a result, numerous English translations of Ayurveda terminologies and accounts of AYUSH practices are published in India as continuing medical education articles for the AYUSH stream, historical translations, or medical textbooks. Albeit, clinical studies always do not support such literature [2]. Many AIDS patients took Ayurvedic or other CAM treatments and biomedical therapy. The initial lacuna of effective antiretrovirals during the emerging epidemic triggered the discussion on integrative medicine or holistic medicine in many North American and European universities.

The Institute of Applied Dermatology (IAD) is among bedside integrative/holistic dermatology leaders. The IAD team has biomedically trained doctors/dermatologists working closely with Ayurvedic and Yoga practitioners, both prominent in India. It records clinical features in detail through written patient notes and photographs, all required details in providing gold-standard care. For example, each patient has 40+ pages of structured case sheets in lymphoedema. The history-taking is detailed, similar to homoeopathy, because it is a system that asks questions about all aspects of a patient's life. Other systems believe that a careful history is essential, but its practitioners rarely give the time necessary, which is about 30–45 min for each chronic patient, as they often come with a heap of old prescriptions. Homoeopathy has its critics but cannot be faulted for the time made available to the patient. Such a detailed recording of the history led to 'dermatology counselling' and tried to answer most questions patients and their family members raised. However, it may be difficult for the biomedical practitioner to understand the relevance of some of the questions because current medical teaching usually suggests that symptoms equate to the presence of pathology. Accordingly, many doctors cannot recognise symptoms that do not suit the understanding in straightforward pathological terms.

A few such medically unexplained symptoms find their reasoning in Ayurveda. For example, although chronic gastritis (CG) patients could be asymptomatic, many patients complain of gastrointestinal discomforts in clinical practice, such as stomach aches, bloating, nausea, vomiting, and loss of appetite. CG could be due to multiple factors, including eating habits. Therefore, CAM doctors adjust the diet habits of CG patients, such as excessive consumption of sweets, salty foods, meat, spices, and fried foods. In addition, reverting to *regular* eating habits is a crucial factor in improving CG. Ayurveda describes food digestion and assimilation as *agni* (sometimes termed *Jatharagni*; *Jathara* = duodenum). *Agni* depends on three energy principles (humor) of Ayurveda involved in physiological balance. These are *motion* (*Vatha*, comparable to the wind in action and properties), *metabolism* (*Pitta*, comparable to combustion with heat production), and *structure* (*Kapha*, meaning 'oily' and stable). If the three energy principles are balanced, with regular food intake and thirst, the person experiences usual bowel habits, a feeling of 'lightness' (not feeling lethargic), and the time to digest food is approximately 3 hours. This state is termed *Sama agni* (*Sama* = equal) and indicates that food gets digested properly.

However, digestion is disturbed when one energy principle is predominantly expressed rather than a balance of all three. When dominated by *vatha*, food intake is erratic (*Vishama*), and the patient struggles to have an eating 'routine'. When dominated by *pitta*, it is excessive (*Theekshna*), and the patient becomes hungry less than 3 hours after the meal. When *Kapha* dominates, the digestion process becomes slow (*Manda*), meaning that a patient might require an increased length of time to become hungry after food. Derangements in *agni* produce additional clinical features such as skin dryness, exhaustion, poor work tolerance, fainting episodes, and rarely phonophobia [3]. The *agni* imbalance causes faltered nourishing of the patient's essential body tissues (*Dhathu*) by the assimilated food. The control of assimilation of the 'essences of digestion' (comparable to nutrients) is *Dhathu agni*.

Ayurveda describes seven of these essences. Ayurveda described the clinical features of each *Dhathu agni* pathology.

The Ayurvedic term *ama* describes food absorbed into the body without being digested adequately due to the patient's digestion being overall reduced (*Manda agni*) or excessive (*Theekshna agni*). *Ama* has a broader comparable meaning of intermediary products of metabolism and toxic substances arising from the diet. Undigested food, according to Ayurveda, is in a 'fermented state' in the stomach, where it contains harmful elements if absorbed, that might cause disease. After absorption, circulating *ama* could reside in sites of altered physiology (described as *Khavaigunya*), such as damaged joints and aggravate such pathology. *Ama* blocks *Dhathu agni* channels, causing more symptoms. *Ama* caused by pathological body tissue (*Dosha*) is known as *Sama*. *Vatha* associated with *ama* presents with abdominal pain and distension, indicating intestinal pathology (*Pakwashaya*, *pakwa* = digested food, *ashaya* = channel). Due to *Pitta* derangement, *ama* presents with an oral foul smell, bitter taste, and excessive salivation. The sensation of an oral 'coating' is due to *Kapha*, which originates from the stomach. Both the stomach and intestine, therefore, may be sites of disease creation. Biomedicine is beginning to recognise that both nutrients and non-nutritional components of a diet are essential to gastrointestinal health; they also may cause or influence the development of gut pathology (e.g., inflammatory bowel disease, dietary intolerance, or sensitivity and/or allergy). The appropriate diet may profoundly affect intestinal recovery and the successful management of chronic gastrointestinal diseases [4]. A proper nutritional assessment and 'diet therapy' are essential in such cases. In determining what dermatology patients should eat, a common question by patients, a lengthy and structured interview with a dietician is required, who should be working with the multi-system team to understand the diseases and the patients.

Ama occurring during treatment could increase disease activity and make medications less effective if such medications require normal digestion for their therapeutic effect. In this situation, the indicated medicines have to be temporarily withdrawn. *Ama* is treated with carminatives (*pachana*). If *ama* is caused by slowed digestion (*Manda agni*), appetisers (*deepana*) could be added to the regimen. Ayurvedic medicine should be restarted after the clinical features of *ama* subside and normal *agni* features manifest. In the above situation, biomedical treatment would add more drugs to control digestion-related symptoms. Figure 25.1 shows the benefit of recognising and treating *ama* during the treatment of vitiligo.

Integrally linked to *agni* is *kosta*, meaning bowel movements. 'Normal' bowel movements (*samakosta*) are defined as opening bowels once daily with semi-solid faeces that pass quickly. Regularly not passing the stool and are hard and dry, is constipated (*krurakosta*) bowel. Constipation (*krura*) is due to erratic *agni* (*vatha* vitiation). If the patients need to open their bowels after drinking a small quantity of milk (*mrudukosta*), this represents excessive *agni* (predominant expression of *pitta*, also known as vitiation). *Kosta* must be corrected prior to prescribing ayurvedic medicines because it can modify the effect of the medicines. For example, high-potency drugs, which take a long time to digest, are not given to *Mrudu kosta* patients. Constipation is a common complaint of patients including those with skin,

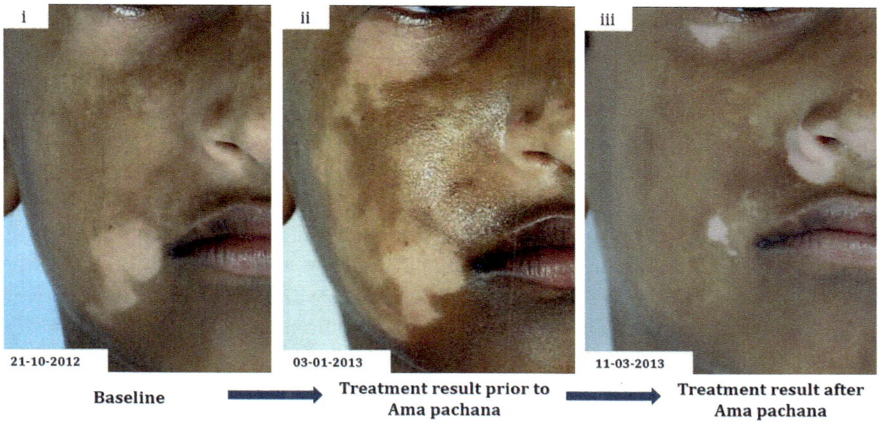

Fig. 25.1 Holistic dermatology: (**i**) Vitiligo patient presenting with biomedically unexplained or non-specific symptoms that could be equated to the ayurvedic diagnosis of *ama* (21-10-2012). (**ii**) Treatment outcome without treating *ama* (03-01-2013). (**iii**) Later, all vitiligo treatments were stopped, and *ama* was managed using the ayurvedic treatment called *ama pachana* and then treated for vitiligo (11-03-2013)

neurological, and kidney diseases and is managed by daily laxatives (*anulomana*). Bowel movements are related to *agni* and can reflect a digestive system abnormality, and Ayurveda recommends looking for its causation. In addition, eating food at a regular time (*kala bhojana*), skipping meals (*abhojana*), the number of meals consumed per day, and symptoms of proper digestion (*jeernalakshana*) are part of ayurvedic clinical evaluation. All these assessments give an idea about the patient's digestive problems, and their correction using herbal medications is part of the regimen to solve the patient's disease condition. So, CAM attributes certain 'biomedically unexplained symptoms' to the clinical features not described in dermatology or internal medicine books; thus, working with AYUSH practitioners brings the patient's perspective to the treatment. Integrative medicine protocols include patient's features and disease-specific management described for gut evaluation. Dysbiosis and gut–brain axis studies are receiving funding, and new publications are emerging every day. We, in our setup, receive many patients who have often been treated in many reputed institutions. Their prescriptions often contain histamine blockers and proton-pump inhibitors, and despite such treatments, patients continue to experience uneasiness, bloating of the abdomen, loss of taste, and lethargy. Integrative Medicine treatment helps relieve such patients, which has been measured by quality-of-life indicators [5].

Novel interventions frequently use health-related quality of life (HRQoL) as an outcome measure to monitor the efficacy of the intervention [6]. HRQoL can be measured by tools such as the World Health Organization Disability Assessment Schedule 2.0 (WHODAS 2.0) and the Dermatology Life Quality Index (DLQI). The qualitative studies focus on patient-reported outcomes (PROMs). Often generic measures miss relevant HRQoL contents reflecting local cultures and patients' beliefs. Hence, disease-specific tools are used, for example, to capture the issues faced by lymphoedema patients (Lymphatic Filariasis Quality of Life Questionnaire-LFSQQ [7]) because the psychometric properties of health status measures help determine the appropriateness of a particular tool in a specific population. LFSQQ guides the care team to treat patients along with their disease. It is administered routinely to all patients by a nurse counsellor. It inquires about many facets of life affected by the disease, often ignored by biomedical doctors. Life domains used to assess the HRQoL of lymphoedema patients include the following: mobility (sitting and getting out of the chair, sitting down and standing up from the floor, travelling by public transport), self-care (dressing, bathing, washing clothes, difficulty in using the toilet), usual activities (difficulty in gardening, doing agrarian work), disease burden (foul smell-odor, itching (eczema/discharge from limb), pain/discomfort (pain in the joints or of the body parts), psychological health (feeling neglected by friends and family members), and social participation (problems in moving around freely without feeling self-conscious, approaching people in the community). LFSQQ, as a PROM introduced to the routine treatment, helped develop patient-centric care for lymphoedema [8]. LFSQQ performed better than other HRQoL tools (WHODAS 2.0, DLQI) in the Lymphatic Filariasis population in the age- and gender-matched control group [6]. LFSQQ, which inquires into seven life domains, had missing value rates lower than 10%, suggesting high feasibility, high internal consistency, and discriminant validity. However, one must be careful because the tick-box approach often does not build rapport and fails to reveal why patients consult doctors or patients' level of satisfaction.

Nurse counsellors' rapport with patients improved when tools to measure PROMs were used routinely in practice and their treatment adherence. Adherence to treatment with a complex and demanding self-help regimen burdens the individual and the family member who participate in giving their support [3, 8]. Home-based self-care requires the support of skilled and time-consuming counselling. Every detail of the proposed therapy is discussed, and an understanding of lymphoedema and its management is ascertained. Close family members also attend the counselling sessions. The nurse emphasises that therapy is lifelong, and the patient could opt out. The nurse counsellor in the treatment team greatly supports the medical consultation. Non-verbal communication, such as body postures, eye contact, facial expressions, and other communication skills, comes from training and experience and wins over patients. The first rule in communication is to shut up and listen; the second is to encourage the debate [9]. Listening to the patient without interruption for at least half a minute is essential whenever they arrive for consultation. They tend to narrate most of their symptoms in that period. The clinical communication should elicit why a patient is trying to consult the doctor. Based on that information, medical treatments could be individualised.

Counselling chronic patients using specialised tools or disease-specific PROMs is likely to bring discussion of their health beliefs that may defy scientific reasoning. In such a patient-centric approach, the healthcare team always listens to the patients and the objective of the patient's visit to the centre is elicited before drawing up the treatment protocol. The health care culture for chronic diseases among great physicians is to listen to the patient, empathise with them through verbal and body language, and do *at least* an organ-specific clinical examination. In addition, reliance on advanced healthcare technology and evidence-based medicine should always be carefully balanced with clinical experience or findings. While in acute care, the goal of the health care team and patients align, and both are happy when patients walk back home.

Nevertheless, this is not the story for chronic care. Chronic patients require training in self-care. Doctors with few treatment options should become advisers rather than being prescriptive. Ayurveda advocates the concept of '*gruhopachara*' a Sanskrit word meaning 'caring for patients at home' or 'giving treatment at home'. It aims at attaining significant symptomatic control at a low cost. '*Gruhopachara*' is the tradition of India and many developing nations to respect the wish of patients to give home care to the sick and elderly to nurse them until death. Many dying patients wish to breathe last in their homes. Families sometimes try palliative care utilising the locally available indigenous medicines. Integrative medicine treatment of lymphoedema is home-based, and family members assist self-care in providing a continuum of care at a low cost (Fig. 25.2) [8]. It incorporates all recommendations of the International Society of Lymphology. India has an estimated 25 million lymphoedema patients. Being a low resource country, *gruhopachara* model implemented after 2 weeks of training at the Institute of Applied Dermatology, Kerala, is accepted widely. The centre draws patients from 26 provincial Indian states and several nations from abroad. We recently audited the follow-up pattern of our lymphoedema patients. Table 25.1 shows the follow-up pattern, and Fig. 25.3 shows the reduction in the disease severity, which is not dependent on the follow-up

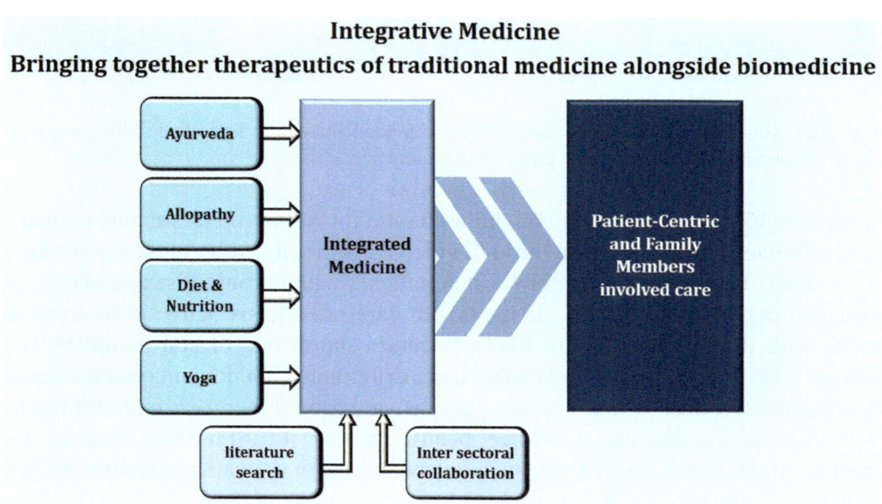

Fig. 25.2 The perfect blend of biomedicine and traditional medicine system requires intensely engaging patient-centric approaches of patient-oriented researchers and multi-disciplinary collaboration and a non-inferiority multi-system health care team

Table 25.1 Percentage reduction in volume at the time of discharge from baseline values and at different follow-ups of 1570 lymphoedema patients from the clinical audit of data (2010–2019) from the Institute of Dermatology, Kasaragod, Kerala, India

At the time of discharge		First follow-up		Second follow-up	
Days of treatment	% Reduction**	Interval	% Reduction**	Interval	% Reduction*
≤14 days	23.48^{a}	≤48 days	23.63^{a}	≤112 days	39.65^{a}
>14 days	29.55^{b}	48–70 days	28.08^{b}	112–203 days	44.00^{b}
		>70 days	28.00^{b}	>203 days	39.28^{a}

Values with the common alphabet as superscript within a column are not significantly different, and different alphabets suggest different groups. It is not possible to reduce the leg volume to nil
One-way ANOVA: *Significant at 5% level, **significant at 1% level

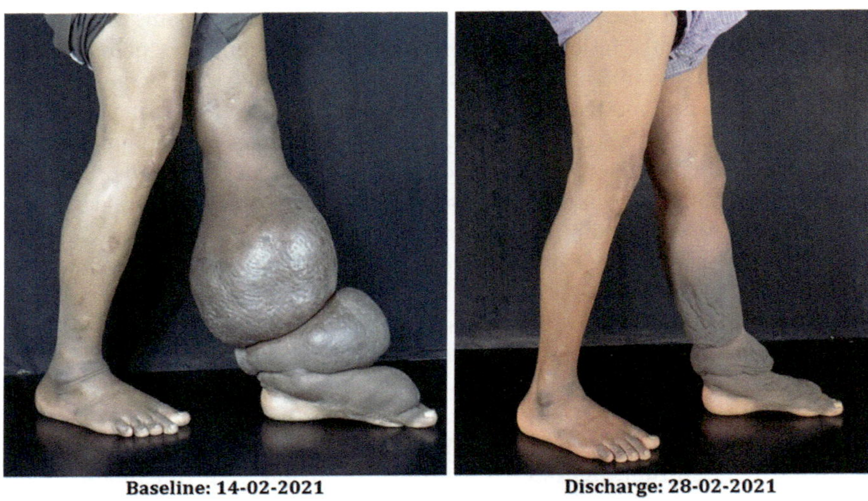

Fig. 25.3 Response to integrative medicine in lymphoedema due to Lymphatic Filariasis; baseline to discharge from the intensive phase of treatment

schedule [10]. Many patients who did not come for follow-up treatments regularly are on WhatsApp consultation through video calls facilitated by nurse counsellors. This brings to the question of how often patients with chronic diseases should be asked to come for the review. If the health care provider is active in intervening more with illness, patients are likely to return more; one reason would be that adverse effects begin to manifest when more drugs are given. Patient reviews should balance the felt-need of the doctors, patients, and family members and aim to prevent disease aggravation, reinforce health literacy regarding the disease, and improve the HRQoL. Over time, such behaviours from the nation's healthcare system would influence the health-seeking behaviour of the people.

The patient-centric approach, as described above, requires dedicated time, at least 45–60 min, with the patient. Additionally, answering their questions when they get back home requires a dedicated healthcare worker to support them through WhatsApp consultation until patients return to their routine or adjust to the changed routine that the disease forces them. Inspired by the international skincare nursing group and the International Society of Dermatology's Task Force for Skin Care for All (Community Dermatology) [11], the IADVL developed a dermatology nursing syllabus in India to train nurses to care for patients suffering from chronic skin diseases as part of the holistic dermatology care system. Cosmetology, dermato-surgery and dermatology service clinics also require nursing support for their dermatology practice. Wound care, performing minor dermatologic procedures, and patient counselling requires deep engagement with patients. With a smiling face and not a hard long one, nurses' involvement is essential to providing better patient services. The nursing practices suit the culture of stakeholders, particularly patients and health delivery practices; nurses should become a vital part of the chronic care delivery team. Over two decades, the IAD developed a holistic care model for lymphoedema; in biomedical hospitals as the nurse-led (as in Japan). In Ayurveda Medical Colleges and AYUSH clinics, treatment is led by Ayurveda doctors, a funded programme of the Bill and Melinda Gates Foundation [12]. When nurses and AYUSH doctors take leadership in bedside care, they automatically bring the patient-centric approaches because both get intense bedside training with patients. They give importance to issues like methods of drug administration, close follow-up, and what the patients tell and believe about their illness.

25.4 Can One Learn a Patient-Centric Approach from the Literature, or Is the Skill Innate?

It is possible if doctors approach each disease with an open mind. Doctors should internalise skills to construct a decision tree for structuring the problem so that alternative courses are defined for each chronic patient. Look at the national guidelines and explore why the national guidelines or institute's protocols might not be followed for the patient. Analyse the diagnostic uncertainty by eliciting specific physical factors for a particular patient and finding reasons in AYUSH/CAM for biomedically unexplained symptoms or patients' individual choices. In addition to the PubMed database, health care providers could look up the AYUSH research portal. Most publications listed in the AYUSH research portal write about comparable biomedical diagnoses. Ayurveda journals publish an overview of patient-centric approaches in AYUSH. A little information is available in the literature on managing Neglected Tropical Diseases. A simplistic and reductionist approach to medical practice fails to recognise the complexities of illness, beliefs, behaviors, and the total requirement of the patients to return to their previous routine (Fig. 25.4). The patient-centric regimens lead to less medicalisation of consultations, lesser investigations, prevention of polypharmacy, identifying associated comorbidities, drug–drug and drug–diet interactions and optimal treatment. It comforts the sick irrespective of the ability to provide the cure.

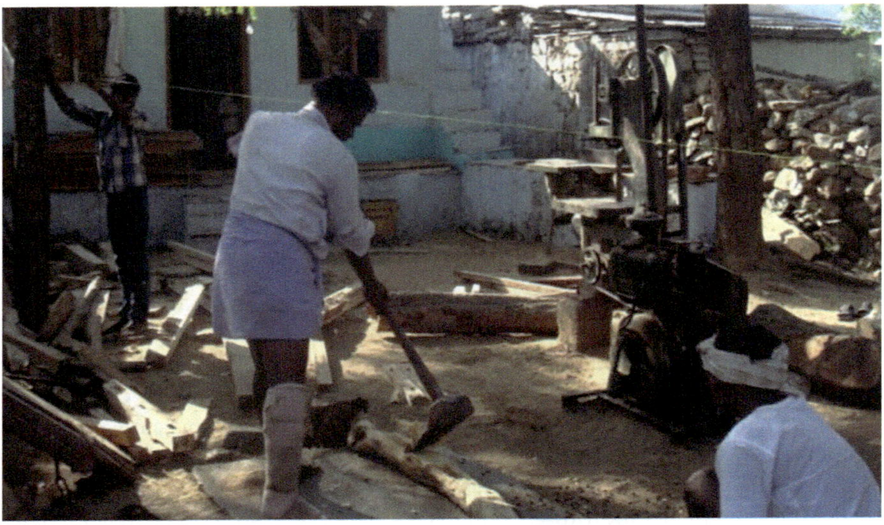

Fig. 25.4 Wellness aims at the total requirement of the patients to return to their previous routine. In the picture, a carpenter returns to his business following integrative medicine received at the primary health centre, Malkhed, in the Lymphatic Filariasis endemic district of Kalaburagi, Karnataka state in south India. The project was supported by the Central Council for Research in Ayurvedic Sciences, Ministry of AYUSH, Government of India

Once patients realise that chronic disease means a permanent disease, they begin speaking to their peers on social media platforms. Doctors should also maintain an online working relationship with the patients in this digitalised world. Their questions should trigger a deviation from the patterned thinking of the doctors. Learning from their problems and experiences shows the way forward and might lead to evolving integrative medicine treatment regimens. Patients need relief no matter which system of medicine they take. Such a philosophy promoted biomedicine's development. However, the compartmentalised systems of medicine and even specialities within biomedicine do not always heed this fundamental principle. As patients' health literacy improves, they remind the Indian proverb that *an old patient is better than a new doctor*. Managing them would require a multi-disciplinary approach, and one system's knowledge may not be sufficient to explain all their symptoms. As patients come with more information from other systems of medicine, doctors can choose to ignore the patient or begin learning from them.

Prof Terence Ryan, the curator of 13 Norham Gardens, Oxford, the home of Sir William Osler, an emeritus professor of dermatology in Oxford, is arguing to use the currently available knowledge for improving the care as a way to reduce the cost of medical treatments and providing better care to the world population. He advocates for '**Do K(no)w Harm**' for both biomedical and CAM systems. Giving clear recommendations about the best course of action, which comes from biomedicine and constantly improving their trust. The communication between the medical care team and patients is central to patient-centric approaches. So, the disconnect between the patients and the health care team must be avoided because that leaves patients dissatisfied despite the advances made by technology-driven medicine, while care teams tend to respect evidence-based protocols putting aside their experience-driven insights in patient management. The patients' chapters of Oxford Medicine point to the reality that evidence-based medicine has not yet collected data in many areas of patients' well-being. It gives the analogy of the parable of 'The Emperor Has No Clothes' for highly disease-driven and protocol-adhered practices leading to doctors thinking what patients are telling cannot be accurate.

The WHO Global Centre for Traditional Medicine at Jamnagar, Gujarat, India, is a global knowledge centre for traditional medicine [13]. The Government of India supports it; it aims to unravel the potential of CAM worldwide through modern science and technology. It has four strategic areas: evidence and learning, data and analytics, sustainability and equity, and innovation and technology to optimise the contribution of CAM to global health and sustainable development. One hundred seventy (87.6%) of the 194 WHO Member States use traditional medicine, and their governments are requesting WHO's support in evidence-based data on traditional medicine practices and drugs. The National AYUSH Mission (NAM) is the country-wide public health programme of the Ministry of AYUSH, Government of India, to promote traditional medicine through cost-effective AYUSH services. The Indian Government has approved financial sanctions to operationalise 12,500 Health and Wellness Centres under *Ayushman Bharat* (the national health insurance) in a phased manner under NAM. The vision is to establish a holistic wellness model to reduce the disease burden, provide informed choices to the needy public, and minimise out-of-pocket expenditure on health care. The initiative, popularly known as AYUSH Wellness centres, stems from the concept of Ayurveda to preserve and retain wellness when one has it, enrich and strengthen when it is diminishing rather than searching for the same after losing it. The mind-body literature advocates for confidence and caution for prudent health management. The term patient denotes the health seeker's healthy mindset against unhealthy physical conditions. A patient bears the suffering and waits for a cure with the power of hope.

25.5 What Are the Responsibilities of the Health Seekers and the Attendants?

They are balancing the Googled knowledge about the disease and its severity with clarity on health hazards and healing, confidence in the doctor, medicine, and their own body's response based on immunity (known as *bala* in Ayurveda; congenital, seasonal, and acquired). Patients should be aware that prescription and lifestyle disciplines are two sides of a cure tool. Sustainable relief from the disease is possible by combining the right doctor, diagnosis, and drug with adherence to treatment and self-care and lifestyle. Doctors' medication gets its life only through endorsement by the patient's commitment. Holistic medicine should strive to bring mental calm to patients. Stress worsens the disease effects and decelerates the drug effects. During the convalescence period, patients need total rest. Rest does not mean being idle round the clock. It is the proper dosage of the preferred dimension of work, such as diversion from routine work, pleasant and customised engagements, and strain-free health-compatible occupations.

There is a role for attendants and care-ambience in patients' speedy recovery. Attendants should spend more time with health seekers and appear brisk, appealing, and inspiring. Often, attendants' presence and personalities bring peace and instil confidence in patients. In addition, attendants trained in patient-friendly language and communication methods function as architects of warmth and wellness and accelerate treatment tolerance levels. Hospital care staff should aim to send off patients with a renewed lease of life, driven by positive energy. The health care team should classify and customise attention to patients according to the latter's mindsets and therapeutic compatibilities, responses, and resources. An ideal wellness centre provides homeliness and exclusiveness in a curing environment and nourishes well-being through comfort and solace. Such an approach could reverse the domination of cry, sorrow, seriousness, and silence often seen in drugs- and device-driven modern hospital buildings.

सत्वमात्माशरीरंचत्रयमेतत्त्रदिंडवत् ।.
लोकस्तष्ठितसिंयोगात्तत्रसर्वंप्रतष्ठितिम् ॥.

(Writing from the chapter on *living a longer life* of the ancient textbook of Ayurveda; *SatwamathmaShariram Cha TrayametathTridandavath*: mind, energy, and body are an individual's tripod [14]).

References

1. Conlon CP, Cox TM. In: Firth J, editor. Oxford textbook of medicine. 6th ed. New York: Oxford University Press; 2020.
2. Narahari SR, Ryan TJ, Bose KS, Prasanna KS, Aggithaya GM. Integrating modern dermatology and Ayurveda in the treatment of vitiligo and lymphedema in India: modern dermatology and Ayurveda in vitiligo. Int J Dermatol. 2011;50:310–34.
3. Narahari SR, Aggithaya MG, Morrow SE, Ryan TJ. Developing an integrative medicine patient care protocol from the existing practice of Ayurveda dermatology. Curr Sci. 2016;111(2):3021–7.
4. Li Y, Su Z, Li P, Li Y, Johnson N, Zhang Q, et al. Association of symptoms with eating habits and food preferences in chronic gastritis patients: a cross-sectional study. Evid Based Complement Alternat Med. 2020;5:197–201.
5. Neri L, Iovino P, Laxative Inadequate Relief Survey (LIRS) Group. Bloating is associated with worse quality of life, treatment satisfaction, and treatment responsiveness among patients with constipation-predominant irritable bowel syndrome and functional constipation. Neurogastroenterol Motil. 2016;28:581–91.
6. Thomas C, Narahari SR, Bose KS, Vivekananda K, Nwe S, West DP, et al. Comparison of three quality of life instruments in lymphatic filariasis: DLQI, WHODAS 2.0, and LFSQQ. PloS Negl Trop Dis. 2014;8(2):e2716.
7. Aggithaya MG, Narahari SR, Vayalil S, Shefuvan M, Jacob NK, Sushma KV. Self care integrative treatment demonstrated in rural community setting improves health related quality of life of lymphatic filariasis patients in endemic villages. Acta Trop. 2013;126:198–204.
8. Narahari SR, Bose KS, Aggithaya MG, Swamy GK, Ryan TJ, Unnikrishnan B, et al. Community level morbidity control of lymphoedema using self care and integrative treatment

in two lymphatic filariasis endemic districts of South India: a non randomised interventional study. Trans R Soc Trop Med Hyg. 2013;107:566–77.
9. Spiegelhalter D. The art of statistics: learning from data. London: Pelican; 2020.
10. Narahari SR, Aggithaya MG, Ryan TJ, Muralidharan K, Franks PJ, Moffatt C, et al. Self-care treatment for lymphoedema of lymphatic filariasis using integrative medicine. Br J Dermatol. 2023;190:94–104.
11. Ryan TJ. The International Society of Dermatology's task force for skin care for all: community dermatology. Int J Dermatol. 2011;50:548–51.
12. Gibson L, Moffatt CJ, Narahari SR, Kabiri L, Ikhile D, Nchafack A, et al. Global knowledge gaps in equitable delivery of chronic edema care: a political economy case study analysis. Lymphat Res Biol. 2021;19:447–59.
13. Global Centre for Traditional Medicine. https://en.wikipedia.org/wiki/Global_Centre_for_Traditional_Medicine. Accessed on February 18, 2024.
14. Caraka.Deerghamjeevitheeyamadhyayam. In: Caraka, Dridhabala, eds. Caraka Samhita. Varanasi: Chowkhamba Sanskrit Series Office, 2002; verse 46.

Social Medicine in Dermatology Must Remain Center Stage

26

Robert Norman

Over the last 4 years I completed a biography of Rudolf Virchow. The book is called *Rudolf Virchow: Father of Pathology*. Rudolf Virchow's approach to medicine was characterized by his ability to examine life with a simultaneous focus on microscopic details and a broader cultural and public health perspective. His renowned statement, "Medicine is a social science, and politics is nothing more than medicine on a grand scale," encapsulates his belief in the interconnectedness of medicine and societal well-being. Virchow viewed medicine as a metaphor for understanding the entirety of society, considering it as an ailing patient in need of remedy.

Virchow's approach extended beyond the traditional bounds of medical science; he treated society as a whole using a disease model. As his career progressed, he incorporated insights from anthropology and social science, broadening his understanding of the factors influencing health on a societal level. His holistic perspective emphasized the importance of considering not only the microscopic aspects of diseases but also their broader cultural, political, and social contexts.

By treating society as a patient and applying a disease model to understand and address societal issues, Virchow left a lasting legacy that continues to influence the way we approach medicine, public health, and social challenges today. His ability to bridge the gap between microscopic observations and societal dynamics highlights the importance of a comprehensive and interdisciplinary approach to understanding and improving health on both an individual and societal level. I learned a tremendous amount during my time with Virchow, and certainly it informs my life and this chapter. As we look at the future of dermatology, we must cast a wide net and consider public health, acute and chronic illness, health care disparity, climate change, and skin of color education. I will focus on these issues. Much also needs to be done to prevent and repair the disfiguring effects brought on by nicotine and

R. Norman (✉)
Center for Geriatric Dermatology, Integrative Dermatology and Neuro-Dermatology, Nova Southeastern, Fort Lauderdale, FL, USA

S. Gupta et al. (eds.), *Critical Thinking in Contemporary Dermatology: Cognitive Essays*, https://doi.org/10.1007/978-981-97-0411-8_26

alcohol, excess weight, mobility and exercise difficulties, dysfunctional nutrition, improper hygiene, lack of immunizations, poor reading and comprehension skills, financial issues, social media influences on body dysmorphia, and many other problems.

26.1 Public Health

Christopher Hamlin's insights, as outlined in the Oxford Handbook of the History of Medicine, emphasize the intricate relationship between public health and political philosophy and practice [1]. The historical context is crucial for understanding the evolution of public health and its impact on societies. Hamlin underscores that the evaluation of health status is inherently a historical problem, as the effects of various influences on populations can only be accurately measured over extended periods. Public health, according to Hamlin, is a significant yet often under-recognized element in the grand moral narratives of history—the struggles of people striving for better lives. The pursuit of health is intertwined with broader societal issues, reflecting the moral and ethical dimensions of human existence. Hamlin also raises essential questions about happiness, prosperity, and self-determination in the context of public health. Considering the future, he suggests that discussions about a healthy population inevitably implicate these broader issues. The advancement of public health is not merely about physical well-being but also about enhancing the overall quality of life, happiness, and the ability of individuals and communities to determine their own destinies. In essence, Hamlin's perspective highlights the multidimensional nature of public health, its embeddedness in historical narratives, and its intersection with fundamental aspects of human existence and societal progress. Understanding the historical context of public health becomes crucial in navigating contemporary challenges and envisioning a future where health is not only a physical state but also a reflection of societal well-being and human flourishing.

In the foreseeable future, the two prominent figures influencing our narrative of health and happiness are likely to remain politics and money. In the United States, there's a notable failure to grapple with the ethical necessity of implementing a single-payer system. The glaring disparities in healthcare access contribute to a significant amount of wastefulness in the daily routines of practitioners, marked by arduous processes like prior authorizations, navigating prescription eligibilities, and coping with delays and denials of treatments. It's conceivable that insurance companies engage in a form of legalized gambling or, some might argue, "legalized" theft. However, the preference should unequivocally be for top-tier healthcare rather than witnessing insurance company and bank edifices dominating the urban American skyline.

A significant number of healthcare practitioners entered the field seeking intellectual engagement, yet the day-to-day reality of medicine is saturated with an unusually high level of interference from insurance and governmental entities, sapping our enthusiasm and vitality. While a single-payer system might pose fewer challenges in an afterlife scenario, the prospect of a comprehensive single-payer system could be the real-world challenge if current conditions persist.

26.2 Chronic Illness

The World Health Organization provides the following key facts related to chronic diseases: chronic diseases have become the primary cause of death and disability on a global scale. Specifically, half of these chronic disease-related deaths, amounting to 17 million annually, are associated with cardiovascular diseases, with heart disease and stroke being the predominant contributors.

Heart attacks and strokes claim the lives of approximately 12 million individuals annually, while an additional 3.9 million succumb to hypertensive and other heart conditions. Over one billion adults globally are overweight, with around 300 million classified as clinically obese. The majority of cardiovascular disease (CVD), accounting for about 75%, can be attributed to key risk factors such as high cholesterol, high blood pressure, inadequate fruit and vegetable consumption, a sedentary lifestyle, and tobacco use. Persistent behavioral interventions have proven effective in reducing these population risk factors. The rise in chronic diseases as the leading cause of death and disability worldwide affects both developing and developed nations, marking a shift influenced by industrialization, urbanization, economic development, and increased globalization of the food market. Changing to a healthier diet, increasing physical activity, and ceasing smoking can prevent up to 80% of coronary heart disease cases, 90% of type 2 diabetes cases, and one-third of cancer cases, demonstrating the substantial impact of lifestyle modifications in a relatively short period.

The World Health Organization's (WHO) World health statistics report of 2021 is the annual compilation of the most recent available data on health and health-related indicators for its 194 Member States and features the latest data for 50+ health-related indicators from the Sustainable Development Goals (SDG) and WHO Triple Billion targets. The 2021 report additionally focuses on the human toll and impact of the coronavirus disease 2019 (COVID-19) pandemic. Despite making up less than 1% of the nation's population, people living in nursing homes and other long-term-care facilities account for at least 35% of the United States COVID-19 deaths. Having multiple chronic diseases greatly increases the COVID-19 mortality rate.

Examining these facts from the WHO should prompt an awareness of the choices available. We navigate a world between expectation and reality, aiming to shed light on the challenges and explore solutions for this growing societal burden.

Chronic illness poses a multifaceted challenge in our society. The desire for a high-quality life has never been greater, yet we inhabit bodies prone to ailments. Over 10,000 individuals are entering their 50s daily, with many believing their best years lie ahead. However, a significant portion of those aged 50 and above will either carry chronic illnesses into their later years or develop such issues as they age.

The focus on chronic illness gained traction in the 1950s, following the widespread use of antibiotics, immunizations, and public health measures that successfully combated many acute illnesses threatening the population. However, the medical field is producing fewer primary care and geriatric physicians equipped with the comprehensive knowledge needed to care for those with chronic illnesses. Only recently has there been a passionate effort to address chronic illness, recognizing its substantial impact on society—financially, socially, and spiritually—revealing the imperative to learn more and seek clear and viable solutions.

26.3 Carcinogens and Chronigens

What should we focus our limited resources on? Given that diseases keeps us inventive, what diseases should we prioritize treating?

We certainly can do our best to provide the ultimate in personalized medicine but we must keep in mind that among the key factors for our future health is how we value our environments, and how we deal with increasing onslaught of carcinogens and chronigens. (Chronigen is a term I created). We've long been aware of carcinogens and have swiftly comprehended endocrine disruptors. But what about chronigens? Any chemical trigger that leads to chronic illness is deemed a chronigen.

Linda Reuscher, a prominent chronic illness expert, expressed concerns about the omnipresence of plastic, stating, "Plastic is everywhere, and it's a problem." The accumulation of plastic water bottles and bags in landfills is a well-known issue, persisting for thousands of years without breaking down. Reuscher highlights the challenge of finding a piece of food that has never touched plastic, emphasizing that plastics leach chemicals into the food and beverages they come into contact with. Moreover, heating plastics exacerbates the release of molecules, intensifying the issue. Particularly problematic is bisphenol A (BPA), an industrial chemical used to make certain plastics and resins since the 1950s. BPA is found in polycarbonate plastics that are often used in containers that store food and beverages, such as water bottles. They may also be used in other consumer goods, although manufacturers are creating more and more BPA-free products [2].

The Food and Drug Administration (FDA) and the Environmental Protection Agency (EPA) assess toxins and establish permissible limits based on their research to prevent immediate illness. However, they often overlook what Janet Jackson-Nakazawa, in her book *The Autoimmune Epidemic* refers to as the "barrel effect" [3]. The cumulative impact of numerous assaults over time can cause the metaphorical barrel to overflow, resulting in illness. This concept applies not only to human health but also to the health of the Earth. When the delicate balance is upset just a little, we self-correct. When the delicate balance is bombarded, it is more difficult to make things right.

Our food is laden with toxins, many of which qualify as chronigens. The concentration of toxins increases up the food chain, exemplified by mercury in fish and pesticides in animals that consume contaminated crops. Livestock routinely receive growth hormones and antibiotics, contributing to the overall toxic load.

Beyond our plates, toxins in the air and water are absorbed by plants and animals, amplifying the environmental burden. Even seemingly innocuous actions like drinking a glass of water expose us to chlorine, pesticides, heavy metals, and pharmaceuticals. The disposal of medications (people flushing pills down the toilet), coupled with incomplete drug metabolism in individuals, contributes to pharmaceuticals entering the water supply. Conventional water filtering methods often fail to remove these drugs, meaning that substances like hormones, contraceptives, antidepressants, and tranquilizers may persist in our water. As these contaminants move up the food chain, their concentration intensifies, posing a potential threat to both human and environmental health.

26.4 Health Care Disparity

Healthcare disparity remains a significant challenge, particularly for individuals with limited financial resources. The economically disadvantaged often lack access to routine screenings and struggle to afford regular visits to a family doctor. Consequently, they frequently resort to using the emergency room as their primary source of care. This delayed and emergency-driven approach to seeking medical attention can result in critical health issues that may have been preventable with timely intervention, such as obesity, heart disease, diabetes, and cancers.

The consequences of this healthcare disparity are further exacerbated by the irreversible toll of chronological aging. As individuals age, the effects become increasingly visible, impacting their most recognizable features. The aging baby boomer population is experiencing a surge in chronic illnesses, necessitating more comprehensive and accessible healthcare solutions to address their evolving healthcare needs.

26.5 Climate Change

In an article about climate change in Dermatology Times by Morgan Petronelli, Associate Editor, it was noted that climate change is significantly affecting the world in general and dermatology in particular, leading to an increase in specific skin diseases and a heightened need for sun protection. Dermatologists are increasingly acknowledging the impact of climate change on global skin health. Vector-borne infectious diseases transmitted by organisms like ticks and mosquitoes are spreading, and instances of skin cancer are rising due to climate change. Changes in climate patterns influence the prevalence of these diseases, with warmer temperatures expanding the geographic range of ticks, with humans being natural or incidental hosts [4]. Additionally, alterations in UV radiation levels contribute to skin cancer risk. During a talk at the 2021 AAD, Caroline Nelson, MD, FAAD, medical director of dermatology inpatient consultative service at Yale School of Medicine, New Haven, Connecticut, specifically mentioned the rise in Lyme disease in the United States. Lyme disease, caused by *Borrelia burgdorferi* and other Borrelia species, can lead to skin manifestations like erythema migrans and acrodermatitis chronica atrophicans. Dr. Caroline Nelson highlighted a significant increase in Lyme disease incidence in the eastern and midwestern United States from 2001 to 2014. She attributed this rise to three primary factors [5]. Firstly, warmer winter temperatures enabled tick vectors like *Ixodes scapularis* (East coast) and *Ixodes pacificus* (West coast), known to be responsible for Lyme disease transmission, to spread farther north between 1996 and 2015. Secondly, the prevalence of *B. burgdorferi* infection in ticks increased, linked to the expansion of the white-footed mouse's range northward, parallel with the tick. Lastly, changes in land use, such as reforestation and residential development, brought humans into closer contact with ticks, white-footed mice, and deer as Ixodes ticks seek hosts when temperatures exceed approximately 7 °C [5].

Dirk Elston, MD, FAAD, professor and chairman of the Department of Dermatology and Dermatologic Surgery at the Medical University of South Carolina, Charleston, discussed the rise of diseases linked to climate change [6]. Among them are anaplasmosis, a tick-borne illness from Ixodes ticks; dengue virus (genus Flavivirus) and chikungunya (togavirus), both transmitted by mosquitoes; and a new tick-borne illness causing severe fever with thrombocytopenia syndrome. Elston also noted an increase in tick bites and red meat allergy; "after Amblyomma tick bites, you can become sensitized where you eat red meat and you develop anaphylaxis," he said. With the increase in global temperatures, *Amblyomma americanum* ticks, which typically are seen in the southern United States, are now being seen in the Midwest, Eastern Seaboard, and Canada, with researchers subsequently seeing a rise in red meat allergies throughout these areas. Additionally, the incidence of Chagas disease has been rising globally as triatomine bugs, carriers of Chagas, expand beyond Latin America. In Tucson, Arizona, 42% of bugs around homes tested positive for *Trypanosoma cruzi* [7].

Elston emphasized that climate change leads to a northward shift in the distribution of disease vectors and arthropods, as species move to new environments [8, 9]. Climate change not only affects vector-borne infectious diseases but also contributes to rising skin cancer rates. Eva Parker, MD, FAAD, assistant professor of dermatology at Vanderbilt University Medical Center, in Nashville, Tennessee, discussing skin cancer's global increase, pointed out its association with climate change and environmental impacts [10]. "Skin cancer is one of the most common diseases that we deal with on a daily basis as dermatologists," she said. In the United States, over five million skin cancer cases occur annually. Parker highlighted a 4–5% yearly increase in melanoma incidence, emphasizing that UV radiation is a complete carcinogen (meaning it causes mutations that lead to skin cancer without the need for additional promoters or initiators), and hence a major factor. Ambient sunlight consists of 90–95% UV-A and 5–10% UV-B. The ozone acts as a protectant against UV-C and a portion of UV-B to create a way for plants and animals to survive on Earth. The ozone layer is a region of the Earth's stratosphere containing high levels of trioxygen, which effectively blocks much of the sun's most harmful ultraviolet radiation from reaching the planet's surface. The rise in UV radiation and skin cancer cases is linked to the depletion of stratospheric ozone. The reduction in ozone levels allows more UV-B radiation to reach the Earth's surface, resulting in increased DNA damage and higher rates of skin cancer. Dr. Eva Parker emphasized that even a 10% decrease in stratospheric ozone is estimated to cause an additional 300,000 skin cancers. Since the 1970s, scientists had pushed for the regulation of chlorofluorocarbons, chemicals found in everyday items like air conditioners and aerosol sprays, bromine-containing halons and methyl bromide, hydrochlorofluorocarbons (HCFCs), carbon tetrachloride (CCI4), and methyl chloroform due to their adverse effects on this layer. In the scientific journal *Nature* on May 16, 1985, three scientists from the British Antarctic Survey announced their detection of abnormally low levels of ozone over the South Pole. Their discovery, commonly known as the Ozone Hole, became a palpable example of mankind's ability to damage the Earth's atmosphere as well as one of the most famous success stories in the history of climate activism [11].

Although there is a lot of controversy over the causes of climate change, it is undeniable that changes in our ecological system have a direct impact on human health. The medical community must deal with the consequences of an ever-changing environment.

26.6 Skin of Color

According to an article in Cutis, the US population is becoming more diverse; by 2044, it is predicted that there will be a majority minority population in the United States [12]. The authors write, "Therefore, it is imperative to continue to develop educational mechanisms for all dermatologists to increase and maintain competency in skin of color dermatology, which will contribute to the achievement of health equity for patients with all skin tones and hair types [13]. "Not only is clinical skin of color education necessary, but diversity, equity, and inclusion (DEI) education for dermatologists also is critical," state the authors. "Clinical examination, diagnosis, and treatment of skin and hair disorders across the skin of color spectrum with cultural humility is essential to achieve health equity. If trainees, dermatologists, other specialists, and primary care clinicians are not frequently exposed to patients with darker skin tones and coily hair, the nuances in diagnosing and treating these patients must be learned in alternate ways" [14].

26.7 Summary

"Physicians," Virchow wrote, "are the natural attorneys of the poor." As a physician, writer, and public health advocate who has primarily served the poor, the "chronically subordinated human mired in the corrosive psychosocial stress of poverty," as Robert Sapolsky wrote, I can claim Virchow's quote as a raison d'etre for my own career [15]. I am certain many of my readers will agree with Virchow's sentiment and we could readily add that we are natural attorneys for those dealing with chronic illness, carcinogens and toxicities, imbalance in racial and health equity and climate change. I have included many challenges in this essay that we must overcome to keep medicine and dermatology alive and well. I believe most importantly we must keep focusing on social medicine in dermatology while we progress in personalized medicine and other exciting opportunities in our future.

References

1. Hamlin C. Public health. In: Jackson M, editor. The Oxford handbook of the history of medicine. Oxford University Press; 2013.
2. Norman RA, Ruescher L. 100 Questions and answers about chronic illness. Jones and Bartlett; 2011.
3. Nakazawa DJ. The autoimmune epidemic. Atria Books; 2009.
4. Petronelli M. Climate change takes toll on skin health. Dermatology Times. 42(8);2021.
5. Nelson C. Infectious diseases, vectors, and climate change. In: Presented at: American Academy of Dermatology Virtual Meeting Experience 2021.
6. Elston D. What's changing in the environment? In: Presented at: American Academy of Dermatology Virtual Meeting Experience 2021.
7. Reisenman CE, Lawrence G, Guerenstein PG, Gregory T, Dotson E, Hildebrand JG. Infection of kissing bugs with *Trypanosoma cruzi*, Tucson, Arizona, USA. Emerg Infect Dis. 2010;16(3):400–5. https://doi.org/10.3201/eid1603.090648.
8. Barker CM, Reisen WK. Epidemiology of vector-borne diseases. In: Mullen GR, Durden LA, editors. Medical and veterinary entomology. Elsevier; 2019. p. 33–49.
9. Beard CB, Eisen RJ, Barker CM, et al. Chapter 5: Vector-borne diseases. In: The impacts of climate change on human health in the United States: a scientific assessment. U.S. Global Change Research Program; 2016.
10. Parker E. Climate change and skin cancer. In: Presented at: American Academy of Dermatology Virtual Meeting Experience 2021.
11. History.com Editors. https://www.history.com/this-day-in-history/discovery-of-antarctic-ozone-hole-announced. Accessed 29 Oct 2021.
12. Colby SL, Ortman JM. Projections of the size and composition of the U.S. population: 2014–2060. United States Census Bureau website. 2015. https://www.census.gov/content/dam/Census/library/publications/2015/demo/p25-1143.pdf. Accessed 11 Aug 2021.
13. Heath C, DeLeo V, Taylor S. Increasing skin of color publications in the dermatology literature: a call to action. Cutis. 2021;108(03):155–7. https://doi.org/10.12788/cutis.0343.
14. Grayson C, Heath C. An approach to examining tightly coiled hair among patients with hair loss in race-discordant patient-physician interactions. JAMA Dermatol. 2021;157:505–6. https://doi.org/10.1001/jamadermatol.2021.0338.
15. Sapolsky R. My personal hero: Robert Sapolsky on Rudolf Virchow. Nautilus; 2016.

Epilogue: Exciting Emerging Trends and Technologies in Dermatology

27

Nikhil Mehta, Mansak Shishak, and Somesh Gupta

Medical science is evolving rapidly, and clinicians are left catching up. The way dermatology was practiced 20 years ago is significantly different from today, and with the current pace of development, we expect a similar quantum of change less than a decade from now. However, many developments can be just fads, or just overhyped at a time, till they find a niche. Here we opine about the trends and technologies we are most excited about in dermatology, and hope that they stay and evolve further.

27.1 Targeted Agents: Biologics and Smaller Molecules

Although being in vogue for the past 20 years, especially in psoriasis, we still expect this trend to continue. We expect more biologicals, which are more targeted, having lesser risk of infections hence safer in patients. We also hope that molecules with a longer interval between two doses for psoriasis and chronic spontaneous urticaria are developed. We also hope for successful use of biologics and other targeted agents for newer indications, in the same line as adalimumab for hidradenitis suppurativa, and for autoinflammatory syndromes and other orphan diseases.

N. Mehta · S. Gupta (✉)
Department of Dermatology and Venereology, All India Institute of Medical Sciences, Delhi, India
e-mail: someshgupta@aiims.edu

M. Shishak
ISIC Multispecialty Hospital and Dr. Mansak Skin Clinic, Delhi, India

S. Gupta et al. (eds.), *Critical Thinking in Contemporary Dermatology: Cognitive Essays*, https://doi.org/10.1007/978-981-97-0411-8_27

27.2 Newer Broad Spectrum Immunosuppressive Agents

JAK inhibitors have a broad use and have a moderately fast onset of action, albeit slower than systemic steroids. They can be used in many indications where systemic steroids are relatively contraindicated, and lack the adverse effects of hypothalamic-pituitary axis suppression, diabetes, hypertension, osteoporosis, and cataract. However, they have their own gamut of adverse effects. A significant drawback is that the diseases for which they are used relapse rapidly once they are stopped. We expect them to find their niche in specific indications, and for them to go down the biologic way, where newer, stronger, safer, more targeted next generation agents will have their specific indications, although the newer agents will stay expensive and out of reach for many patients for quite some time.

27.3 Artificial Intelligence

Motion pictures depicting deep conversations and attentive interactions between chatbots and humans is often labeled "fictional." Having come to life much earlier than expected, it is on a scale impossible to ignore. Generative large language models (LLMs) such as ChatGPT, even in its infantile stage of evolution, and yet to evolve into far more powerful systems, has the potential to usurp healthcare delivery mechanisms including doctors. Delivering personalized answers and unlimited attention remains the cornerstone of LLMs, a stark contrast from the more commonly encountered less-enthused, overburdened and heuristic healthcare worker, who is not necessarily a skilled communicator. The machine, meanwhile, is devoid of sleep requirements: constantly and consistently consuming digital data.

The Gell-Mann Amnesia Effect explains how an expert may forget the inaccuracies within a medium, when exposed to an unknown topic, even after knowing the fallacies that the medium contains. An example of which is medical journalism. Au contraire, LLMs have been perceived as non-experts yet possess technical accuracy, ability to pass specialty examinations and have an empathy score higher than human subjects. It's far more powerful and accurate than we had expected.

With next generation chatbots poised to integrate auditory, visual and other special sensory experiences, this era of cooperation and coexistence with virtual systems is here, in the now. Attempting to regulate it in healthcare is complex. Are we ready to efficiently handle cybercrime in digital healthcare and intercept different checkpoints? Deep fakes and data duplication in research remains an increasingly concerning matter. Reality is definitely more complex than fiction!

27.4 Cameras and Photography Technology

Not just medical tech, but tech in general has improved a lot. The images from the cameras of current flagship smartphones are practically indistinguishable from those by a digital single-lens reflex (DSLR) camera in the eyes of a layperson. Total body 3D photography, thermography, Ultraviolet (UV) photography, infrared photography, and single camera integrating functions of close-up imaging, UV imaging and dermoscopic imaging have been developed, although they have not been widespread in use. We hope these devices to be smaller, more portable, cheaper, and with multiple photography modalities in a single device. We expect them to have newer indications in clinical use and research. We expect the software tech in them to be more automated, user-friendly, with better and consistent image processing, and with Artificial Intelligence-based data analytics to enable objective analysis and user-friendly ghost overlaying to enable better pre and post comparisons. We expect more advances in image capture and analysis, with more accurate software for objective measurement of wound dimensions, body surface area etc.

27.5 Dermoscopy

Despite many recent advances, the current generation of dermoscopes still suffer from many disadvantages. There is a dichotomy in hand-held vs. digital dermoscopes. Dermatologists should not need adaptors to fix cameras or smartphones on dermoscopes for imaging, and wireless connectivity to devices such as phone or laptop even without internet should be an option even in entry level dermoscopes, without compromising on the lens or picture quality. We feel that a manufacturer designing a low-cost device with features currently considered "premium," opting for a shift from a high-margin low-volume model to a low-margin per device but high-volume overall will capture a sizeable market and collect decent profits. We hope rapid viewing as well as simultaneous documentation and picture archiving through dermoscopy devices is made much more rapid and convenient. We expect next generation dermoscopy devices to have built-in analytics and artificial intelligence, to give parameters such as size of lesions, hair count and density, proportion of leucotrichia, and superimposition with previous dermoscopy pictures over the same site with automated spatial adjustment. We hope they are able to intelligently adjust the pressure applied by the dermoscope, the distance between the skin and the center of lens, and illumination, or be able to take batches of multiple photos in quick succession with variations of these parameters. In parallel to whole-body 3-D photography, we expect whole body dermoscopy, along with AI analysis, to assist in or replace the tedious task of manual examination and photography of each individual lesion.

27.6 Newer Imaging Techniques

High frequency skin sonography, optical coherence tomography, and reflectance confocal microscopy have been shown useful in many studies but have not been widespread in use. They have a huge potential for noninvasive diagnosis, monitoring, and guiding procedures. We hope that these devices become portable, cheaper, and more accepted. We hope that they develop more indications for use in inflammatory and infectious diseases. With the development of combinations of reflectance confocal microscopy with optical coherence tomography, and confocal mosaic stitching of images and processing to mimic hematoxylin and eosin slides, along with AI-based diagnosis of the images, these newer imaging techniques have the potential to significantly alleviate the need of pathology services.

27.7 Newer Research Methods

A robust meta-analysis needs head-to-head trials of various modalities. This strict requirement limits the level of evidence of treatment for many diseases with multiple modalities. Many institutes and regulatory guidelines have strict requirements for head-to-head comparison to support prescription practices. Network meta-analysis is a modality which enables us to get a hierarchy of treatments without a head-to-head comparison between all individual treatments, and we expect to see much more of them in the future.

We also expect patient-reported outcome measures to take a center stage, and to be included as very important, if not essential, secondary outcome measures in interventional trials. Also, with the advent of big data and rigorous recordkeeping, we expect studies with much larger sample size, census-based rather than sample-based, with more variables per patient and more follow-up data, with visual records. Artificial Intelligence-based data analytics will lead to rapid almost real-time availability of trends, enabling us to closely monitor and intervene rapidly during epidemics.

27.8 Procedures and Aesthetics

Procedural dermatology, including cosmetic dermatology and aesthetics, is the branch with maximum innovations recently. Although it has the potential of maximum innovations, it is also the one with maximum fads and overhyped procedures. We hope more evidence-based procedures are developed, and more procedure–procedure combinations are evaluated. We hope that the existing way to evaluate evidence, which is significantly biased towards drug interventions, develops enough modifications to allow evaluation of procedural interventions, and for them to be considered higher in the hierarchy of management. We expect newer procedures to be less invasive, be easily available, and be possible as add-on on previous procedures.

27.9 Precision Medicine

We have made significant advances in mapping the genes and individual variations for various genodermatoses and polygenic inflammatory diseases. Excellent genotypic–phenotypic correlation models have been developed for ichthyosis, and variations for psoriasis and vitiligo have been established. With big data, AI, and the ever-reducing cost of sequencing, we expect the field of precision medicine and pharmacogenomics to grow, and to be used in clinical practice more frequently even in fields other than dermato-oncology. We hope to be able to predict more accurately which patients of a particular disease are likely to respond better to a particular targeted agent.

27.10 Gene Therapy and Gene Editing

Genodermatoses lead to significant morbidity and mortality. Previous attempts at gene therapy in Epidermolysis Bullosa have been moderately successful in the short run, and newer topical gene therapies like the FDA-approved topical gene therapy in form of modified herpes virus seem more promising. However, it is expensive and out of reach for most patients. With the advent of CRISPR-Cas9 based gene editing, we expect gene therapy to become much cheaper in the future. Repurposing of older drugs like gentamicin for correcting frameshift mutations is also a significantly cheaper form of gene therapy, and we hope that more such therapies and uses are discovered.

27.11 Sensors and Wearables

Despite interest and enthusiasm from various sensors and wearables, they haven't caught up explosively, neither in the technological world nor in the field of dermatology. However, they hold the potential to offer data not harnessed before. For example, the continuous 24 × 7 real-time monitoring of total epidermal water loss is likely able to offer more insights in atopic dermatitis patients compared to the current way of assessing it transiently during a visit. With big data and analytics, it is possible to meaningfully analyze such data and hopefully drive clinically meaningful results. Sensors and wearables are likely to offer better research tools and data compared to the one we have currently.

27.12 3-D Printing

3-D printing has been used successfully to design footwear customized to individual leprosy patients to enable proper off-loading of their ulcers. However, further refinement is warranted. In the tech world, it seems limited to hobbyists and small do-it-yourself projects. In dermatology, we hope that it is able to develop meaningful clinical applications, not limited to customized dressings but also drug delivery and bioprinting, i.e., in the realm of synthetic skin substitutes.

27.13 Mobile Phone Apps

Dermatologists have had their share of apps based on residency training, quizzes, case-based review, board testing, etc. We expect better picture archiving applications to make saving pictures easy through smartphones, wound and lesion dimension monitoring which is accurate, consistent, reliable, and doesn't require frequent calibration, body surface area measurement apps, dermoscopy integrated apps including those for hair counting, etc.

27.14 Metaverse

Although regarded as a hype by many, metaverse is considered to be an ideal platform to demonstrate cosmetic and aesthetic procedures by the few. It has the potential to improve teledermatology services, provide an immersive surgical planning platform, and better virtual training using 3D skin models. Hopefully it will be able to find its niche in dermatology.

27.15 Conclusion

These are exciting times in dermatology. With science and technology progressing exponentially, we need to keep up our pace. The future holds tremendous potential, and it is collectively up to us to strive to realize it! A note of caution: technology cannot replace the significance of personal support, empathy, and genuine human interaction. It is crucial that we persistently enhance the humanistic dimensions of medicine.

GPSR Compliance

The European Union's (EU) General Product Safety Regulation (GPSR) is a set of rules that requires consumer products to be safe and our obligations to ensure this.

If you have any concerns about our products, you can contact us on ProductSafety@springernature.com

In case Publisher is established outside the EU, the EU authorized representative is:

Springer Nature Customer Service Center GmbH
Europaplatz 3
69115 Heidelberg, Germany

Batch number: 10726133

Printed by Printforce, the Netherlands